Illustrative Handbook of General Surgery

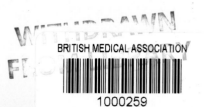

Herbert Chen
Editor

Illustrative Handbook of General Surgery

Second Edition

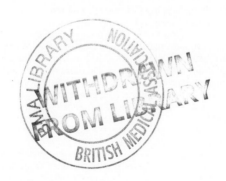

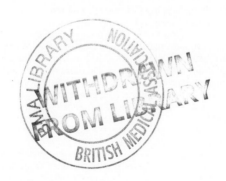

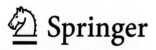

Springer

Editor
Herbert Chen
University of Wisconsin
Madison, Wisconsin
USA

ISBN 978-3-319-24555-3   e-ISBN 978-3-319-24557-7   (eBook)
DOI 10.1007/978-3-319-24557-7

Library of Congress Control Number: 2016931617

Springer Cham Heidelberg New York Dordrecht London
© Springer International Publishing Switzerland 2016

Springer International Publishing AG Switzerland is part of Springer Science+Business Media (www.springer.com)

Contents

Contents   vii

Contributors

Cameron D. Adkisson, MD Division of Endocrine Surgery, Department of Surgery, University of Pittsburgh, Pittsburgh, PA, USA

Jacquelynn D. Arbuckle, MD Department of Surgery, University of Wisconsin School of Medicine and Public Health, Madison, WI, USA

Jocelyn F. Burke, MD Department of General Surgery, University of Wisconsin Hospital and Clinics, Madison, WI, USA

Guilherme M. Campos, MD, FACS Division of Bariatric and Gastrointestinal Surgery, Department of Surgery, Virginia Commonwealth University, Richmond, Virginia, USA

Clifford S. Cho, MD Department of Surgery, University of Wisconsin School of Medicine and Public Health, Madison, WI, USA

Marquita Renee Decker, MD, MPH Department of Surgery, University of Wisconsin Hospital and Clinics, Madison, WI, USA

Dina M. Elaraj, MD, FACS Department of Surgery, Section of Endocrine Surgery, Northwestern University Feinberg School of Medicine, Chicago, IL, USA

Alain Elian, MD Department of Surgery, University of Wisconsin, University of Wisconsin School of Medicine and Public Health, Madison, WI, USA

Abbey L. Fingeret, MD Department of General Surgery, New York-Presbyterian Hospital, Columbia University Medical Center, New York, NY, USA

Division of Gastrointestinal and Endocrine Surgery, Department of Surgery, College of Physicians and Surgeons of Columbia University, New York, NY, USA

Laura E. Fischer, MD, MS Department of Surgery, University of Wisconsin, University of Wisconsin School of Medicine and Public Health, Madison, WI, USA

Department of General Surgery, University of Wisconsin Hospitals and Clinics, Madison, WI, USA

Luke M. Funk, MD, MPH Department of Surgery, University of Wisconsin School of Medicine and Public Health, University of Wisconsin, Madison, WI, USA

Department of Surgery, University of Wisconsin Hospitals and Clinics, Madison, WI, USA

Michael J. Garren, MD Department of Surgery, University of Wisconsin, Madison, WI, USA

Jacob A. Greenberg, MD, EdM Department of Surgery, University of Wisconsin Hospital and Clinics, Madison, WI, USA

Rebecca Gunter, MD Department of General Surgery, University of Wisconsin Hospital and Clinics, Madison, WI, USA

Nicholas A. Hamilton Department of General Surgery, Washington University, St. Louis, MO, USA

William G. Hawkins Department of General Surgery, Washington University, St. Louis, MO, USA

Department of Surgery, Washington University in St Louis, St Louis, MO, USA

Charles P. Heise, MD, FACS Department of Surgery, University of Wisconsin Hospital and Clinics, Madison, WI, USA

University of Wisconsin School of Medicine and Public Health, Madison, WI, USA

Mary Beth Henry, RN, MS, CS, APNP Department of Surgical Oncology, University of Wisconsin Health System, Madison, WI, USA

Sara E. Holden, MD Department of General Surgery, University of Wisconsin Hospital and Clinics, Madison, WI, USA

Gregory D. Kennedy, MD, PhD Department of Surgery, University of Alabama at Birmingham, Birmingham, AL, USA

Jad Khoraki, MD Department of Surgery, University of Wisconsin School of Medicine and Public Health, Madison, WI, USA

James A. Lee, MD Department of Endocrine Surgery, New York-Presbyterian Hospital, Columbia University Medical Center, New York, NY, USA

Division of Gastrointestinal and Endocrine Surgery, Department of Surgery, College of Physicians and Surgeons of Columbia University, New York, NY, USA

Christina W. Lee, MD Department of Surgery, University of Wisconsin School of Medicine and Public Health, Madison, WI, USA

Charles M. Leys, MD, MSCI Department of General Surgery, University of Wisconsin Hospital and Clinics, Madison, WI, USA

Ryan A. Macke, MD Section of Thoracic Surgery, Division of Cardiothoracic Surgery, Department of Surgery, University of Wisconsin, University of Wisconsin School of Medicine and Public Health, Madison, WI, USA

David M. Melnick, MD, MPH Department of Surgery, University of Wisconsin School of Medicine and Public Health, Madison, WI, USA

Clinton T. Morgan, MD, PhD Department of Surgery, University of Wisconsin, University of Wisconsin School of Medicine and Public Health, Madison, WI, USA

Lilah F. Morris, MD Department of Surgery, Northwest Medical Center, Northwest Allied General Surgery, Tucson, AZ, USA

Heather B. Neuman, MD, MS Department of Surgery, University of Wisconsin School of Medicine and Public Health, Madison, WI, USA

Francesco Palazzo, MD, FACS Department of Surgery, Thomas Jefferson University, Philadelphia, PA, USA

Christina M. Papageorge, MD Department of Surgery, University of Wisconsin Hospital and Clinics, Madison, WI, USA

Terrah J. Paul Olson, MD Department of General Surgery, University of Wisconsin Hospital and Clinics, Madison, WI, USA

Scott N. Pinchot Department of Surgery, University of Wisconsin, Madison, WI, USA

Matthew R. Porembka Section of HPB Surgery, Department of Surgery, Washington University in St Louis, St Louis, MO, USA

Charlotte Rabl, MD, FACS Department of Surgery, Paracelsus Medical University, Salzburg, Austria

Andrew J. Russ, MD Department of Surgery, University of Tennessee Graduate School of Medicine, University of Tennessee Medical Center, Knoxville, TN, USA

M. Shirin Sabbaghian, MD Riverside Surgical Group, Department of Surgery, Lexington Medical Center, Columbia, SC, USA

Surgical Oncology and General Surgery, Private Practice, Louisiana State University Health Sciences Center, Suite D Crowley, LA, USA

Sarah C. Schaefer, MS, ANP-BC Department of Surgery, University of Wisconsin School of Medicine and Public Health, Madison, WI, USA

Patrick J. Shabino, MD Department of Surgery, University of Wisconsin, Wisconsin School of Medicine and Public Health, Madison, WI, USA

Wen T. Shen, MD, MA Endocrine Surgery Section, Department of Surgery, University of California, San Francisco, UCSF Medical Center—Mount Zion, San Francisco, CA, USA

Stanley B. Sidhu, PhD, FRACS Endocrine Surgery Unit, University of Sydney, St. Leonards, NSW, Australia

Endocrine Surgery Unit, University of Sydney and RNSH, St. Leonards, NSW, Australia

Department of Endocrine and Oncologic Surgery, Royal North Shore Hospital, St. Leonards, NSW, Australia

Rebecca S. Sippel, MD Department of General Surgery, University of Wisconsin School of Medicine and Public Health, Madison, WI, USA

Sarah E. Smith, RN, MS, ANP-BC, APNP Department of General Surgery, University of Wisconsin, University of Wisconsin-Madison, Madison, WI, USA

Jennifer G. Steiman, MD Department of Surgery, University of Wisconsin, Madison, WI, USA

Steven M. Strasberg Section of HPB Surgery, Department of Surgery, Washington University in St Louis, St Louis, MO, USA

Cord Sturgeon, MD, MS Department of Surgery, Section of Endocrine Surgery, Northwestern University Feinberg School of Medicine, Chicago, IL, USA

Insoo Suh, MD Endocrine Surgery Section, Department of Surgery, University of California, San Francisco, UCSF Medical Center—Mount Zion, San Francisco, CA, USA

Lauren J. Taylor, MD Department of Surgery, University of Wisconsin Hospital and Clinics, Madison, WI, USA

Sarah E. Tevis, MD Department of General Surgery, University of Wisconsin, Madison, WI, USA

Allan Tsung, MD Division of Hepatobiliary and Pancreatic Surgery, UPMC Liver Cancer Center, Montefiore Hospital, University of Pittsburgh Medical Center, Pittsburgh, PA, USA

Sharon M. Weber Department of Surgery, University of Wisconsin, Madison, WI, USA

Lee G. Wilke, MD Department of Surgery, University of Wisconsin Hospital and Clinics, Madison, WI, USA

Jennifer B. Wilson, PA Department of General Surgery, University of Wisconsin Hospital and Clinics, Madison, WI, USA

Jason T. Wiseman, MD, MSPH Department of Surgery, University of Wisconsin School of Medicine and Public Health, Madison, WI, USA

Department of Surgery, University of Wisconsin Hospitals and Clinics, Madison, WI, USA

Michael W. Yeh, MD Department of Surgery, Section of Endocrine Surgery, UCLA David Geffen School of Medicine, Los Angeles, CA, USA

Linwah Yip, MD, FACS Division of Endocrine Surgery, Department of Surgery, University of Pittsburgh, Pittsburgh, PA, USA

Division of Endocrine Surgery, University of Pittsburgh School of Medicine, Pittsburgh, PA, USA

Nisar A. Zaidi, MD Endocrine Surgical Unit, University of Sydney, Royal North Shore Hospital, St Leonards, NSW, Australia

Part I
Endocrine Surgery

Rebecca S. Sippel

Chapter 1
Total Thyroidectomy and Thyroid Lobectomy

Insoo Suh and Wen T. Shen

Abstract   The key to a safe thyroidectomy is to dissect in the correct cervical planes using absolutely meticulous, bloodless technique. This optimizes the surgeon's ability to identify and preserve delicate perithyroidal structures such as the recurrent laryngeal nerve and parathyroid glands, as well as minimize the risk of life-threatening postoperative neck hematoma. This chapter describes the technique of a conventional thyroidectomy performed via an anterior cervical incision. An overview of preoperative workup and postoperative care is also included.

Keywords Thyroid • Thyroidectomy • Thyroid nodule • Thyroid cancer • Goiter • Hyperthyroidism • Hypothyroidism • Recurrent laryngeal nerve • Parathyroid

I. Suh, MD • W.T. Shen, MD (✉)
Endocrine Surgery Section, Department of Surgery,
UCSF Medical Center – Mount Zion, University of California,
San Francisco, Campus Box 1674, San Francisco,
CA 94115, USA
e-mail: insoo.suh@ucsf.edu; wen.shen@ucsfmedctr.org

H. Chen (ed.), *Illustrative Handbook of General Surgery*,
DOI 10.1007/978-3-319-24557-7_1,
© Springer International Publishing Switzerland 2016

Indications

The indications for thyroidectomy encompass a wide spectrum of thyroid disorders, but the majority fall under three categories:

1. Hyperthyroidism or thyroiditis refractory to nonsurgical management [1, 2]
2. goiters with or without local compressive symptoms [3, 4], and
3. thyroid nodules and cancers [5].

The decision to perform a total thyroidectomy versus unilateral lobectomy or other more limited procedure depends on the underlying disease, the patient's clinical profile, suspicion of intraoperative recurrent laryngeal nerve injury, and in some instances on surgeon or patient preference.

Preoperative Preparation

All patients undergoing thyroidectomy should have preoperative biochemical thyroid function tests as well as a neck ultrasound with fine-needle aspiration biopsies of suspicious nodules [6]. Depending on the type and extent of disease, selected patients may require further imaging studies such as CT, MRI, thyroid scintigraphy, and endoscopy [7]. Patients should ideally be euthyroid at the time of operation, either with antithyroid medication and/or Lugol's solution for hyperthyroidism or exogenous thyroid hormone supplementation for hypothyroidism.

Preoperative laryngoscopy must be performed on any patient with hoarseness or a prior history of neck operations in order to assess preoperative vocal cord function. Preanesthetic evaluation should be a routine step prior to any procedure requiring general anesthesia.

Positioning and Anesthesia

Most thyroidectomies are performed under general anesthesia with endotracheal intubation. The patient is placed supine in a 20° reverse Trendelenburg position, with both arms tucked. The neck is extended by placing a beanbag or soft roll behind the scapulae and a foam ring under the head. This places the thyroid in a more anterior position. The head must be well-supported to prevent neck hyperextension and postoperative posterior neck pain.

The use of intraoperative nerve monitoring (IONM) for recurrent laryngeal nerve (RLN) function has become increasingly common in many endocrine surgical practices despite ongoing controversy over the true effectiveness of IONM in reducing the incidence of RLN injury and vocal cord palsy [8]. Proponents of IONM use cite its value in, among other things, tracing the anatomic course of nerves (particularly for challenging situations such as reoperations), more sensitively detecting injury in the intraoperative setting, and enabling the detection of vagal and superior laryngeal nerve function. If the use of IONM is planned, an appropriate endotracheal tube with contact electrodes for the vocal cords is used, and grounding and return surface electrodes are applied per the individual manufacturer's instructions. The remainder of this chapter will assume and describe the use of IONM during the relevant steps of the operation.

We routinely perform a bilateral superficial cervical anesthetic block with 0.25 % bupivacaine, as this provides excellent anesthesia in the postoperative setting [9]. In addition, prior to surgical prep, we routinely perform our own intraoperative neck ultrasound in order to (1) confirm the findings of the preoperative study, (2) identify any new findings, and (3) assess the overall anatomy of the gland to facilitate incision placement and operative planning. The surgical area is prepared with 1 % iodine or chlorhexidine and sterilely draped.

Description of Procedure

In general, thyroid operations should be performed in a bloodless field so that vital structures can be identified. Bleeding obscures the normal color of the parathyroids and RLN, placing these important structures at greater risk for injury. If bleeding does occur, application of manual pressure is the preferred hemostatic maneuver; vessels should be clamped only if they are precisely identified, or shown to not be in close proximity to the RLN.

A centrally placed, 4–5 cm Kocher transverse incision is made typically 1 cm caudad to the cricoid cartilage, paralleling the normal skin lines of the neck (Fig. 1.1). The incision is

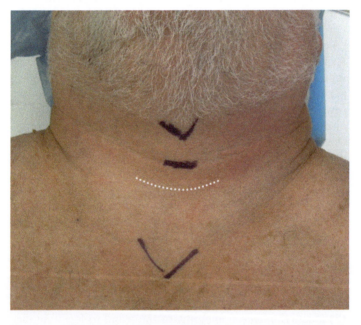

Figure 1.1 Skin incision. The pen marks, from top to bottom, denote the thyroid cartilage, cricoid cartilage, and suprasternal notch, respectively. A centrally placed, 4–6 cm Kocher transverse incision is made 1 cm caudad to the cricoid cartilage, paralleling the normal skin lines of the neck (*white dotted line*)

extended through the platysma, and subplatysmal flaps are raised, first cephalad to the level of the thyroid cartilage and then caudad to the suprasternal notch. Five straight Kelly clamps placed on the dermis of each flap aid in retraction for this dissection.

In a cancer operation, dissection of the thyroid gland is generally begun on the side of the suspected tumor, since problems with the dissection on this side (e.g. concern for RLN injury) could allow the surgeon the option to perform a less-than-total thyroidectomy on the contralateral side in order to avoid bilateral injury and resultant complications. One exception is the large bulky tumor, in which case the surgeon may choose to resect the contralateral side first in order to more easily mobilize the larger lobe.

The strap muscles are separated in the midline via an incision through the superficial layer of the deep cervical fascia starting at the suprasternal notch and extending cephalad to the thyroid cartilage. On the side of the suspected tumor, the more superficial sternohyoid is separated from the deeper sternothyroid muscle by blunt dissection, proceeding laterally until the ansa cervicalis is visible at the lateral border of the sternothyroid muscle. The sternothyroid is then dissected from the underlying thyroid capsule until the middle thyroid vein is encountered laterally. The thyroid is retracted anteromedially, and the carotid sheath and strap muscles are retracted laterally. A peanut sponge can be used to facilitate retraction and exposure of the area posterolateral to the thyroid. The middle thyroid vein is optimally exposed for division at this time (Fig. 1.2). For those that use IONM, a pre-RLN dissection vagus signal (denoted V1) is obtained by stimulating the vagus nerve which is typically located posterolateral to the carotid.

In the case of thyroid lobectomy, the isthmus is usually divided early in the dissection to facilitate mobilization. The isthmus is clamped and divided lateral to the midline, taking care to not leave residual tissue anterior to the

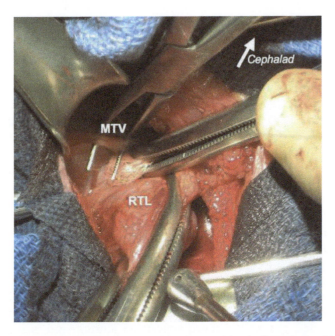

FIGURE I.2 Identification of the middle thyroid vein (MTV). On this side, the right thyroid lobe (RTL) is retracted antero-medially to expose the MTV, which is isolated in preparation for division and ligation

trachea to minimize the chances of hypertrophy of the thyroid remnant. Energy sealing devices such as the Ligasure (Covidien, New Haven, CT) or Harmonic scalpel (Ethicon, Cincinnati, OH) are useful for dividing the thyroid parenchyma in a hemostatic manner; alternatively, the isthmus can be divided with a scalpel between clamps and the thyroid remnant oversewn at the cut edge. The pyramidal lobe, present in 80 % of patients, drapes cephalad over the anterior midline just right or left of the cricoid cartilage, and can extend as superiorly as the hyoid bone. It is dissected until it tapers into a fibrous band, divided, and ligated.

The superior pole is dissected mostly in a blunt fashion with a small peanut sponge on a clamp. The dissection is carried out superolaterally and posteriorly, with counter-traction of the thyroid inferomedially. This exposes the superior thyroid vessels, as well as some connective tissue lateral to the superior pole. These tissues are carefully mobilized below the level of the cricothyroid muscle, since the RLN passes through Berry's ligament and dive deep to the inferior constrictor muscle at the level of the cricoid cartilage. The superior pole is similarly separated from the cricothyroid muscle medially with gentle blunt sweeping (into the so-called avascular space of Reeve). The superior pole vessels are dissected, double- or triple-clamped, and ligated (Fig. 1.3); again, the use of energy sealing devices may augment or replace manual ligation. They are then divided close to the surface of the thyroid in order to prevent injury to the external branch of the superior laryngeal nerve as it traverses the anterior surface of the cricothyroid muscle. Division of these vessels allows for easy sweeping of the remaining filmy tissues away from the posterior aspect of the superior pole via blunt dissection. The superior parathyroid gland is often identified behind the superior pole during this dissection, at the level of the cricoid cartilage (Fig. 1.3).

The mobilization of the lateral and inferior aspects of the thyroid lobe includes the definitive identification of the inferior parathyroid gland (Fig. 1.4). With the inferior thyroid lobe retracted anteromedially and the carotid sheath laterally, dissection should proceed cephalad along the lateral edge of the thyroid. Fatty and lymphatic tissues immediately adjacent to the thyroid are swept laterally with a peanut sponge, and small vessels are ligated with clips. The inferior parathyroid is usually encountered during this lateral mobilization, and care must be taken to not transect any tissues in this area until these vital structures are identified. The location of the inferior parathyroid gland is less constant than that of the superior gland, but it is invariably located anterior

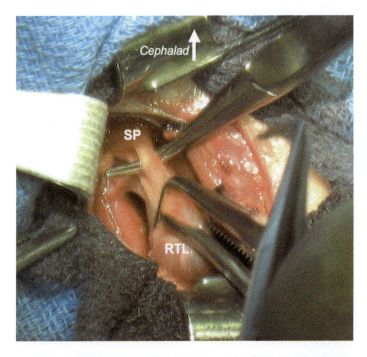

FIGURE 1.3 Dissection of the superior pole (*SP*). In the image, counter-traction of the right thyroid lobe (*RTL*) infero-medially exposes the SP vessels, which are individually skeletonized, clamped, and ligated

to the RLN and inferior to the inferior thyroid artery as it crosses the RLN. In its "normal" location, it is often adherent to the posterolateral surface of the inferior lobe. All normal parathyroid glands should be carefully swept away from the thyroid on as broad a vascular pedicle as possible to prevent devascularization, since this would necessitate autotransplantation of the gland.

Once the superior pole and inferior aspect of the lobe are dissected and mobilized, the majority of the gland aside from its tracheal attachments and ligament of Berry can be delivered out of the incision with anteromedial retraction. This

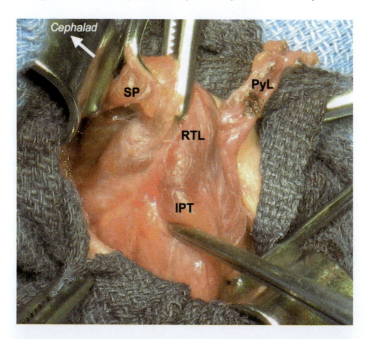

FIGURE 1.4 Identification of the inferior parathyroid (*IPT*). After the superior pole (*SP*) has been dissected and mobilized, the right thyroid lobe (*RTL*) is retracted supero-medially to begin the inferior pole dissection. The IPT is often variable in position, but is invariably anterior to the recurrent laryngeal nerve. The pyramidal lobe (*PyL*) is also seen medially

judicious retraction (either with a finger or with an atraumatic sponge) is imperative for controlled dissection and protection of the RLN. Care must be taken not to use excessive force, which may place the nerve under stretch and increase the risk of injury. The course of the right and left RLN can vary considerably. The left RLN is usually situated deeper and more medially, running in the tracheoesophageal groove, while the right RLN takes a more superficial and oblique course and may pass either anterior or posterior to the inferior thyroid artery. Two commonly-used rules of thumb are used for RLN identification: (1) it is located within

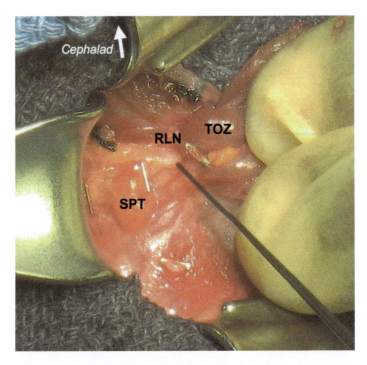

FIGURE 1.5 Identification of the superior parathyroid gland (*SPT*) and recurrent laryngeal nerve (*RLN*). The SPT is usually posterolateral to the RLN (shown here with the nerve monitoring probe), at the level of the cricoid cartilage. The right thyroid lobe, including the tubercle of Zuckerkandl (*TOZ*), is retracted medially for optimal exposure of the RLN

1 cm anteromedial to the superior parathyroid, at the level where the nerve crosses the inferior thyroid artery; and (2) its course through the ligament of Berry is also situated just posteromedial to a small posterolateral protuberance of the thyroid lobe known as the tubercle of Zuckerkandl (Fig. 1.5). Once the nerve is dissected and visually identified, the IONM may be used to obtain an initial signal (denoted R1).

Once the parathyroids and RLN are identified and preserved, the remainder of the thyroid is easily dissected in a more superficial plane off of the trachea. Occasionally, the course of the RLN at the ligament of Berry is intimately associated with the thyroid tissue at the tubercle of Zuckerkandl; in these circumstances, it would be appropriate to leave a small amount of thyroid tissue behind in the interest of protecting the nerve. The entire thyroid lobe should now be completely freed.

Meticulous hemostasis is obtained, and post-resection RLN and vagus signals (denoted R2 and V2, respectively) are confirmed with the IONM system. If a total thyroidectomy is to be performed, the same steps described above apply for the contralateral lobe.

For closure, the sternothyroid and sternohyoid muscles are re-approximated with 3-0 absorbable sutures, with a small opening left in the midline at the suprasternal notch to allow any blood to exit. The platysma layer is approximated with similar sutures, and the skin is closed with a 4-0 subcuticular monofilament absorbable suture.

Postoperative Care

Though relatively uncommon in experienced centers, significant complications can occur after thyroidectomy, including RLN injury, hypoparathyroidism, bleeding and neck hematoma leading to life-threatening airway compromise, injury to the external branch of the superior laryngeal nerve, infection, seroma, and keloid formation. Because of the small but serious risk of neck hematoma, postoperative patients are usually admitted overnight to the hospital ward for observation. They are positioned in a low Fowler position with the head and shoulders elevated 10–20° for the first 6–12 postoperative hours, in order to maintain negative pressure in the veins. Eating is resumed within 4 h. For patients who have undergone bilateral exploration, serum calcium levels are measured 6 h after operation and again the next morning; a serum phosphorus level is also measured at the latter time point. Since calcium levels may not nadir for several days after surgery, a parathyroid hormone level may be obtained post-operatively to help assess the risk of hypocalcemia. Patients who have undergone unilateral first-time exploration do not require biochemical evaluation. Oral calcium supplements are administered for signs of biochemical and/or symptomatic hypocalcemia.

The vast majority of patients are discharged on the first postoperative day; they are given a prescription for thyroid hormone supplementation if the procedure was more extensive than a lobectomy, and are instructed to take calcium tablets for symptoms of hypocalcemia. Most patients can return to work or full activity within 1 week. They are seen in the outpatient clinic within 2 weeks after discharge, at which time further management is discussed in light of the pathology findings as well as the results of any relevant follow-up laboratory evaluation.

References

1. Alsanea O, Clark OH. Treatment of Graves' disease: the advantages of surgery. Endocrinol Metab Clin North Am. 2000;29: 321–37.
2. Farwell AP, Braverman LE. Inflammatory thyroid disorders. Otolaryngol Clin North Am. 1996;29:541–56.
3. Samuels MH. Evaluation and treatment of sporadic nontoxic goiter—some answers and more questions. J Clin Endocrinol Metab. 2001;86:994–7.
4. Shen WT, Kebebew E, Duh QY, Clark OH. Predictors of airway complications after thyroidectomy for substernal goiter. Arch Surg. 2004;139:656–9. discussion 9–60.
5. The American Thyroid Association (ATA) Guidelines Taskforce on Thyroid Nodules and Differentiated Thyroid Cancer. Revised American thyroid association management guidelines for patients with thyroid nodules and differentiated thyroid cancer. Thyroid. 2009;19(11):1167–214.
6. Yassa L, Cibas ES, Benson CB, et al. Long-term assessment of a multidisciplinary approach to thyroid nodule diagnostic evaluation. Cancer. 2007;111:508–16.

7. King AD. Imaging for staging and management of thyroid cancer. Cancer Imaging. 2008;8:57–69.
8. Pisanu A, Porceddu G, Podda M, et al. Systematic review with meta-analysis of studies comparing intraoperative neuromonitoring of recurrent laryngeal nerves versus visualization alone during thyroidectomy. J Surg Res. 2014;188(1):152–61.
9. Shih M, Duh QY, Chung BH, et al. Bilateral superficial cervical plexus block combined with general anesthesia administered in thyroid operations. World J Surg. 2010;34(10):2338–43.

Chapter 2
Central Neck Dissection

Dina M. Elaraj and Cord Sturgeon

Abstract   The central compartment of the neck, also known
as level VI, is bounded by the carotid arteries laterally, the
hyoid bone superiorly, and the suprasternal notch or innominate artery inferiorly. Papillary thyroid cancer, derived from
follicular cells, and medullary thyroid cancer, derived from
parafollicular cells, commonly metastasize to the cervical lymph nodes. Therapeutic central neck dissection for
papillary thyroid cancer is clearly indicated, while routine
prophylactic central neck dissection for papillary thyroid
cancer is controversial. Pre-operatively, all patients should
undergo comprehensive neck ultrasound with fine needle
aspiration biopsy of any suspicious lymph nodes. To perform
a central neck dissection, the patient is positioned supine
with the neck extended. Total thyroidectomy is performed
in the standard fashion. The thin fascial layer overlying the
recurrent laryngeal nerve is incised and the nerve then dissected away from the fibrofatty lymph node-bearing tissue
of the paratracheal space extending from the point of the

D.M. Elaraj, MD, FACS (✉) • C. Sturgeon, MD, MS, FACS
Department of Surgery, Section of Endocrine Surgery,
Northwestern University Feinberg School of Medicine,
676 N St Clair St., Suite 650, Chicago,
IL 60611, USA
e-mail: delaraj@nm.org; csturgeo@nm.org

H. Chen (ed.), *Illustrative Handbook of General Surgery*,   17
DOI 10.1007/978-3-319-24557-7_2,
© Springer International Publishing Switzerland 2016

nerve's insertion into the criocthyroid muscle superiorly to the thoracic inlet inferiorly and between the carotid arteries laterally. The pretracheal tissue is dissected inferiorly to the suprasternal notch. The lower parathyroid gland is frequently devascularized during this procedure and should be autotransplanted if its blood supply is in doubt. Drains are not usually necessary. Patients are usually discharged home the following day.

Keywords Papillary thyroid cancer • Medullary thyroid cancer • Delphian lymph node • Lymph node metastases • Central neck dissection • Level 6 lymph nodes

Indications

Lymph nodes in the neck are classified by their location (Levels I-VI). Level VI, also known as the central compartment of the neck, is bounded by the carotid arteries laterally, the hyoid bone superiorly, and the suprasternal notch or innominate artery inferiorly [1, 2]. It contains the Delphian (precricoid), pretracheal, and paratracheal lymph nodes. Level VII nodes, although not technically located in the neck, are often included when describing lymph node groups/levels in the neck. They are located in the anterior superior mediastinum between the suprasternal notch and brachiocephalic vessels, and lymph nodes in Level VII can be resected en bloc with those in Level VI [1]. Some references define the inferior boundary of the central neck as the innominate artery on the right and the corresponding axial plane on the left [2]. If using this definition, the level VII lymph nodes superior to the innominate artery will be included in level VI.

Thyroid cancer is classified by cell of origin. Differentiated thyroid cancers of follicular cell origin include papillary, follicular, and Hürthle cell cancers.

Medullary thyroid cancer is derived from the calcitonin-producing parafollicular cells and has a different biology than cancers of follicular cell origin. Eighty percent of thyroid cancers are of the papillary subtype, which first metastasize to the cervical lymph nodes [3]. Medullary thyroid cancer also tends to first metastasize to the cervical lymph nodes [4]. Follicular and Hürthle cell cancers have a propensity for hematogenous metastases and rarely spread to cervical lymph nodes.

Lymph node metastases from papillary and medullary thyroid cancer are very common, and they have been observed to have an adverse impact on prognosis, with the possible exception of patients with papillary thyroid cancer who are younger than 45 years [5]. Cervical nodal metastases usually occur in a stepwise fashion, first involving lymph nodes of the ipsilateral central neck, then involving lymph nodes of the ipsilateral lateral neck (Levels II-IV), followed by lymph nodes on the contralateral side. Skip metastases, while unusual, can occur.

Central neck dissection for differentiated thyroid cancer is clearly indicated when central compartment lymph nodes are grossly involved with cancer. This is termed therapeutic central neck dissection. Therapeutic central neck dissection is also indicated if an enlarged or suspicious lymph node in the central neck is found to contain metastatic thyroid cancer on frozen section analysis. The role of routine, prophylactic central neck dissection for papillary thyroid cancer is controversial. The American Thyroid Association (ATA) guidelines and the National Comprehensive Cancer Network (NCCN) guidelines both recommend considering routine prophylactic central compartment neck dissection for patients with papillary thyroid cancer [5, 6]. The possible benefit to reducing cancer recurrence, however, must be balanced with the possible increased risk of morbidity associated with this procedure [7]. In contrast to papillary thyroid cancer, routine, bilateral prophylactic central neck dissection is recommended in the treatment of medullary thyroid cancer [4].

Preoperative Preparation

All patients with a diagnosis of thyroid cancer should have a preoperative ultrasound of the central and lateral compartments of the neck, with fine needle aspiration biopsy of any suspicious lymph nodes [5, 6]. If positive in the lateral neck, then the patient will require a modified radical neck dissection in addition to total thyroidectomy and central neck dissection.

Position

The patient is positioned supine on the operating table with the neck extended and the arms tucked at the sides. A beanbag or shoulder role is used to help extend the neck. A foam ring is helpful to pad the head and hold it in place. All pressure-points are padded. Semi-Fowler's or reverse Trendelenberg positioning is helpful to decompress the veins in the neck.

Description of Procedure

A curvilinear incision is made in a natural neck crease overlying the thyroid isthmus and carried through the subcutaneous tissue and platysma. Subplatysmal flaps are raised superiorly to the notch in the thyroid cartilage and inferiorly to the sternal notch. The strap muscles are separated vertically in the midline in an avascular plane. It is usually not necessary to divide the strap muscles for exposure. Total thyroidectomy is then performed in the standard fashion. Once the thyroid has been removed, the lymph nodes in the central compartment of the neck can then be addressed. The Delphian (precricoid) lymph node is located overlying the cricothyroid membrane and is often encountered and resected during the dissection of the thyroid isthmus and pyramidal lobe (if present).

Central compartment lymph node dissection involves resection of the fibrofatty lymph node-bearing tissue in the paratracheal and pretracheal spaces. The boundaries of this dissection are:

1. Hyoid bone – superiorly
2. Carotid artery – laterally
3. Midportion of the anterior trachea – medially
4. Suprasternal notch or innominate artery – inferiorly
5. Prevertebral fascia – deep

Structures at risk during this dissection include the parathyroid glands (particularly the lower glands) and the recurrent laryngeal nerves.

The technique of central compartment lymph node dissection first starts by defining the medial and lateral boundaries of the dissection [8]. A distinction can also be made between unilateral central neck dissection, which includes the precricoid/prelaryngeal, pretracheal, and unilateral paratracheal lymph nodes, and bilateral central neck dissection, which adds dissection of the contralateral paratracheal space [2]. Medially, the fibrofatty tissue overlying the trachea is incised to the level of the suprasternal notch, exposing the anterior surface of the trachea. Laterally, the medial border of the carotid artery is dissected down to the prevertebral fascia. The thin fascial layer overlying the recurrent laryngeal nerve is then opened along its length and the nerve dissected away from the fibrofatty tissue of the central neck and gently retracted laterally. This dissection, which can usually be done sharply, extends from the point of the nerve's insertion into the cricothyroid muscle superiorly to the thoracic inlet inferiorly. Figure 2.1 illustrates the left recurrent laryngeal nerve partially dissected out at the beginning of the central neck dissection. The fibrofatty lymph node-bearing tissue of the paratracheal space is then taken off the prevertebral fascia in a cephalad-to-caudad and lateral-to-medial fashion, lastly freeing it from the trachea and esophagus. Figure 2.2 illustrates the appearance of the left central neck at the conclusion of the dissection and Fig. 2.3 shows the

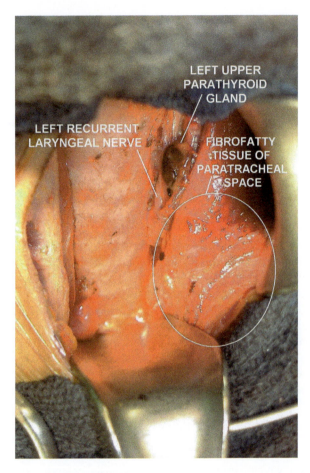

FIGURE 2.1 Left central neck dissection. The left recurrent laryngeal nerve is partially dissected, and the left upper parathyroid gland is visible in its normal position posterior to the nerve. The fibrofatty lymph node-bearing tissue of the paratracheal space is seen within the ellipse

resected specimen. Care must be taken to preserve the upper parathyroid gland on its vascular pedicle. The lower parathyroid gland is frequently devascularized during a formal central

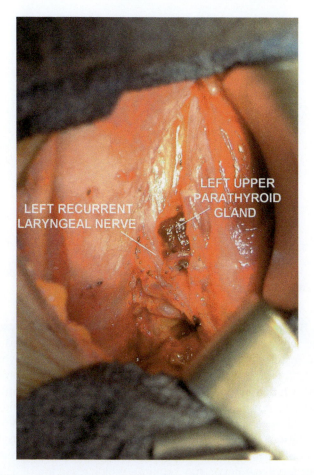

FIGURE 2.2 Left central neck dissection. The left recurrent laryngeal nerve has been skeletonized, and the fibrofatty lymph-node bearing tissue of the central neck has been removed

compartment neck dissection and should be autotransplanted if its blood supply is threatened. Hemostasis is assured and closure is performed in the standard fashion. Drains are usually not necessary.

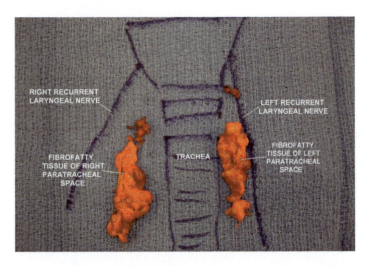

FIGURE 2.3 Post-resection specimens from a patient who required bilateral central neck dissections

Bulky central compartment nodal metastases that invade the recurrent laryngeal nerve should be managed based on the histology of the primary tumor and preoperative vocal cord function. Papillary thyroid cancer should be "shaved off" a functioning recurrent laryngeal nerve in an attempt to preserve vocal cord function on that side, and these patients should receive postoperative adjuvant radioactive iodine. Because there are no good adjuvant treatment options for patients with medullary thyroid cancer, invasion of the recurrent laryngeal nerve may require en-bloc resection of a segment of the nerve. Primary reanastomosis, nerve graft reconstruction, or anastomosis to the ansa cervicalis can be performed to preserve muscle bulk on that side.

Postoperative Care

Patients are observed in the hospital overnight. The head of the bed is elevated 30°. Clear liquids are given initially, and the diet advanced as tolerated. Recurrent laryngeal nerve function is assessed clinically by evaluating voice quality and aspiration of thin liquids. A serum calcium and parathyroid hormone level is checked the morning after surgery, or sooner if there are symptoms of hypocalcemia. Oral calcium supplementation is given to patients at risk of perioperative hypocalcemia.

References

1. Robbins KT, Clayman G, Levine PA, Medina J, Sessions R, Shaha A, et al. Neck dissection classification update: revisions proposed by the American Head and Neck Society and the American Academy of Otolaryngology-Head and Neck Surgery. Arch Otolaryngol Head Neck Surg. 2002;128(7):751–8.
2. Carty SE, Cooper DS, Doherty GM, Duh QY, Kloos RT, Mandel SJ, et al. Consensus statement on the terminology and classification of central neck dissection for thyroid cancer. Thyroid. 2009;19(11):1153–8. Epub 2009/10/29.
3. Hay ID, Thompson GB, Grant CS, Bergstralh EJ, Dvorak CE, Gorman CA, et al. Papillary thyroid carcinoma managed at the Mayo Clinic during six decades (1940–1999): temporal trends in initial therapy and long-term outcome in 2444 consecutively treated patients. World J Surg. 2002;26(8):879–85.
4. Kloos RT, Eng C, Evans DB, Francis GL, Gagel RF, Gharib H, et al. Medullary thyroid cancer: management guidelines of the American Thyroid Association. Thyroid. 2009;19(6):565–612. Epub 2009/05/28.
5. Cooper DS, Doherty GM, Haugen BR, Kloos RT, Lee SL, Mandel SJ, et al. Revised American Thyroid Association management guidelines for patients with thyroid nodules and differentiated thyroid cancer. Thyroid. 2009;19(11):1167–214. Epub 2009/10/29.
6. Tuttle R, Ball D, Byrd D, Dickson P, Duh Q, Ehya H, et al. National Comprehensive Cancer Network Clinical Practice Guidelines in oncology: thyroid carcinoma v.2.2013. 2013. Available from: http://www.nccn.org/professionals/physician_gls/pdf/thyroid.pdf.
7. Mazzaferri EL, Doherty GM, Steward DL. The pros and cons of prophylactic central compartment lymph node dissection for papillary thyroid carcinoma. Thyroid. 2009;19(7):683–9. Epub 2009/07/09.
8. Grodski S, Cornford L, Sywak M, Sidhu S, Delbridge L. Routine level VI lymph node dissection for papillary thyroid cancer: surgical technique. ANZ J Surg. 2007;77(4):203–8.

Chapter 3
Modified Radical Neck Dissection

Cord Sturgeon and Dina M. Elaraj

Abstract All patients with a diagnosis of thyroid cancer should have a complete preoperative ultrasound of the central and lateral compartments of the neck, with a clear documentation of the description and location of suspicious lymph nodes using the standard nomenclature. Fine needle aspiration biopsy of suspicious lymph nodes should be performed preoperatively in order to guide the extent of surgery. Papillary and medullary thyroid cancers frequently metastasize to the cervical lymph nodes. Thyroid cancer nodal metastases are best treated with formal compartmental clearance. For metastatic thyroid cancer within the lateral neck, the authors perform a formal nodal clearance of levels IIA, III, IV, and VB. The standard nomenclature, preoperative preparation, steps of the dissection, and postoperative care are described.

Keywords Neck dissection • metastatic thyroid cancer • surgical technique

C. Sturgeon, MD, MS (✉) • D.M. Elaraj, MD
Department of Surgery, Section of Endocrine Surgery,
Northwestern University Feinberg School of Medicine,
676 North Saint Clair Street, Suite 650, Chicago,
IL 60611, USA
e-mail: csturgeo@nmh.org; delaraj@nmh.org

H. Chen (ed.), *Illustrative Handbook of General Surgery*,
DOI 10.1007/978-3-319-24557-7_3,
© Springer International Publishing Switzerland 2016

27

Indications

The neck is divided into seven lymph node-bearing compartments, the nomenclature of which was originally described by the Memorial Sloan Kettering Head and Neck Service [1] and has been standardized and modified several times by the Committee for Neck Dissection Classification of the American Head and Neck Society and the American Academy of Otolaryngology-Head and Neck Surgery [2–4]. The seven nodal compartments are defined as follows:

I. Submental (IA) and submandibular (IB) triangle nodes.
II. Upper third jugular nodes located between the skull base and the hyoid bone. This compartment is subdivided into IIA (anterior) and IIB (posterior) based on the relationship to the spinal accessory nerve (CN XI).
III. Middle third jugular nodes located between the hyoid bone and the cricoid cartilage.
IV. Lower third jugular nodes located between the cricoid cartilage and the clavicle.
V. Posterior triangle nodes located between the anterior border of the trapezius muscle, the posterior border of the sternocleidomastoid muscle (SCM), and the clavicle. This group is subdivided into spinal accessory (VA) and supraclavicular (VB) nodes by a horizontal plane defined by the lower border of the cricoid cartilage.
VI. Central neck nodes located between the carotid sheaths extending from the hyoid bone to the suprasternal notch.
VII. Upper mediastinal nodes located between the suprasternal notch and the innominate artery.

The radical neck dissection, as originally described by Crile in 1906, entailed removal of all of the node-bearing tissue in Levels I–V along with the SCM, internal jugular vein and CN XI. The radical neck dissection is not considered a standard operation for thyroid cancer. Numerous modifications of the original operation have been described, however, that do have a significant role in the surgical management of thyroid cancer [5]. A "modified radical neck dissection" (MRND) is defined as an operation that involves the preservation of one or more non-lymphatic structures that were routinely removed in the radical neck dissection, but still results in the formal compartmental clearance of levels I–V [3]. Some experts have referred to an operation that formally clears compartments I–V and preserves the SCM, CN XI, and internal jugular vein as a "functional neck dissection". Expert guidelines would classify a procedure as a "selective neck dissection" (SND) when one or more of the lymph node levels is preserved during a formal neck dissection, and is usually depicted in the medical record as SND with the levels removed following in parentheses [2, 3]. An "extended neck dissection" is defined as a neck dissection that includes the removal of additional lymph node groups or structures beyond those included in the radical neck dissection.

The term "therapeutic neck dissection" implies that nodal metastases are clinically apparent at the time of the neck dissection. The terms "prophylactic neck dissection" or "elective neck dissection" imply that there are no clinical or radiographic findings to suggest that there are nodal metastases at the time of the dissection.

Papillary and medullary thyroid cancers frequently metastasize to the cervical lymph nodes. Thyroid cancer nodal metastases are best treated with formal compartmental clearance. There is no role for the selective removal of individual metastatic lymph nodes ("berry picking") [6]. For metastatic thyroid cancer, the authors perform a formal nodal clearance of levels IIA, III, IV, and VB, and in the text that follows we will refer to clearance of these node-bearing regions as a MRND. We recognize that some authors include levels I and IIB, and may perform a more extensive clearance of level V than what is described herein [2]. The SCM, internal jugular vein and CN XI are preserved, except in rare cases of directly invasive thyroid cancers, where a decision can be made to sacrifice one of these structures to allow resectability.

Therapeutic MRND is indicated for biopsy-proven lateral neck metastases from thyroid cancer [6–8]. Prophylactic MRND is not indicated in the treatment of patients with papillary thyroid cancer. The role and extent of prophylactic MRND in the treatment of medullary thyroid cancer (MTC) is controversial, with some authors advocating prophylactic MRND based on clinical parameters and intraoperative findings [9, 10]. The National Comprehensive Cancer Network recommends considering prophylactic ipsilateral MRND in the treatment of MTCs that are ≥1 cm (>0.5 cm if Multiple Endocrine Neoplasia [MEN] 2B) or with adjacent central compartment metastases [11], while other consensus guidelines for the treatment of patients with MEN recommend MRND for patients with MEN 2 only if there is clinical or radiographic evidence of involved lymph nodes in the lateral neck [12]. The 2009 American Thyroid Association (ATA) guidelines on the management of medullary thyroid cancer recommend dissection of the lateral neck including levels IIA, III, IV and V for patients with clinically apparent lateral neck nodal metastases [13]. It should also be noted that a minority of members on the ATA panel favored prophylactic ipsilateral MRND when lymph node metastases were present in the adjacent central compartment [13].

Preoperative Preparation

All patients with a diagnosis of thyroid cancer should have a complete preoperative ultrasound of the central and lateral compartments of the neck, with a clear documentation of the description and location of suspicious lymph nodes using the standard nomenclature described above. Fine needle aspiration biopsy of suspicious lymph nodes should be performed in order to guide the extent of surgery [6]. The patency of both internal jugular veins should be assessed and documented. A thorough neurologic examination should be done to assess the baseline function of the nerves at risk during

MRND. Preoperative laryngeal exam is recommended in cases of voice alteration or for revision surgery, although many clinicians perform this routinely to evaluate baseline vocal cord function in thyroid cancer patients. Patients should be counseled on the risks, benefits and alternatives to the proposed procedure(s), and the details of the discussion and the patient's understanding thereof should be documented.

Description of Procedure

The neck is extended and the head turned to expose the lateral aspect of the neck. A beanbag or shoulder role is used to help extend the neck. A foam ring is helpful to pad and immobilize the head. The patient is placed in semi-Fowler's position to decompress the neck veins. The entire neck extending from the chin, corner of the mouth, and pinna of the ear, laterally to the shoulders, and down onto the upper chest is prepped and draped. In order to visually assess the function of the marginal mandibular branch of the facial nerve, the corner of the mouth can be kept visible with the use of clear sterile draping.

Many skin incisions have been described for the MRND [14]. An incision from the mastoid process carried inferiorly along the posterior border of the SCM, then curved medially in a Langer's line towards the midline yields excellent exposure with an acceptable cosmetic result. For simplicity, only the MRND through this hemi-apron or "hockey-stick" incision will be described herein.

The skin is marked in the proposed line of the incision and infiltrated with 1 % lidocaine with epinephrine to allow for sharp dissection in a relatively bloodless field. The skin, subcutaneous tissues and platysma are incised sharply. Subplatysmal flaps are raised sharply towards the midline, taking care to preserve the greater auricular nerve and external jugular vein as the dissection proceeds over the surface of the SCM. The marginal mandibular nerve is preserved at the medial aspect of the subplatysmal flap.

Levels II and III

Dissection is begun in Level II. The second layer of deep cervical fascia along the anterior aspect of the SCM is incised along its entire length and the internal jugular vein exposed and traced cephalad to the posterior belly of the digastric muscle. CN XI is usually identified as it crosses the internal jugular vein from medial to lateral, or as it enters the posterior aspect of the SCM. There can be anatomic variation in the course of CN XI, with it coursing posterior to the internal jugular vein rather than superficial to it in one third of patients. Within the apex of the triangle bordered by the internal jugular vein and CN XI lies the fibrofatty tissue containing the level IIA nodes (Fig. 3.1). This node-bearing tissue located anterior and inferior to CN XI is opened sharply and

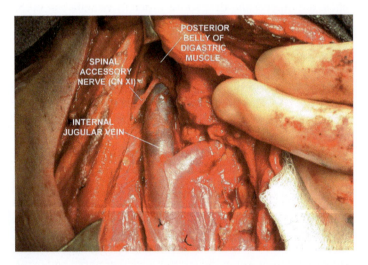

FIGURE 3.1 Right modified radical neck dissection. The dissection is started in Level IIA at the apex bounded by the internal jugular vein, and the spinal accessory nerve (CN XI)

swept inferiorly. Level IIB nodes (found superior and posterior to CN XI) should also be included when there is evidence of their involvement. The dissection proceeds caudad
and the fibrofatty tissue packet is sharply dissected from the
posterior aspect of the SCM and the anterior surface of the
scalene muscles. The lateral border of the level II dissection
is the posterior border of the SCM. The dissection is continued caudad past the hyoid bone into Level III, and inferiorly
to the omohyoid muscle, which is an alternative surgical
landmark for the inferior extent of level III (Fig. 3.2). The
omohyoid muscle is mobilized and preserved, although can
be divided without any consequence. The sensory branches of
the cervical plexus are preserved when possible.

Levels IV and VB

The dissection is continued caudad along the posterior border of the SCM until the clavicle is reached. There is often
additional node-bearing tissue inferior to the clavicle extending to the subclavian vein that should also be resected.
Furthermore, the node-bearing supraclavicular (Level VB)
tissue can be resected en-bloc with Level IV by extending the
dissection lateral to the posterior border of the SCM.

Medial Dissection

The fibrofatty bundle is retracted medially and completely dissected off the deep cervical fascia overlying the scalene muscles. This third layer of deep cervical fascia is usually preserved.
The medial border of the dissection is the carotid sheath. The
phrenic nerve, vagus nerve (Fig. 3.3), transverse cervical artery,
and brachial plexus are identified and preserved. Lymphatics
joining the thoracic duct are individually ligated. The internal
jugular vein is rolled medially to access the lymph nodes deep
to the carotid sheath. The internal jugular vein can be sacri-

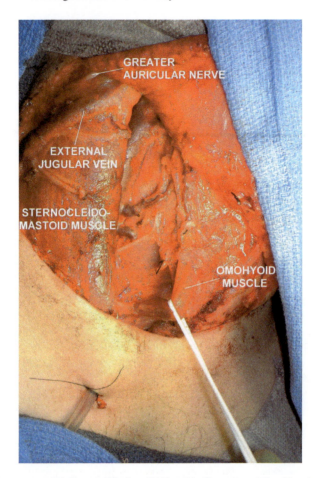

FIGURE 3.2 Right modified radical neck dissection. The fibrofatty lymph node-bearing tissue of Levels IIA and III have been cleared. The omohyoid muscle is being retracted inferomedially. The external jugular vein and greater auricular nerve are visible on the anterior surface of the sternocleidomastoid muscle

ficed unilaterally for gross invasion when the contralateral vein is patent. Dissection of the fibrofatty tissue packet is then completed sharply over the surface of the carotid sheath. Hemostasis is assured and closure performed in the standard fashion. Many experts routinely drain the dissection bed.

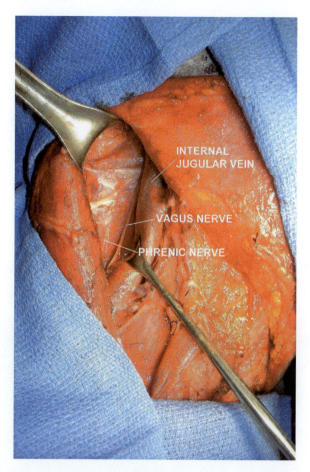

FIGURE 3.3 Right modified radical neck dissection. The internal jugular vein is being retracted medially and the sternocleidomastoid muscle is being retracted laterally. The vagus nerve is visible posterior to the internal jugular vein, and the phrenic vein is visible on the surface of the anterior scalene muscle

Postoperative Care

When the patient has regained consciousness, a neurological exam should be performed and the results documented. A chest radiograph can be performed in the recovery room to rule out pneumothorax or elevated hemidiaphragm if there is concern that the dissection could have violated the pleura or injured the phrenic nerve. Not all surgeons routinely drain the dissection bed, however, a common practice is to continue closed suction drainage until output is less than 25–30 mL in 24 h and non-chylous. Vocal cord paresis is a rare complication of MRND, and is usually temporary. Routine laryngoscopy following head and neck surgery is controversial, but is practiced by some experts. There is general agreement that laryngeal exam should be performed for suspected vocal cord paresis when early diagnosis and intervention would improve outcome (i.e. in cases of dysphagia, impaired pulmonary toilet, aspiration or potential airway compromise). Physical therapy is usually prescribed for patients with CN XI paresis.

References

1. Shah JP, Strong E, Spiro RH, Vikram B. Neck dissection – current status and future possibilities. Clin Bull. 1981;11(1):25–33.
2. Robbins KT, Medina JE, Wolfe GT, Levine PA, Sessions RB, Pruet CW. Standardizing neck dissection terminology. Official report of the academy's committee for head and neck surgery and oncology. Arch Otolaryngol Head Neck Surg. 1991;117(6):601–5.
3. Robbins KT, Clayman G, Levine PA, Medina J, Sessions R, Shaha A, et al. Neck dissection classification update: revisions proposed by the American Head and Neck Society and the American Academy of Otolaryngology-Head and Neck Surgery. Arch Otolaryngol Head Neck Surg. 2002;128(7):751–8.
4. Robbins KT, Shaha AR, Medina JE, Califano JA, Wolf GT, Ferlito A, et al. Consensus statement on the classification and terminology of neck dissection. Arch Otolaryngol Head Neck Surg. 2008;134(5):536–8.
5. Bocca E, Pignataro O. A conservation technique in radical neck dissection. Ann Otol Rhinol Laryngol. 1967;76(5):975–87.
6. Cooper DS, Doherty GM, Haugen BR, Kloos RT, Lee SL, Mandel SJ, et al. Management guidelines for patients with thyroid nodules and differentiated thyroid cancer. Thyroid. 2006; 16(2):109–42.

7. Cooper DS, Doherty GM, Haugen BR, Kloos RT, Lee SL, Mandel SJ, et al. Revised American Thyroid Association management guidelines for patients with thyroid nodules and differentiated thyroid cancer. Thyroid. 2009;19(11):1167–214.
8. Tuttle RM, Ball DW, Byrd D, Dilawari RA, Doherty GM, Duh QY, et al. Thyroid carcinoma. J Natl Compr Canc Netw. 2010;8(11):1228–74.
9. Moley JF, DeBenedetti MK. Patterns of nodal metastases in palpable medullary thyroid carcinoma: recommendations for extent of node dissection. Ann Surg. 1999;229(6):880–7; discussion 7–8.
10. Evans DB, Shapiro SE, Cote GJ. Invited commentary: medullary thyroid cancer: the importance of RET testing. Surgery. 2007;141(1):96–9.
11. Tuttle RM, Ball DW, Byrd D, Daniels GH, Dilawari RA, Doherty GM, et al. Medullary carcinoma. J Natl Compr Canc Netw. 2010;8(5):512–30.
12. Brandi ML, Gagel RF, Angeli A, Bilezikian JP, Beck-Peccoz P, Bordi C, et al. Guidelines for diagnosis and therapy of MEN type 1 and type 2. J Clin Endocrinol Metab. 2001;86(12):5658–71.
13. Kloos RT, Eng C, Evans DB, Francis GL, Gagel RF, Gharib H, et al. Medullary thyroid cancer: management guidelines of the American Thyroid Association. Thyroid. 2009;19(6):565–612.
14. Uchino S, Noguchi S, Yamashita H, Watanabe S. Modified radical neck dissection for differentiated thyroid cancer: operative technique. World J Surg. 2004;28(12):1199–203.

Chapter 4
Parathyroidectomy

Lilah F. Morris and Michael W. Yeh

Abstract Parathyroidectomy is definitive treatment for sporadic, primary hyperparathyroidism with cure rates as high as 98 % at expert centers. We explore the predictive value of preoperative localizing studies including ^{99m}Tc-sestamibi scan, ultrasound, and four-dimensional CT scan. Operative technique for bilateral neck exploration is described with special attention given to anatomic principles. While there are multiple techniques for limited exploration — defined as a unilateral, image-directed parathyroidectomy involving an incision measuring 2.5 cm or less — we describe the lateral mini-incision approach. Although uncommon, complications of parathyroidectomy include hematoma, hypocalcemia, permanent hypoparathyroidism, nerve injury, and operative

L.F. Morris, MD (✉)
Department of Surgery, Northwest Allied General Surgery,
Northwest Medical Center, 6130 N. La Cholla Blvd,
Ste 210, Tucson, AZ 85741, USA
e-mail: Lilah.morris@northwestmedicalcenter.com

M.W. Yeh, MD
Department of Surgery, Section of Endocrine Surgery,
UCLA David Geffen School of Medicine,
10833 Le Conte Ave. 72-228 CHS, Los Angeles,
CA 90095, USA
e-mail: myeh@mednet.ucla.edu

H. Chen (ed.), *Illustrative Handbook of General Surgery*,
DOI 10.1007/978-3-319-24557-7_4,
© Springer International Publishing Switzerland 2016

failure. Finally, we address the advantages, disadvantages, and controversies of four-gland versus limited exploration.

Keywords Sporadic primary hyperparathyroidism • Parathyroid adenoma • Bilateral neck exploration • Minimally invasive parathyroidectomy

Indications

Primary hyperparathyroidism (pHPT) is diagnosed biochemically by hypercalcemia in the presence of elevated or inappropriately normal parathyroid hormone (PTH) levels. Eighty-five percent of cases of sporadic pHPT are caused by a parathyroid adenoma – a single enlarged, hyperfunctioning gland. Four-gland hyperplasia represents about 10 % of cases, while double adenomas constitute 4 % and parathyroid carcinoma <1 %. While parathyroidectomy is the recommended treatment of patients with symptomatic pHPT, the need for surgical intervention in patients with asymptomatic disease is less clear. The Fourth International Workshop consensus statement, last updated in 2014, recommended surgical intervention for patients with asymptomatic primary hyperparathyroidism who meet a defined set of criteria (Table 4.1) [1].

Preoperative Preparation: Imaging Studies

Preoperative localizing studies may be performed after confirmation of the biochemical diagnosis and once the decision for surgery has been made. The most commonly used study is the ^{99m}Tc-sestamibi scan, which can correctly identify the site of abnormal parathyroid tissue with 78.9 % accuracy and a 90.7 % positive predictive value (PPV) in a pooled meta-analysis. Parathyroid ultrasound, an increasingly used method of pre-operative localization, has a pooled accuracy rate of 76.1 % and PPV 93.2 % [2]. Four-dimensional CT scan, a newer technique for localizing parathyroid adenomas, relies on the differential contrast enhancement between the

TABLE 4.1 The Fourth International Workshop updated 2013 consensus statement for recommending parathyroidectomy in patients with asymptomatic primary hyperparathyroidism

Age <50 years

Serum calcium > 1.0 mg/dL above normal

Creatinine clearance < 60 mL/min; 24-h urinary calcium > 400 mg/dL and increased calcium containing stone risk by biochemical stone risk analysis; radiologic evidence of nephrolithiasis or nephrocalcinosis

Osteoporosis (reduction in bone density > 2.5 standard deviations below peak bone mass at lumbar spine, total hip, femoral neck, or distal 1/3 radius) and/or radiologic evidence of vertebral fracture

Medical surveillance not desired or possible

thyroid and parathyroid glands (perfusion over time is the fourth dimension). Though several scanning protocols have been published, all include an early arterial phase followed by a delayed venous phase. Parathyroid adenomas display avid early arterial contrast enhancement and rapid washout, and can thus be differentiated from the thyroid gland which has less avid early contrast enhancement (Fig. 4.1) [3]. Pooled accuracy rates for localization of parathyroid adenomas are 89.4 % and PPV 93.5 % [2].

Surgical Positioning and Anesthesia

The patient should be positioned supine on the operating table with the neck hyperextended using a horizontal shoulder roll and both arms tucked. For bilateral neck exploration, general anesthesia using an endotracheal tube or laryngeal mask airway is commonly used. For limited exploration, some centers use general anesthesia while others employ local/regional anesthesia with sedation (monitored anesthetic care or MAC). Regardless of the planned procedure, the surgical area should be prepped and draped to accommodate a bilateral neck exploration.

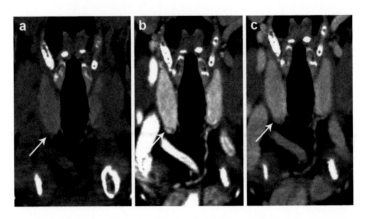

FIGURE 4.1 4D CT images for parathyroid localization help distinguish parathyroid adenomas from normal thyroid. These multiple imaging phases demonstrate the lower density parathyroid gland (indicated by an *arrow*) compared to the thyroid on pre-contrast (**a**) and venous phase (**c**) but is similar to the thyroid on arterial phase scan (**b**) (Images courtesy Dr. Ali Sepahdari, Department of Radiology, UCLA David Geffen School of Medicine)

Description of Procedure

Four-Gland Exploration

Bilateral neck exploration, with identification of all four parathyroid glands, has long been the standard approach to parathyroid surgery. A 2.5–4 cm central, transverse cervical (Kocher) incision is made along a skin crease 1 cm below the cricoid cartilage. After the creation of subplatysmal flaps, the strap muscles are separated in the midline (Fig. 4.2). The plane between the sternothyroid muscles and the thyroid capsule is developed. The middle thyroid veins are divided to allow rotation of the thyroid gland anteriomedially, as the majority of the parathyroid glands lie posterior to the thyroid. The elements of the carotid sheath are then retracted laterally away from the thyroid. A critical maneuver in parathyroid exploration is

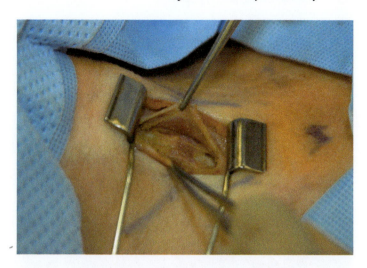

FIGURE 4.2 Initial dissection for bilateral neck exploration. A central, transverse cervical incision lies 2 cm above the suprasternal notch (marked in *purple*, far right). Subplatysmal flaps are being retracted and forceps are elevating the divided strap muscles. The thyroid isthmus is visible

exposure and palpation of the prevertebral space that lies posterior to the esophagus. Indeed, failure to adequately interrogate the posterior (paraesophageal and retroesophageal) spaces of the neck is the most common cause of failed initial parathyroid exploration [4].

Normal parathyroid glands are yellow-tan in color. They are 5 mm in diameter, flattened or discoid in shape, and weigh between 30 and 50 mg. They are generally housed in a thin fatty envelope, giving them a classic "fried egg" appearance. Open exploration begins with interrogation of the superior parathyroid territory. Because of their shorter path of embryologic migration, the superior parathyroids are more consistent in their location than the inferior parathyroids, with the majority located within a 1.5 cm radius of the tubercle of Zuckerkandl, a postero-lateral prominence of the thyroid gland. Other important nearby structures include the terminus

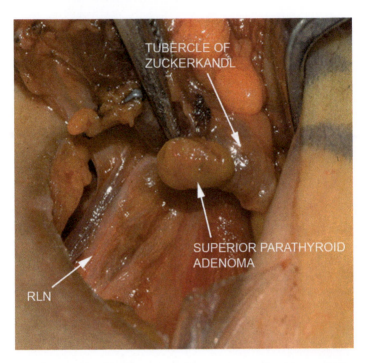

FIGURE 4.3 Relationship of structures surrounding the superior parathyroid gland during a bilateral neck exploration. The superior parathyroid adenoma abuts the thyroid's tubercle of Zuckerkandl. The recurrent laryngeal nerve (*RLN*) can be seen traversing anterior-medially to the gland

of the recurrent laryngeal nerve, arborization of the inferior thyroid artery, and the cricoid cartilage (Fig. 4.3).

As superior parathyroid adenomas enlarge, they often slide inferiorly along the paraesophageal space. By definition, the superior parathyroids are located postero-laterally to the plane of the recurrent laryngeal nerve (Fig. 4.4) [5].

Though routine identification of the recurrent laryngeal nerve is not considered mandatory during parathyroid exploration, the surgeon must be extremely wary of avoiding nerve injury while operating near the superior parathyroids.

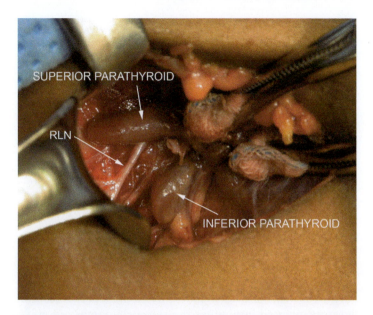

FIGURE 4.4 Relationship of the recurrent laryngeal nerve (*RLN*) to the parathyroid glands during bilateral neck exploration for renal hyperparathyroidism. The thyroid gland has been retracted medially toward the patient's left

A small fraction of parathyroid glands lie partially or completely embedded in the thyroid gland parenchyma; these may be either superior or inferior parathyroids.

The inferior parathyroid glands are located anteromedially to the plane of the recurrent laryngeal nerve (Fig. 4.4). The territory of the inferior parathyroid is relatively large, ranging from the superior pole of the thyroid to the anterior mediastinum. The majority of inferior parathyroid glands lie on the surface of the inferior pole of the thyroid, often near the inferior pole veins that demarcate the top of the thyrothymic tract. Inferior parathyroid adenomas can frequently be found by following the thyrothymic tract down into the chest. Ectopic inferior parathyroids are most commonly located in the thymus, and can almost always be removed transcervically.

If three glands appear normal and one gland is enlarged, the diagnosis is a single parathyroid adenoma. The safest method of dissecting out a parathyroid adenoma is to start away from the vascular pedicle, mobilizing the lateral and inferior aspects while avoiding violation of the gland capsule. The vascular pedicle is isolated last and ligated. Frozen section may be employed to confirm that resection of hypercellular parathyroid tissue has been achieved. After irrigation and hemostasis, the strap muscles and platysma are reapproximated. The skin is then closed in a subcuticular fashion.

If a four-gland exploration reveals hyperplasia (four enlarged glands), a subtotal parathyroidectomy is generally performed. This involves complete removal of the three most abnormal-appearing glands and partial resection of the fourth gland, leaving 40–50 mg of normal appearing tissue on an intact vascular pedicle. Should the remnant become devascularized, it can be excised, morcellated, and autotransplanted into either the sternocleidomastoid muscle or the brachioradialis muscle of the forearm.

Limited Exploration

Limited exploration is defined as a unilateral, image-directed parathyroidectomy involving an incision measuring 2.5 cm or less. These operations may involve inspection of a single gland or two glands on the same side. Frequently, intraoperative parathyroid hormone (IOPTH) monitoring is used to confirm completeness of resection. Described techniques include: (1) videoscopic, (2) video-assisted, (3) direct view central mini-incision, and (4) direct view lateral mini-incision [6]. We will describe the lateral mini-incision approach, which provides the most direct exposure of the parathyroid-bearing regions (Fig. 4.5). The incision site is placed directly over the parathyroid adenoma using ultrasound guidance. Alternatively, placement of the incision approximately 5 mm inferior to the cricoid cartilage will typically offer adequate exposure. A 2 cm

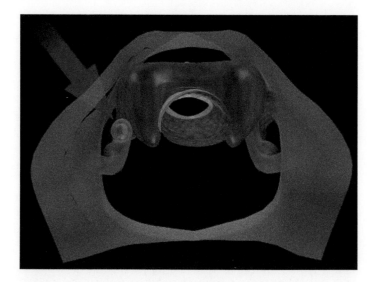

FIGURE 4.5 An axial representation of the direct access to the parathyroid obtained using the lateral mini-incision technique

transverse incision is placed along a skin crease, centered over
the anterior border of the sternocleidomastoid muscle. Small
subplatysmal flaps are created. The sternocleidomastoid muscle is retracted laterally and the strap muscles are retracted
medially. The thyroid is rotated anteriomedially and the
carotid sheath elements retracted laterally. After identification of the abnormal gland, dissection proceeds as in open
exploration (Fig. 4.6). At the surgeon's preference, exploration of the territory of the non-excised ipsilateral gland can be
undertaken at this point to evaluate for multiple gland
disease.

IOPTH Monitoring

IOPTH monitoring is used to confirm complete removal of
hyperfunctioning parathyroid tissue during limited exploration. Fall of the 10 min post-excision PTH value to less than

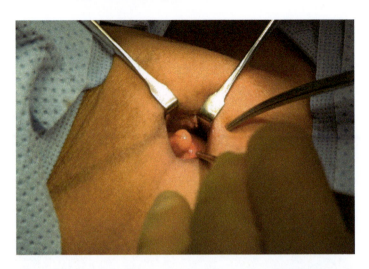

Figure 4.6 Identification of an inferior parathyroid adenoma via lateral mini-incision technique. The adenoma was localized preoperatively with a functional ^{99m}Tc-sestamibi scan. Immediately prior to incision, the position of the gland was confirmed with surgeon-performed ultrasound and a 2 cm incision was made on overlying skin

50 % of the highest pre-excision value is highly predictive of long-term cure [7]. Failure to meet this criterion may prompt the surgeon to convert to bilateral neck exploration.

Is Four-Gland Exploration or Limited Exploration Preferred?

The relative merits of four-gland exploration and limited exploration have been debated for more than 30 years [8, 9]. Four-gland exploration allows for identification of all parathyroid glands, may lead to discovery of occult multigland disease, and permits conclusion of the case without IOPTH monitoring. Its disadvantages include increased operative time, placing two recurrent laryngeal nerves at risk, and the theoretical risk of permanent hypoparathyroidism. Limited exploration is generally faster and involves fewer risks; however, it generally requires waiting for an IOPTH result and may, in the opinion of some authors, lead to a slightly higher rate of operative failure from missed multiple gland disease. While this controversy is ongoing, the only reliable predictor of successful parathyroid surgery is surgeon experience [10, 11]. At present, no convincing data exist to support the superiority of one operative approach over another.

Post-operative Care

Parathyroid surgery has typically been followed by an overnight hospital stay, though a number of centers have moved to a same day discharge approach. Complications of parathyroidectomy are uncommon [12]. Hematoma occurs in approximately 0.3 % of patients, and requires emergent reexploration. Post-operative hypocalcemia may occur due to either iatrogenic hypoparathyroidism after four gland manipulation or, more commonly, high-turnover bone disease and suppression of remaining parathyroid tissue in patients with biochemically severe disease. Symptoms should be assessed and treated with supplemental calcium as needed. Permanent hypoparathyroidism is only a risk for patients undergoing bilateral neck exploration and should occur in <1 % of patients. The rate of permanent recurrent laryngeal nerve paresis is 1 % or less in expert hands. The most common complication of parathyroid exploration is operative failure (persistent hyperparathyroidism), defined as hypercalcemia occurring within 6 months of operation. These patients require reoperation. The overall frequency of operative failure ranges from 2 % in expert centers to 20 % or more in low-volume centers [8, 9].

References

1. Udelsman R, Åkerström G, Biagini C, Duh QY, Miccoli P, Niederle B, Tonelli F. The surgical management of asymptomatic primary hyperparathyroidism: Proceedings of the Fourth

International Workshop. J Clin Endocrinol Metab. 2014;99:3595–606.

2. Cheung K, Wang TS, Farrokhyar F, Roman SA, Sosa JA. A meta-analysis of preoperative localization techniques for patients with primary hyperparathyroidism. Ann Surg Oncol. 2012;19:577–83.

3. Vu TH, Guha-Thakurta N, Harrell RK, Ahmed S, Kumar AJ, Johnson VE, Perrier ND, Hamberg LM, Hunter GJ, Schellingerhout D. Imaging characteristics of hyperfunctioning parathyroid adenomas using multiphase multidetector computed tomography: a quantitative and qualitative approach. J Comput Assist Tomogr. 2011;35:560–7.

4. Shen W, Düren M, Morita E, Higgins C, Duh QY, Siperstein AE, Clark OH. Reoperation for persistent or recurrent primary hyperparathyroidism. Arch Surg. 1996;131:861–7.

5. Thompson N, Eckhauser FE, Harness JK. The anatomy of primary hyperparathyroidism. Surgery. 1982;92:814–21.

6. Palazzo F, Delbridge LW. Minimal-access/minimally invasive parathyroidectomy for primary hyperparathyroidism. Surg Clin North Am. 2004;84:717–34.

7. Carniero D, Solorzano CC, Nader MC, Ramirez M, Irvin GL. Comparison of intraoperative iPTH assay (QPTH) criteria in guiding parathyroidectomy: which criterion is the most accurate? Surgery. 2003;134:973–81.

8. Wang CA. Surgery of hyperparathyroidism: a conservative approach. J Surg Oncol. 1981;16:225–8.

9. Tibblin S, Bondeson AG, Ljungberg O. Unilateral parathyroidectomy in hyperparathyroidism due to single adenoma. Ann Surg. 1982;195:245–52.

10. Yeh MW, Wiseman JE, Chu SD, Ituarte PH, Liu IL, Young KL, Kang SJ, Harari A, Haigh PI. Population-level predictors of persistent hyperparathyroidism. Surgery. 2011;150:1113–9.

11. Abdulla AG, Ituarte PH, Harari A, Wu JX, Yeh MW. Trends in the frequency and quality of parathyroid surgery: analysis of 17,082 cases over 10 years. Ann Surg. 2015;261(4):746–50.

12. Carty S. Prevention and management of complications in parathyroid surgery. Otolaryngol Clin North Am. 2004;37:897–907.

Chapter 5
Open Adrenalectomy

Nisar A. Zaidi and Stanley B. Sidhu

Abstract Though laparoscopic adrenalectomy has become the gold standard for management of benign adrenal tumours, open adrenalectomy remains the standard of care for large tumours or tumours suspicious for malignancy. In this chapter we will detail the indications for open adrenalectomy. Preoperative considerations, particularly indicators of malignancy, will be discussed. A thorough description of open right and left adrenalectomy will be separately described, along with important post-operative considerations for patients undergoing open resection.

Keywords Open adrenalectomy • Adrenocortical cancer • Transperitoneal adrenalectomy

N.A. Zaidi, MD
Endocrine Surgical Unit, Royal North Shore Hospital,
University of Sydney, St Leonards, NSW Australia

S.B. Sidhu, PhD, FRACS (✉)
Endocrine Surgical Unit, University of Sydney,
St. Leonards, NSW Australia

Department of Endocrine and Oncologic Surgery, Royal North Shore Hospital, Reserve Rd, St. Leonards, NSW 2065, Australia

Endocrine Surgery Unit, University of Sydney and RNSH,
St. Leonards, NSW Australia
e-mail: stansidhu@nebsc.com.au

H. Chen (ed.), *Illustrative Handbook of General Surgery*,
DOI 10.1007/978-3-319-24557-7_5,
© Springer International Publishing Switzerland 2016

51

Indications

Laparoscopic adrenalectomy has become the standard of care for the surgical management of functional and non-functional adrenal tumours [1, 2]; open adrenalectomy is utilized in the following situations:

1. Large adrenal tumours, usually over 10 cm in diameter [2].
2. Known, or high suspicion of adrenocortical carcinoma pre-operatively [3].
3. Conversion after laparoscopic inspection of an adrenal tumour and suspicion of malignancy intraoperatively. Such features include abnormally large tumour blood vessels, local invasion and tumour thrombus inside the adrenal vein [4].

Suspicion of adrenocortical carcinoma is raised with a number of clinical, biochemical, and radiographic findings summarized below.

Clinical	Pain, palpable mass, rapid growth, IVC compression or obstruction.
Biochemical	Mixed hormone secretion, virilizing hormone secretion, elevated levels of hormone precursors (i.e., DHEA).
Radiographic	Size > 4–6 cm, > 10 Hounsfield units on non-contrast CT, < 50 % washout on contrast CT, irregular borders, lymphadenopathy, presence of calcification or necrosis, evidence of invasion, >3.4 SUV on PET-CT.

There are a number of approaches for open adrenalectomy including the retroperitoneal, thoracoabdominal and the anterior or lateral transperitoneal approach. In our unit, we favour the lateral transperitoneal approach (Fig. 5.1).

Preoperative Preparation

Pre-operative workup is essential to diagnose a functional adrenal tumor. The common syndromes that require evaluation are Conn's syndrome, pheochromocytoma, Cushing's

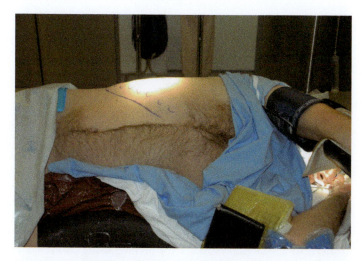

FIGURE 5.1 The patient is placed in the lateral position. The operating table is then broken to maximize the space between the costal margin and the iliac crest. The bean bag is then aspirated to firmness to secure the patient in place

syndrome, and functional adrenocortical carcinoma, which usually has Cushing-virilizing features. Open adrenalectomy is usually reserved for large pheochromocytomas or functional and non-functional adrenocortical carcinomas [5, 6].

A full preoperative workup for hyperaldosteronism, Cushing's syndrome and pheochromocytoma is reviewed in detail by Young [5] and Sidhu et al. [7].

At induction, patients should have DVT prophylaxis with subcutaneous fractioned heparin or equivalent, pneumatic calf compressors as well as an indwelling bladder catheter and a nasogastric tube.

Positioning

The patient is placed in the lateral position with the operating table placed in maximal flexion to accentuate the space between the costal margin and the iliac crest. A bean bag is useful to secure the patient in position and appropriate strapping is provided (Fig. 5.1).

Description of Procedure

Right Sided Adrenalectomy

The costal margin is palpated and a subcostal incision two fingerbreadths below the costal margin is performed from the mid-clavicular line medially to the mid-axillary line posteriorly. This incision can be extended down to the midline anteriorly if required. The skin and underlying fat along this line are incised. The external oblique, internal oblique and transverse abdominal muscles are divided using cautery. The peritoneum is then entered sharply exposing the peritoneal cavity. At this point, full palpation of the peritoneal cavity is required to exclude metastatic disease.

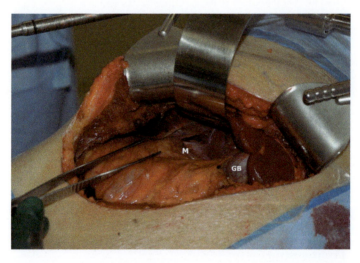

FIGURE 5.2 A subcostal incision is made, the muscle layer is divided and the peritoneal cavity entered. The triangular ligament is divided, the liver retracted superiorly and the peritoneum of the hepatorenal pouch is divided to gain access to the upper border of the adrenal tumor (*M*). *GB* gallbladder

The hepatic flexure of the colon is mobilized and retracted inferiorly. The duodenum can then be kocherized to allow better access to the IVC. The liver is mobilized medially and superiorly by dividing the right triangular ligament (Fig. 5.2). Morrison's pouch is then entered by incising the peritoneum below the liver and overlying the adrenal gland. The superior margin of the adrenal tumor is identified. The lower margin of the tumor and the renal vein are identified inferiorly (Fig. 5.3). Medial to the tumor, the IVC can then be identified by a combination of sharp and blunt dissection after incising the overlying peritoneum. We aim to triangulate the dissection onto the adrenal vein from below and above (Fig. 5.4). With the patient in the lateral position, the adrenal vein is encountered as the IVC is passing under the liver. Once the adrenal vein is secured, the tumor is lifted off from the retroperitoneum and the feeding arteries, which

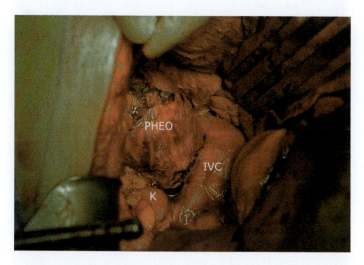

FIGURE. 5.3 Open adrenalectomy for a right sided adrenal pheochromocytoma. Dissection is carried out along the lateral margin of the IVC, triangulating from above and below to encounter the adrenal vein (not shown). *PHEO* pheochromocytoma, *K* kidney, *IVC* inferior vena cava

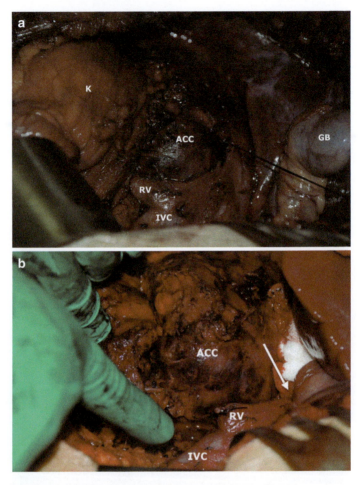

FIGURE 5.4 Open adrenalectomy for a large ACC invading the right kidney. (**a**) Right renal vein is identified below the inferior margin of the tumor. (**b**) The renal vein has been divided. The *arrow* shows the putative position of the right adrenal vein. *ACC* adrenal tumor, *RV* renal vein, *IVC* inferior vena cava, *K* kidney, *GB* gallbladder

arise from the inferior phrenic, the aorta and the renal arteries are ligated and divided with a thermal sealing device.

Left Sided Adrenalectomy

Open adrenalectomy on the left side is completely different to surgery of the right side. A subcostal incision is performed in a similar way with the patient in the right lateral position. The peritoneal cavity is entered and explored. Attention is directed to the splenic flexure of the colon, which should be mobilized along the line of Toldt (Fig. 5.5). The lienorenal ligament is then divided and the spleen and tail of the pancreas are rotated medially (Fig. 5.6). The adrenal tumor can then be inspected and the renal vein is identified on its inferomedial aspect. The adrenal vein is then identified as it

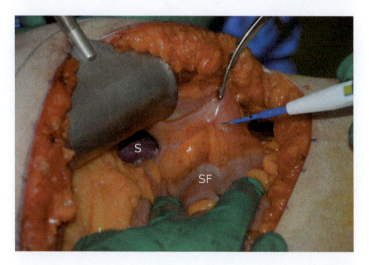

FIGURE 5.5 Open adrenalectomy for a left 4 cm ACC. The splenic flexure of the colon is mobilized to expose the spleen, which is then medialized by dividing the lienorenal ligament. *S* spleen, *SF* splenic flexure

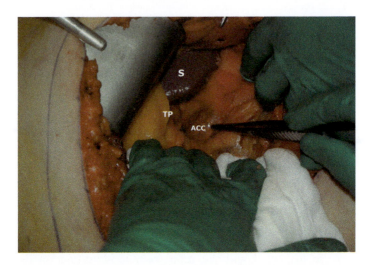

FIGURE 5.6 The spleen and the tail of the pancreas have been medialized to expose the adrenal gland. *S* spleen, *ACC* adrenal tumor, *TP* tail of pancreas

enters the left renal vein; it is often joined by the inferior phrenic vein prior to this point (Fig. 5.7). The adrenal vein is ligated and divided. The tumor is then lifted off from the retroperitoneum and any feeding vessels are ligated and divided.

The use of drains is optional. The muscle layer is closed using a running non-absorbable suture. Skin is then sutured using an absorbable subcuticular stitch.

Postoperative Care

Patients should be observed closely for signs of bleeding and blood pressure should be monitored frequently. Signs of adrenal insufficiency should be addressed immediately especially in patients with Cushing's syndrome. Electrolyte values are checked daily. Patients with Cushing's syndrome should be placed on IV steroids until able to take them orally. The urinary catheter can usually be removed on the first postop-

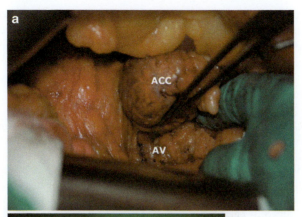

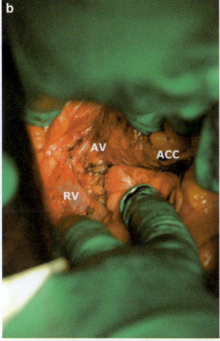

FIGURE 5.7 (**a**) The left adrenal vein is encountered on the inferome-dial aspect of the gland. (**b**) The left renal vein is identified; the adrenal vein is shown here draining into the left renal vein. *AV* adrenal vein, *ACC* adrenal tumor, *RV* renal vein

erative day as well as the nasogastric tube. Diet is recommenced once peristalsis is re-established. Patients are usually able to leave the hospital after the fifth postoperative day.

References

1. Grumbach MM, Biller BMK, Braunstein GD, et al. Management of the clinically inapparent adrenal mass ("Incidentaloma"). Ann Intern Med. 2003;138(5):424–9.
2. Soon PS, Yeh MW, Delbridge LW, Bambach CP, Sywak MS, Robinson BD, Sidhu SB. Laparoscopic surgery is safe for large adrenal lesions. Eur J Surg Oncol. 2008;34(1):67–70.
3. Sidhu S, Sywak M, Robinson B, Delbridge L. Adrenocortical cancer: recent clinical and molecular advances. Curr Opin Oncol. 2003;16(1):13–8.
4. Henry JF, Sebagb F, Iacobone M, Mirallie E. Results of laparoscopic adrenalectomy for large and potentially malignant tumours. World J Surg. 2002;26(8):1043–7.
5. Young WF. The incidentally discovered adrenal mass. N Eng J Med. 2007;356(6):601–10.
6. Alderazi Y, Yeh MW, Robinson BG, Benn DE, Sywak MS, Learoyd DL, Delbridge LW, Sidhu SB. Phaeochromocytoma: current concepts. Med J Aust. 2005;15(4):201–4.
7. Sidhu SB, Gicquel C, Bambach CP, Campbell P, Magarey C, Robinson BG, Delbridge LW. Clinical and molecular aspects of adrenocortical tumourigenesis. ANZ J Surg. 2003;73(9):727–38.

Chapter 6
Laparoscopic Adrenalectomy: Transperitoneal Approach

Abbey L. Fingeret and James A. Lee

Abstract   This chapter discusses laparoscopic transabdominal adrenalectomy. The authors review the indications and contraindications for this procedure. Patient preoperative historical factors, biochemical testing, and operative preparation are presented. The authors describe in detail the operative technique including patient positioning, port placement, and procedural steps with special considerations for left versus right adrenalectomy. Finally, postoperative care recommendations are reviewed.

A.L. Fingeret, MD
Division of Gastrointestinal and Endocrine Surgery,
Department of Surgery, College of Physicians and Surgeons
of Columbia University, New York, NY, USA

Department of General Surgery, New York-Presbyterian Hospital,
Columbia University Medical Center, New York, NY, USA

J.A. Lee, MD (✉)
Division of Gastrointestinal and Endocrine Surgery,
Department of Surgery, College of Physicians and Surgeons
of Columbia University, New York, NY, USA

Department of Endocrine Surgery,
New York-Presbyterian Hospital,
Columbia University Medical Center, 161 Fort Washington Ave,
New York, NY 10032, USA
e-mail: Jal74@columbia.edu

H. Chen (ed.), *Illustrative Handbook of General Surgery*,   61
DOI 10.1007/978-3-319-24557-7_6,
© Springer International Publishing Switzerland 2016

Keywords Laparoscopic • Minimally invasive • Adrenal-ectomy • Adrenal incidentaloma • Aldosterone producing adenoma • Cushing's syndrome • Pheochromocytoma • Adrenocortical carcinoma

Indications

In recent years, there has been a shift from open adrenalec-tomy toward laparoscopic adrenalectomy for the treatment of adrenal tumors due to such factors as decreased post-operative pain and faster recovery. Indeed, the majority of adrenalectomies in high volume centers are performed lapa-roscopically. Indications for an adrenalectomy, whether open or laparoscopic, include a functional tumor, growth of an adrenal mass of 0.5 cm in 6 months based on imaging, adrenal tumor greater than 3–4 cm (since the risk of adrenal carci-noma increases with increasing tumor size), and isolated metastatic disease. The indications for laparoscopic adrenal-ectomy are essentially the same as those for open adrenalec-tomy with the notable exception of adrenocortical cancer, malignant pheochromocytoma, and large metastases. However, as skill and experience with laparoscopy increases, many authors have advocated laparoscopic adrenalectomy even for malignant disease. Contraindications for laparoscopic adrenalectomy also include general contraindications to lap-aroscopic procedures such as severe cardiopulmonary risk and coagulopathy.

Preoperative Preparation

Upon discovery of an adrenal mass, the two main goals are to (1) determine if it is functional and (2) determine the risk of malignancy. History and physical exam may provide useful clues as to whether a tumor is functional, but bio-chemical interrogation is mandatory. If the tumor is non-functional the next task is to determine the risk for cancer. If a patient is found to have an adrenal mass and has a primary tumor elsewhere, he/she should be suspected of having metastatic disease. Patients with adrenal incidentalomas, however, should undergo age- and risk factor-appropriate screening. Aside from the presence of local invasion, the best indication of risk for adrenocortical carcinoma is tumor size. Based on size, the risk for adrenocortical cancer is approximately: less than 3 % for tumors smaller than 4 cm, 7 % for tumors 4–6 cm, and 25 % or greater for tumors larger than 6 cm. The following biochemical evaluation should be performed for the work-up for adrenal tumors.

1. <u>24-h urine metanephrines or plasma metanephrines</u>: pheochromocytoma
2. <u>24-h urine cortisol, midnight salivery cortisol, or low dose dexamethasone suppression test</u>: Cushing's syndrome
3. <u>Plasma aldosterone and renin</u>: primary hyperaldosteronism
4. <u>Cross-sectional imaging (CT or MRI)</u>: localization and operative planning
5. <u>CXR, colonoscopy, mammogram as appropriate</u>: metastatic disease work-up
6. <u>Free testosterone, estradiol, dehydroeipandrosterone</u>: Virilizing functional tumors
7. <u>Urinary 5-HIAA, octreotide scan</u>: Carcinoid

Pre-operative preparation for patients depends largely upon the pathology encountered. For most adrenal tumors, no special precautions are needed. However, with pheochromocytoma and Cushing's syndrome, specific measures are needed due to the tumor pathophysiology. For pheochromocytoma, pre-operative alpha-blockade with repletion of intravascular volume is crucial to a safe and successful operation. Once the patient is adequately alpha-blocked and volume resuscitated, a beta-blocker may be started if the patient is tachycardic. Starting a beta-blocker prior to alpha-blockade may lead to unopposed alpha-mediated vasoconstriction that could precipitate a hypertensive crisis. In addition, it is essential that the anesthesiologist utilize short-acting pharmacologic agents to combat hyper- or hypotension. For patients with Cushing's syndrome, a stress dose of steroids should be given prior to induction of anesthesia. In addition, patients with Cushing's syndrome should receive prophylactic antibiotics since they are more prone to infectious complications due to steroid excess.

Description of Procedure

There are several approaches to laparoscopic adrenalectomy: transabdominal (lateral and anterior) and retroperitoneal (lateral and posterior). The duration of operating time is proportional to the experience of the operating surgeon with both general laparoscopy and laparoscopic adrenalectomies. The laparoscopic lateral transabdominal approach is currently the most common. However, some single-institution observational studies have found the laparoscopic retroperitoneal approach to have several advantages including shorter operative times, fewer complications (such as hernia), less post-operative pain, and shorter duration of hospital of stay. Large meta-analyses have demonstrated that either approach may be performed safely and effectively without difference in morbidity or mortality. The following description is of the laparoscopic lateral transabdominal approach.

Positioning (Fig. 6.1)

Patient positioning is often the hardest and most time consuming part of the operation. Constant communication with the anesthesiologists and staff is critical to prevent mishaps. It is important to place the urinary catheter and to gather all the necessary positioning equipment prior to moving the patient. The patient is placed on a beanbag in the lateral decubitus position with the side of the adrenal tumor up. It is important to place the patient's costal margin 2–3 cm superior to the point

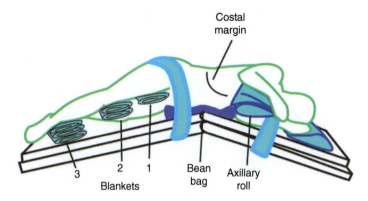

FIGURE 6.1 This figure illustrates the proper decubitus positioning for a laparoscopic transabdominal adrenalectomy. It is very important to ensure that the inferior costal margin is positioned at the "break" in the bed. Used with permission of COACHsurgery.com

where the bed flexes. Positioning here places the junction of the superior pole of the kidney and the adrenal gland at the break, allowing gravity to auto-retract the kidney inferiorly. The bed should be flexed maximally to increase the space between the costal margin and the hip to create more working space. In addition, a kidney rest should be elevated to further accentuate this space. The beanbag is inflated taking care not to push it into the abdomen, as this will decrease the intra-abdominal working space. Rather the beanbag should be conformed to the patient's hip and chest to insure secure positioning. The arms are placed in an ergonomically correct position without tension on the shoulder joints, most often separated by pillows rather than with an arm board. All pressure points are adequately padded and an axillary roll is placed. Pillows are placed between the legs in the usual decubitus positioning.

Port Placement (Fig. 6.2a, b)

We typically enter the abdomen via a Veress needle technique at Palmer's point 2–3 cm inferior to the costal margin

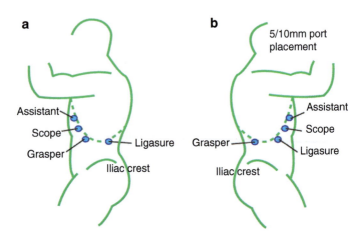

FIGURE 6.2 (**a**) Illustrates the placement of the ports for a laparoscopic transabdominal left adrenalectomy. Often, only 3 ports are used in a left adrenalectomy. Used with permission of COACHsurgery.com. (**b**) Illustrates the placement of the ports for a laparoscopic transabdominal right adrenalectomy. In this case, the fourth port is used to place a liver retractor. Used with permission of COACHsurgery.com

at the midclavicular line. On the left side, we place three ports subcostally about 5–10 cm apart, with the lateral-most port in the midaxillary line. On the right side, we typically place four ports in total with the additional port for a liver retractor. When inserting the ports, it is important to enter obliquely svhat the trochars are pointed toward the adrenal gland, otherwise you will have to work against the abdominal wall the entire case. The camera is placed in the middle port and the surgeon works with a two-handed technique.

Procedure

Although some authors advocate identifying and ligating the adrenal vein first, we do not adopt this strategy for the following reasons: (1) identifying the vein can sometimes be difficult early on, especially in obese patients; (2) after ligating the vein in cases of pheochromocytoma, the friable para-sitic blood vessels characteristic of that disease dilate and lead to increased bleeding. The key to performing this opera-tion successfully is respecting and exploiting the clear planes between structures – the hook cautery as a very precise means of following these planes. A vessel-sealing device is utilized to coagulate and ligate vessels. The operation is divided into a series of steps popularized by Quan-Yang Duh at UCSF:

1. Opening the book – Incising the peritoneum and Gerota's fascia to separate the adrenal gland and peri-adrenal fat from surrounding structures medially
2. Reading from the top down – Opening the plane between the adrenal gland and peri-adrenal fat and the medial structures starting from the peri-adrenal fat tail superiorly and moving to the adrenal vein or renal hilum
3. Identifying and ligating the adrenal vein
4. Separating the adrenal gland from the superior pole of the kidney
5. Freeing the rest of the peri-adrenal attachments

Left Adrenalectomy

First mobilize the splenic flexure by incising the lienorenal and lienophrenic ligaments to allow the spleen to fall medially with gravity. The dissection continues by using the hook cau-tery – stay one centimeter off the splenic capsule to prevent tearing the capsule. Incise the ligament at the superior pole of the spleen, at this point it is important to identify and avoid the stomach, which lies just posteriorly. Once the spleen is dis-sected and reflected medially, the plane between Gerota's fascia and the pancreas becomes readily identified. Retracting the spleen medially accentuates this plane. In obese patients, a fourth port for lateral retraction of the kidney and adrenal is sometimes helpful. The plane between Gerota's fascia and the pancreas is carried inferiorly (Fig. 6.3). The splenic flexure often needs to be mobilized as you come to the superior pole

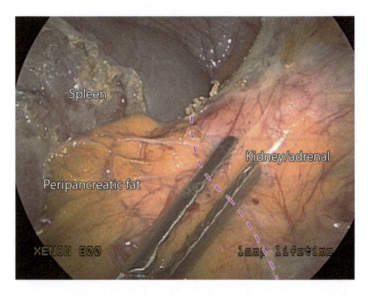

Spleen

Peripancreatic fat

Kidney/adrenal

XENON 300   lamp lifetime

FIGURE 6.3 This figure illustrates the line of dissection between the pancreas/spleen and the left adrenal gland

of the kidney. Once the plane between spleen and Gerota's fascia is developed, open Gerota's fascia superiorly and dissect through the peri-adrenal fat to identify the psoas muscle. Carry this dissection laterally 4–5 cm to allow for lateral and inferior retraction of the adrenal gland as necessary. Then divide the peri-adrenal fat along the medial edge of the adrenal gland and carry this dissection toward the renal hilum. Multiple adrenal arteries will be identified and may be ligated with the electrocautery or vessel-sealing device as suitable. During this dissection the phrenic vein is often encountered and will lead to the adrenal vein (Fig. 6.4). Another rule of thumb is that the splenic vessels "point" to the location of the adrenal vein. The adrenal and phrenic veins are dissected with careful blunt dissection and ligated either with clips or the vessel-sealing device. Once the vessels are divided, identify the plane between the superior pole of the kidney and adrenal gland. When carrying out this dissection, it is important to watch out for a superior pole renal artery and avoid injuring

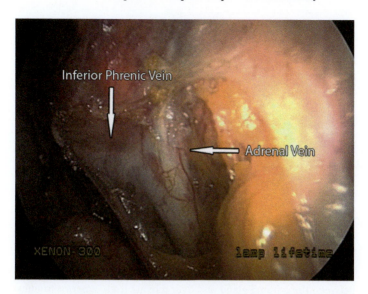

FIGURE 6.4 This figure demonstrates the relative anatomy of the inferior phrenic vein joining the left adrenal vein. The common trunk then drains into the left renal vein

it. The adrenal gland is then separated from the kidney. Then using a combination of blunt and sharp dissection, the adrenal gland is liberated from the psoas muscle and lateral abdominal wall. Hemostasis is obtained with irrigation, aspiration and electrocautery. The specimen is then removed in an impermeable specimen bag through the most anterior trocar. Enlarging the incision may occur for larger specimens. Fascial and skin incisions are closed.

Right Adrenalectomy

First divide the triangular ligament and the filmy attachments in the bare area of the liver to fully mobilize the lateral portion of the liver medially. The inferior leaflet of the ligament will transition into the peritoneum and Gerota's fascia, which is divided carefully up to the lateral edge of the inferior vena

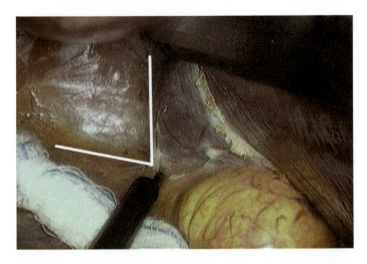

FIGURE 6.5 The "V" illustrates the technique of creating a plane between the adrenal gland and liver moving from superior to inferior. The liver is being retracted anteriorly and medially to expose the anterior surface of the adrenal gland

cava. The dissection is then carefully carried along the lateral edge of the inferior vena cava. Once the Gerota's fascia, peritoneum, and triangular ligaments are widely incised, mobilize the superior peri-adrenal fat pad as with the left side. Dissection is carried along the medial edge of the adrenal gland as described with the left adrenalectomy (Fig. 6.5). Typically a single adrenal vein enters the adrenal and inferior vena cave at the midpoint of the gland and is quite short (Fig. 6.6). The vein is dissected free and divided between clips or with the vessel-sealing device. The rest of the adrenalectomy proceeds as described for the left adrenalectomy.

Postoperative Care

A collaborative effort with the endocrinologists and general medical physicians is important to successful post-operative care. Postoperative follow-up is based on the particular

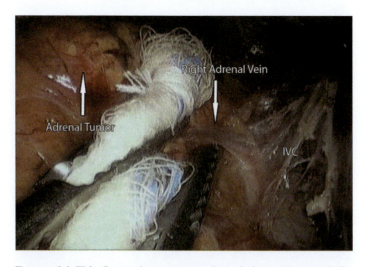

FIGURE 6.6 This figure demonstrates the relative anatomy of the right adrenal vein, which enters the adrenal gland anteriorly. The right adrenal vein is relatively short and comes directly off of the inferior vena cava (*IVC*) into the adrenal gland/tumor

pathology encountered and institutional requirements. The following are general guidelines for follow-up care based on pathology:

1. <u>Aldosterone-producing adenoma</u>: Stop all aldosterone receptor antagonists and potassium supplementation immediately after the operation. Anti-hypertensive medications may be either stopped and added back as needed or halved and adjusted as needed.
2. <u>Cushing's syndrome</u>: A rapid steroid taper to a low dose of oral steroids should be undertaken in conjunction with the endocrinologists. It is crucial to monitor these patients closely for signs and symptoms of adrenal insufficiency or frank Addisonian crisis.
3. <u>Pheochromocytoma</u>: Patients must be monitored for hemodynamic instability, especially hypotension. Post-operative hypotension should be treated with volume resuscitation. Repeat cross-sectional imaging and plasma

metanephrines should be obtained in 6 months to rule out recurrent or metastatic disease.

4. <u>Adrenocortical cancer</u>: Patients should be enrolled in a clinical trial or placed on adjuvant chemotherapy such as mitotane. Repeat cross-sectional imaging should be obtained in 3 months to rule out recurrent or metastatic disease.

Bibliography

Chen W, Li F, Chen D, Zhu Y, He C, Du Y, Tan W. Retroperitoneal versus transperitoneal laparoscopic adrenalectomy in adrenal tumor: a meta-analysis. Surg Laparosc Endosc Percutan Tech. 2013;23(2):121–7.

Constantinides VA, Christakis I, Touska P, Palazzo FF. Systematic review and meta-analysis of retroperitoneoscopic versus laparoscopic adrenalectomy. Br J Surg. 2012;99(12):1639–48.

Duh QY. Laparoscopic adrenalectomy for isolated adrenal metastasis: the right thing to do and the right way to do it. Ann Surg Oncol. 2007;14(12):3288–9.

Gagner M, Assalia A. Laparoscopic adrenalectomy. In: Saunders E, editor. Textbook of endocrine surgery. Philadelphia: Elsevier Inc; 2005. p. 647–62.

Mohammadi-Fallah MR, Mehdizadeh A, Badalzadeh A, Izadseresht B, Dadkhah N, Barbod A, Babaie M, Hamedanchi S. Comparison of transperitoneal versus retroperitoneal laparoscopic adrenalectomy in a prospective randomized study. J Laparoendosc Adv Surg Tech A. 2013;23(4):362–6.

Nigri G, Rosman AS, Petrucciani N, Fancellu A, Pisano M, Zorcolo L, Ramacciato G, Melis M. Meta-analysis of trials comparing laparoscopic transperitoneal and retroperitoneal adrenalectomy. Surgery. 2013;153(1):111–9.

Swanstrom LL. Laparoscopic adrenalectomy. In: Cameron JL, editor. Current Surgical Therapy. 11th edn. Elsevier; 2014.

Tada HTDS, Lee JE. Adrenal tumors. In: Wilkins LW, editor. The M.D. Anderson surgical oncology handbook. Houston: Lippincott Williams & Wilkins; 2003.

Chapter 7
Laparoscopic Adrenalectomy: Retroperitoneal Approach

Cameron D. Adkisson and Linwah Yip

Abstract   Posterior retroperitoneoscopic adrenalectomy has emerged as an alternative operative approach for the laparoscopic removal of non-malignant tumors of the adrenal gland. Retroperitoneoscopic adrenalectomy offers advantages to transperitoneal adrenalectomy and may be the ideal approach in patients with anticipated extensive adhesions from prior abdominal surgery in the same quadrant or in patients requiring bilateral adrenalectomy as this approach avoids patient repositioning. The retroperitoneoscopic approach has been shown to be associated with operative times, complications, and mortality that are equivalent to adrenalectomy via the transperitoneal approach. Partial or cortical-sparing procedures have also been performed with favorable results. In this chapter, we describe the background,

C.D. Adkisson, MD
Division of Endocrine Surgery, Department of Surgery,
University of Pittsburgh, Pittsburgh, PA, USA

L. Yip, MD, FACS (✉)
Division of Endocrine Surgery, University of Pittsburgh
School of Medicine, 3471 5th Ave Suite 101 Kaufmann Bldg,
15213 Pittsburgh, PA, USA

Department of Surgery, University of Pittsburgh,
Pittsburgh, PA, USA
e-mail: yipl@upmc.edu

H. Chen (ed.), *Illustrative Handbook of General Surgery*,   73
DOI 10.1007/978-3-319-24557-7_7,
© Springer International Publishing Switzerland 2016

rationale, indications and contraindications, preoperative preparation, and operative technique.

Keywords   Adrenalectomy • Laparoscopic • Retroperitoneal • Retroperitoneoscopic • Posterior adrenalectomy

Introduction

Laparoscopic adrenalectomy has become the gold standard for removal of non-malignant tumors of the adrenal gland since its introduction by Gagner in 1992 [1–3]. Advantages of the laparoscopic approach include decreased pain and expedited recovery. Indications for adrenalectomy have been reviewed elsewhere and include either the presence of a functional tumor of the adrenal cortex or medulla, or clinical concern for malignancy such as an adrenal nodule that demonstrates interval growth, is ≥ 4 cm in size, or has concerning features on imaging. Isolated metastatic disease in patients who may benefit from metastasectomy is a less common indication for adrenalectomy.

Posterior retroperitoneoscopic adrenalectomy has emerged as an alternative approach to total or partial adrenalectomy, and has demonstrated utility in a variety of adrenal tumors including aldosteronomas, cortisol-secreting tumors, pheochromocytomas, virilizing tumors, benign adenomas, angiomyolipomas, ganglioneuromas, and adrenal metastases [4–6]. First reported in 1995 by Mercan et al., the posterior retroperitoneoscopic approach was not widely adopted until the necessary increased insufflation pressures for improved visualization were deemed safe for patients [7]. Giebler et al. clearly demonstrated that impaired cardiac filling occurred only when peritoneal insufflation pressures exceeded 15 mmHg, but did not occur when retroperitoneal insufflation pressures exceeded 15 mmHg [8].

The retroperitoneoscopic approach to the adrenal gland offers distinct advantages to the transperitoneal approach including direct exposure of the adrenal gland and adrenal vein, avoidance of intraabdominal adhesions, and avoiding the need for adjacent organ displacement including the spleen, colon, and liver. Finally, bilateral adrenalectomies for ACTH-dependent Cushing's or familial pheochromocytoma can be performed through a retroperitoneal approach without patient repositioning. Walz et al. described 560 adrenalectomies in 520 patients utilizing the retroperitoneoscopic approach during a 12 year period with no reported mortalities, a major complication such as myocardial infarction, bleeding requiring transfusion, and pneumonia occurring in 1.3 %, and a conversion rate to open or lateral approach of only 1.7 % [4]. Furthermore, they observed improved operative efficiency with cases performed at a mean of 40 min by the end of their study period [4]. The retroperitoneoscopic approach should be used with caution in patients with (1) severe lung disease or COPD, (2) inadequate working space determined by the distance from the posterior 12th rib margin to the superior border of the iliac crest, (3) suspected adrenocortical cancer or suspected invasion into surrounding structures, (4) inability to tolerated the prone positioning, and (5) BMI > 45. Larger adrenals ≥6 cm should also be approached with caution through a retroperitoneoscopic approach as the malignancy rate is higher and the ability to manipulate large tumors in the retroperitoneal space is limited.

Other groups have described their successful experience with the posterior approach as well. In the largest US series by Perrier et al. 68 patients had retroperitoneoscopic adrenalectomy with a low conversion rate of 9 %, a mean operating time of 121 min, and no mortalities [5]. They further demonstrated the feasibility and safety of the procedure in obese patients (BMI ≥ 30) requiring either unilateral or bilateral adrenalectomy [5]. This finding has been further confirmed in the obese population, noting decreased operative time and blood loss for retroperitoneoscopic compared to transperitoneal adrenalectomy [9]. Partial or cortical-sparing adrenalectomy is also feasible and safe through the retroperitoneoscopic approach [10, 11]. In a meta-analysis comparing 9 studies and 632 patients, the retroperitoneoscopic approach was associated with shorter operative time, less blood loss, and shorter length of hospital stay than patients who had laparoscopic transperitoneal adrenalectomy, with no differences identified in the rates of major complications or conversion to open [12]. Single access posterior approaches and use of robotic-assisted retroperitoneoscopic adrenalectomy have also been described with favorable results [13, 14].

Preoperative Preparation

The pre-operative planning for patients having retroperitoneoscopic adrenalectomy is the same as that for the transperitoneal approach. Prior to surgery, the planned approach and tumor functional status is discussed with the anesthesia and operating room teams. An operating room table is ready and available immediately outside the operative suite during all retroperitoneoscopic adrenalectomies in preparation for emergent open laparotomy if necessary.

Description of Procedure

Positioning

Similar to preparing for laparoscopic transperitoneal adrenalectomy, patient positioning can sometimes be difficult and time-consuming. While the patient is supine on the transporting gurney, general anesthesia with endotracheal intubation, foley catheter and needed IV access including central and arterial lines are placed before prone positioning on the operating table. We frequently inform anesthesia about the potential for CO_2 retention and request mild hyperventilation after intubation to decrease CO_2 levels before positioning. This is particularly helpful in obese patients or those with

COPD as they can have a higher degree of CO_2 retention which may cause challenges with intraoperative hemodynamic instability and extubation. The patient is then rotated into a prone jackknife position. We use a modified table with a thin gel pad placed in the lower ½ of the bed instead of the typical operating table padding, and large gel rolls that are positioned under the breasts and across the pubic symphysis to maximize the working space which is defined as the 12th rib posteriorly to the superior border of the iliac crest on the ipsilateral side (Fig. 7.1). The goal of padding placement is to allow the ventral abdominal wall to hang freely anteriorly. A Cloward table saddle can also be used. The patient's arms are extended to 90° and placed on arms rests with padding in an ergonomic position to ensure no tension on the shoulders or pressure on the cubital tunnel. Manipulation of the surgical table with Trendelenburg positioning and flexing the hips to approximately 90° further maximizes the working space. The patient's legs are positioned without pressure on the

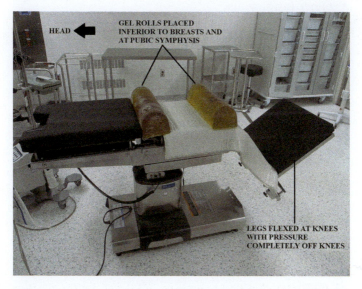

FIGURE 7.1 Operating table modified to facilitate retroperitoneal approach

knees to avoid hip displacement. Two high-definition monitors are placed on either side of the operating table. The flank is then prepared using chlorhexidine or betadine, and draped with blue towels and standard operating sheets from the lower border of the shoulder blades as far laterally as possible to the medial portion of the gluteus maximus inferiorly.

Required Equipment

- Ports:
    - 5 mm bladeless trocar × 2
    - 10 mm disposable Balloon trocar (Autosuture)
    - 5 mm bladeless trocar × 1 (optional)
- Laparoscopic cameras:
    - 10 mm 30° scope
    - 5 mm 30° scope
    - 5 mm 45° scope (optional)
- Other Instruments:

    - 5 mm LigaSure™ (*Covidien Ltd, Mansfield, MA*) or Harmonic Ultrasound Device® (*Ethicon Endo-Surgery, Inc*)
    - Laparoscopic Suction/Irrigation
    - Laparoscopic blunt grasper
    - Laparoscopic peanuts
    - EndoCatch™ (*Covidien Ltd, Mansfield, MA*) for specimen extraction

Insufflation

20–24 mmHg CO_2

Port Placement

An initial 1.5–2 cm incision is made just beneath the tip of the 12th rib transversely and will be used for initial camera placement and specimen extraction. Using a combination of sharp and blunt dissection, the retroperitoneal space is entered. Using the index finger to clear retroperitoneal fat off the postero-medial border (paraspinous musculature) enables creation of a working space. This dissection then is carried to the superior-most extent of the operator's reach medially and inferiorly until enough working space is created for placement of the camera port and the two 5 mm trocars. A 5 mm trocar is then placed 4–5 cm laterally and 2 cm inferior to the tip of the 11th rib angled appropriately to avoid collision with the rib during instrument manipulation. We insert a finger through the initial incision to guide the trocar into the working space and clear any overlying retroperitoneal fat. A second 5 mm trocar is placed at the medial border of the paraspinous muscles usually ~4 cm medial to the 10 mm trocar and 3–4 cm below the 12th rib angled to 45°. The balloon trocar is placed through the initial incision and CO_2 insufflation is achieved to 20–24 mmHg. The surgeon and assistant typically stand on the same (ipsilateral) side of the target gland.

Procedure

Using the 10 mm 30° scope, additional working space in the retroperitoneum is first created using two peanuts/graspers in a sweeping motion. The paraspinous muscle is an important landmark that allows for appropriate orientation in the retroperitoneum, and is first identified and cleared as superiorly as possible towards the adrenal. Starting medially will also prevent entry into the peritoneum which lies laterally and near the plane of dissection particularly in thin patients. Entering the peritoneum during the dissection is suboptimal as CO_2 insufflation into the peritoneal cavity can cause progressive reduction of the retroperitoneal working space as the peritoneal contents are displaced by the CO_2. The superior border of the kidney is then identified as the retroperitoneal fat is swept away. The upper pole of the kidney is identified and Gerota's fascia is sharply entered, aided by pushing the kidney down with the surgeon's opposite hand exposing the adrenal gland. Freeing up the adrenal from the superior pole of the kidney is best accomplished at this point while the

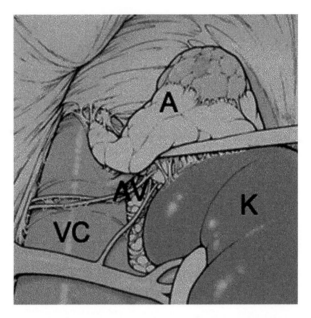

FIGURE 7.2 Intraoperative anatomy of right retroperitoneoscopic adrenalectomy. *A* adrenal gland, *AV* adrenal vein, *k* right kidney, *VC* inferior vena cava (Image from Walz et al. [4], with permission from Elsevier)

adrenal is still attached superiorly and medially. Rarely, if exposure is limited, a 4th 5 mm trocar may be placed inferior to the lateral port to retract the kidney during dissection of the inferior portion of the adrenal gland.

During right adrenalectomy, the adrenal vascular supply is encountered posterior to the vena cava. Further dissection of the medial aspect of the adrenal gland facilitates gentle lateral retraction of the gland and clear visualization of the IVC. The adrenal vein is then typically seen running posterior and lateral at 9–10 o'clock and may be clipped or doubly ligated with the coagulation device (Fig. 7.2). During left adrenalectomy the adrenal vein is encountered running medial to the upper pole of the kidney at approximately 4–5 o'clock and is clipped or doubly ligated with coagulation

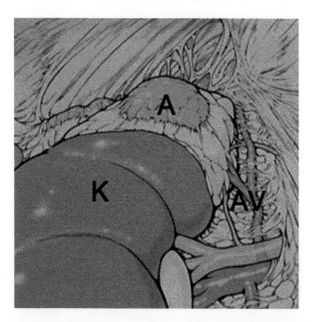

FIGURE 7.3 Intraoperative anatomy of left retroperitoneoscopic adrenalectomy. *A* adrenal gland with adenoma, *AV* adrenal vein, *K* left kidney (Image from Walz et al. [4], with permission from Elsevier)

(Fig. 7.3). An accessory renal artery may be present and is usually located in the 6 o'clock position, and should be preserved. On the left, there is often a limb of adrenal that extends anteriorly and medially into the renal hilum. Care should be taken not to inadvertently transect the adrenal at this location.

Once the vein has been divided, dissection is then carried out laterally, leaving the superior attachments for last. The adrenal gland is then extracted through the 10 mm port using an EndoCatch™ (*Covidien Ltd, Mansfield, MA*). After extraction, the specimen is always inspected carefully on the back table to ensure that the adrenal has been resected in total. The camera is then re-inserted to visualize the adrenal bed for both adequate hemostasis and ensure complete resection. The balloon trocar site fascia is then closed, port sites are reapproximated at the skin, and sterile dressing (either steristrips or surgical glue) is applied.

Postoperative Care

Subcutaneous crepitus may be evident but resolves rapidly. Standard management of incisional pain is administered. Patients are given clear liquids after operation and if well tolerated move quickly to regular diet. The majority of patients are discharged home on postoperative day 1 with follow up in 2–3 weeks. Postoperative follow-up and medication continuation or discontinuation is based on the functional status of the lesion, and is similar to the approach after the laparoscopic transperitoneal approach. A multidisciplinary approach facilitates safe, timely discharge.

References

1. Gagner M, Lacroix A, Bolte E. Laparoscopic adrenalectomy in Cushing's syndrome and pheochromocytoma. N Engl J Med. 1992;327:1033.
2. Schlinkert RT, van Heerden JA, Grant CS, et al. Laparoscopic left adrenalectomy for aldosteronoma: early Mayo Clinic experience. Mayo Clin Proc. 1995;70:844–6.
3. Brunt LM. Minimal access adrenal surgery. Surg Endoscopy. 2006;20:351–61.
4. Walz MK, Alesin PF, Wenger FA, Deligiannis A, Szuczik E, et al. Posterior retroperitoneoscopic adrenalectomy – results of 560 procedures in 520 patients. Surgery. 2006;140:943–50.
5. Perrier ND, Kannamer DL, Bao R, et al. Posterior retroperitoneoscopic adrenalectomy: preferred technique for removal of benign tumors and isolated metastases. Ann Surg. 2008;248:666–74.
6. Alesina PF, Hommeltenberg S, Meier B, et al. Posterior retroperitoneoscopic adrenalectomy for clinical and subclinical Cushing's syndrome. World J Surg. 2010;34:1391–7.
7. Mercan S, Seven R, Ozarmagan S, et al. Endoscopic retroperitoneal adrenalectomy. Surgery. 1995;118:1071–5.

8. Giebler RM, Behrends M, Steffens T, et al. Intraperitoneal and retroperitoneal carbon dioxide insufflations evoke difference effects on caval vein pressure gradients in humans: evidence for the starling resistor concept of abdominal venous return. Anesthesiology. 2000;92:1568–80.

9. Epelboym E, Digesu C, Johnston MG, et al. Expanding the indications for laparoscopic retroperitoneal adrenalectomy: experience with 81 resections. J Surg Res. 2014;187:496–501.

10. Walz MK, Peitgen K, Diesing D, et al. Partial versus total adrenalectomy by the posterior retroperitoneoscopic approach: early and long-term results of 325 consecutive procedures in primary adrenal neoplasias. World J Surg. 2004;28:1323–9.

11. Grubbs EG, Rich TA, Ng C, et al. Long-term outcomes of surgical treatment for hereditary pheochromocytoma. J Am Coll Surg. 2013;216:280–9.

12. Chen W, Li F, Chen D, et al. Retroperitoneal versus transperitoneal laparoscopic adrenalectomy in adrenal tumor: a meta-analysis. Surg Laparosc Endosc Percutan Tech. 2013;23:121–7.

13. Walz MK, Alesina PF. Single access retroperitoneoscopic adrenalectomy (SARA) – one step beyond in endocrine surgery. Langenbecks Arch Surg. 2009;394:447–50.

14. Dickson PV, Alex GC, Grubbs EC, et al. Robotic-assisted retroperitoneoscopic adrenalectomy: making a good procedure even better. Am Surg. 2013;79:84–9.

Part II
Breast Surgery

Lee G. Wilke

Chapter 8
Breast Biopsy

**Lauren J. Taylor, Marquita Renee Decker,
and Jennifer G. Steiman**

Abstract Image guided biopsy techniques are the primary
mechanism for evaluating breast abnormalities and have
largely replaced surgical biopsy as a diagnostic procedure.
The indications for biopsy include findings from screening mammograms which are supplemented with diagnostic
imaging as well as clinical findings such as a palpable mass,
nipple discharge or skin changes. The techniques for biopsy
primarily utilize a core needle device and more rarely fine
needle aspiration, punch biopsy and surgical excision.

Keywords Image guided breast biopsy • Breast abnormality
• Surgical biopsy • Core needle device • Needle aspiration •
Punch biopsy • Surgical excision

L.J. Taylor, MD (✉) • M.R. Decker, MD, MPH
Department of Surgery, University of Wisconsin Hospital
and Clinics, 600 Highland Avenue, Madison, WI 53792, USA
e-mail: ltaylor2@uwhealth.org; marquita.decker@fulbrightmail.org

J.G. Steiman, MD
Department of Surgery, University of Wisconsin,
600 Highland Avenue, H4/724, Madison, WI 53792, USA
e-mail: steiman@surgery.wisc.edu

H. Chen (ed.), *Illustrative Handbook of General Surgery*, 87
DOI 10.1007/978-3-319-24557-7_8,
© Springer International Publishing Switzerland 2016

Introduction

Over the past 15 years, image-guided breast biopsy has nearly replaced open surgical biopsy for the diagnosis of suspicious breast lesions. As a result of this shift in practice, the majority of women with identified breast abnormalities no longer require surgical intervention for diagnosis. This minimally-invasive diagnostic procedure is now also recognized as having equivalent accuracy to open surgical biopsy with fewer complications [1, 2].

With increasing national emphasis on quality and patient-centered outcomes, radiologists and surgeons have focused efforts on credentialing programs to assure high quality outcomes for image-guided breast biopsies. Beginning in the late 1990s, the American College of Radiologists (ACR) and the American College of Surgeons (ACS) worked collaboratively to develop consensus guidelines for the performance and certification of image-guided breast procedures, which included requirements for radiologists and surgeons, as well as the facilities performing the procedures [3, 4]. In recent years, the American Society of Breast Surgeons, in collaboration with the ACS, has also developed and endorsed a certification program specifically for surgeon-performed stereotactic and ultrasound image-guided breast procedures. (http://www.breast-surgeons.org)

One vital component to the accreditation process for breast interventional procedures is having a documentation process for imaging and pathologic concordance. Given the risk for under-diagnosis and sampling error with image-guided breast biopsies, individual case concordance with the imaging and the final pathology is crucial towards avoiding false negatives and pathologic underestimation. Through concordance assessment, decisions can be made regarding the need for open surgical excision, if a false negative result is suspected or if the patient has an atypical lesion that requires a larger excision for definitive diagnosis.

Indications

According to the National Comprehensive Cancer Network (NCCN) Guidelines on Screening and Diagnosis of Breast Cancer, indications for a breast biopsy should be determined by patient age, symptom presentation, and radiographic findings [5]. Algorithms to screen for breast cancer and diagnose suspicious breast lesions begin with mammography and are supplemented by diagnostic breast imaging inclusive of mammography, ultrasound and MRI. For patients with a symptomatic presentation such as a mass or skin or nipple changes, diagnostic imaging is used to further evaluate the areas of concern.

BI-RADS 4 and 5 Lesions

The American College of Radiology developed and maintains the Breast Imaging and Reporting Data System (BI-RADS®) for classifying mammograms by level of suspicion for malignancy [6]. Women of any age who undergo screening or diagnostic mammograms and have findings consistent with BI-RADS 4 classification (suspicious abnormality) or BI-RADS 5 classification (highly suggestive of malignancy) should undergo biopsy of the breast lesion(s). Open surgical biopsy should only be performed if image-guided core needle biopsy is not possible. For patients with BI-RADS 3 lesions (probably benign), diagnostic algorithms for biopsy are then based upon symptom presentation and a shared decision making discussion between the provider and patient for percutaneous biopsy vs close imaging and exam follow-up.

Palpable Breast Mass

A patient appreciated and clinician confirmed or provider identified palpable breast mass should undergo imaging evaluation. The breast imaging procedure will vary based on patient age with women under age 30 more likely to receive an ultrasound as the first imaging procedure. Women over 30 years of age should be assessed with diagnostic mammogram and ultrasound for a palpable mass. Imaging confirmed cysts that are well-circumscribed and non-complex can be aspirated or monitored. Palpable BI-RADS 4 and 5 lesions by either ultrasound, mammography or MRI should undergo image guided biopsy. A biopsy of a palpable breast lesion without image guidance is not recommended. Although a lesion may be palpable and large, directing the biopsy needle to the most diagnostic portion of the tissue under radiographic visualization will significantly reduce the risk of under-diagnosis or false negative pathologic results from the biopsy [1, 2].

Nipple Discharge

Women who present with nipple discharge that appears to drain from a single duct in only one breast, is clear or bloody in appearance, and occurs non-spontaneously should undergo a breast ultrasound with retro-areolar views and a diagnostic mammogram. The most common cause of bloody nipple discharge is an intraductal papilloma; thus, if an intraductal mass is identified, then an image-guided biopsy is warranted to confirm the diagnosis. If no cause is detected on imaging, then an excisional biopsy of the entire duct or a central duct excision is warranted. Nipple discharge from multiple ducts that is spontaneous can often be observed and managed expectantly.

Skin Lesions

Patients with skin changes suspicious for inflammatory breast cancer such as a peau d' orange appearance or significant diffuse erythema of over 1/3 of the breast, can undergo a punch biopsy of the skin to identify dermal lymphatic invasion from a malignancy. While the diagnosis of inflammatory breast cancer is clinical in nature, a biopsy can help to support the diagnosis. A negative test result, however, does not exclude inflammatory breast cancer. A skin biopsy can also be utilized for nipple changes that are different or suspicious of a intra-ductal malignancy such as Paget's disease.

Description of Breast Biopsy Procedures

Several imaging techniques are used to guide breast biopsies, including mammography (conventional and stereotactic), ultra-sound, and magnetic resonance imaging (MRI). The choice of imaging modality depends on a variety of factors including lesion access and visualization, in addition to physician experience and availability of equipment. Lesions located near the chest wall or immediately deep to the areola may not be accessible with percutaneous techniques and may require an open surgical approach but an image guided biopsy should always be discussed and entertained prior to an excisional breast biopsy.

Fine Needle Aspiration

Fine needle aspiration (FNA) has largely been replaced by core needle biopsy for the evaluation of solid lesions. It does not provide histological information and therefore has limited diagnostic capabilities. Currently, FNA is used primarily in the assessment of cystic lesions and is typically performed under ultrasound-guidance. The ACR recommends the use of a high-resolution linear array transducer (frequency of 10 mHz or greater) for optimal breast imaging. The choice of needle should be large enough to aspirate potentially viscous fluid. The operator is advised to keep the needle as parallel to the chest wall and trans-ducer face as possible to avoid penetration of the chest wall.

Core Needle Biopsy/Vacuum Assisted Core Needle Biopsy

Core needle biopsy is a common percutaneous method used to obtain a tissue diagnosis of a breast abnormality. Needle sizes vary from as large as 9 to smaller 16 gauge needles.

Ultrasound guidance is often the preferred approach for lesions visualized equally well on both mammography and sonography. This method allows for the patient to be in the supine position without compression of the breast. Stereotactic biopsy is the next choice for a lesion seen only on mammography. MRI core biopsy is reserved for patients in which the MRI abnormality cannot be seen by mammogram or ultrasound. Placement of a localizing tissue marker following any percutaneous biopsy is mandatory to identify the biopsy site. This also facilitates accurate localization for subsequent surgical excision or for patients undergoing neoadjuvant chemotherapy in which the lesion may not be visible post treatment. A post-biopsy mammogram is strongly recommended to document location of the marker as compared to the identified imaging abnormality.

There are several available options of needle biopsy devices including automated core needles and vacuum-assisted products. While the optimal device and needle size varies by the type of lesion and operator preference, vacuum-assisted products have been shown to be most effective in stereotactic and MRI-guided biopsy and allow multiple passes through the lesion via a single access site. For a stereotactic biopsy, the patient is placed in the prone position, and the breast is compressed between an image receptor and a compression plate. The lesion is identified and computer generated coordinates are calculated to target the skin's entry site. Skin infiltration with local anesthetic is used for any biopsy procedure to limit discomfort and pain. By using a single site, this technique allows for the collection of more specimens during one procedure and is most often used for micro-calcifications. The ACR recommends the use of vacuum-assisted devices of 11 gauge or larger in the performance of stereotactic biopsies for micro-calcifications. Of note, currently stereotactic tables cannot accommodate patients over a weight of 300 pounds and image guided open surgical excision may be necessary in this obese population. For MRI-guided procedures, the patient is prone and the breast is stabilized between grid plates. Pre- and post-contrast

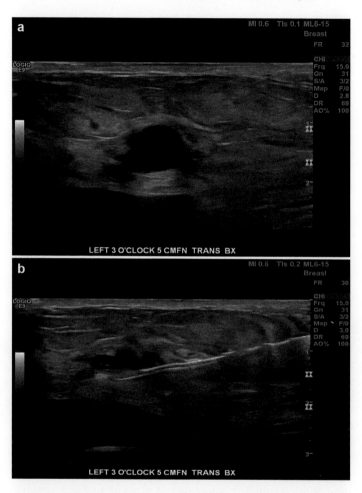

FIGURE 8.1 (a) Ultrasound of a breast mass. (b) Core biopsy of the mass

images are obtained, and the breast is repositioned as necessary so that the lesion of interest is easily accessible. Post
biopsy care includes closure of the core site with strips of tape
and a small compression bandage and intermittent ice use
over the site for the first few hours post procedure. See
Fig. 8.1.

Punch Biopsy

While there are several different methods that may be used to biopsy skin, punch biopsy has the ability to sample the subcutaneous fat. This is a simple office procedure that employs a punch instrument that may range in size from 2 to 8 mm. After adequate local anesthesia is infused, the physician simply holds the skin taught and twists the instrument perpendicular to the skin until it has penetrated the dermis to reach the subcutaneous tissue. The wound may be closed with either adhesive strips or a non-absorbable suture.

Excisional Biopsy

Surgical excision for the purposes of obtaining a tissue diagnosis should only be performed when there is no access via image guidance. The technique performed is the same as for an image localized lumpectomy. The goal should not only be to obtain a tissue diagnosis but to also completely excise the lesion with clear margins. For a complete description of the procedure, please see the chapter of this book on breast lumpectomy.

Complications

As compared to open biopsy, an image-guided minimally invasive approach offers similar accuracy with lower complication rates. While adverse outcomes such as a seroma or hematoma may occur, adequate compression is often all that is necessary following the procedure to ensure hemostasis. More serious complications, including pneumothorax and retained wire fragments, have been described but are quite rare [7].

Follow Up

After any biopsy of a breast lesion, the pathologic findings largely determine next steps in follow up. Patients with benign pathologic findings that are concordant with imaging should be followed with physical exam and regularly-scheduled imaging, if age-appropriate. For lesions that are found to be malignant, planning for surgical excision versus neoadjuvant therapy should be employed. For patients with indeterminate pathology, atypical ductal hyperplasia, lobular carcinoma in situ, flat epithelial atypia, benign pathology with discordant imaging, intraductal papillomas or otherwise pathologically concerning lesions, an open surgical excision for a representative sample of tissue may need to be performed.

Summary

In summary, when performing a diagnostic procedure of a breast lesion, the specific method should be determined by patient age, symptom presentation, and breast imaging characteristics. Given the rapid growth of technological advances in breast cancer treatment, it is best to consult the most recent consensus guidelines on appropriate choices for diagnostic modalities and image guided biopsy technology.

References

1. Bruening W, Fontanarosa J, Tipton K, Treadwell JR, Launders J, Schoelles K. Systematic review: comparative effectiveness of core-needle and open surgical biopsy to diagnose breast lesions. Ann Intern Med. 2010;152:238–46.
2. Verkooijen HM, Core Biopsy After Radiological Localisation (COBRA) Study Group. Diagnostic accuracy of stereotactic large-core needle biopsy for nonpalpable breast disease: results of a multicenter prospective study with 95 % surgical confirmation. Int J Cancer. 2002;99:853–9.
3. American College of Radiology. Stereotactic breast biopsy accreditation program requirements. 2013. http://www.acr.org/~/media/ACR/Documents/Accreditation/SBB/Requirements.pdf.
4. American College of Radiology. ACR practice guideline for the performance of stereotactically guided breast interventional procedures, Amended 2014 (Resolution 6). http://www.acr.org/Quality-Safety/Standards-Guidelines/Practice-Guidelines-by-Modality/Breast-Imaging.

96   L.J. Taylor et al.

5. National Comprehensive Cancer Network Clinical Practice Guidelines in Oncology (NCCN Guidelines®). Breast Cancer Screening and Diagnosis, Version 1.2014. http://www.nccn.org/.
6. American College of Radiology. BI-RADS® – mammography. 2013. http://www.acr.org/Quality-Safety/Resources/BIRADS/Mammography.
7. Bates T, Davidson T, Mansel RE. Litigation for pneumothorax as a complication of fine needle aspiration of the breast. Br J Surg. 2002;89:134–7.

Chapter 9
Breast Conservation Surgery (Surgical Biopsy, Lumpectomy, Nipple Exploration, Partial Mastectomy)

Lee G. Wilke and Jennifer G. Steiman

Abstract Breast conservation surgery for a benign or malignant breast lesion remains the cornerstone operation for the oncologic and general surgeon. Localization of non palpable lesions is performed with either a wire or radioactive seed but intraoperative ultrasound can be utilized for those with training to employ this approach. Oncoplastic techniques are becoming increasingly popular for excision of a breast malignancy.

Keywords Lumpectomy • Partial mastectomy • Oncoplastic • Localization

L.G. Wilke, MD (✉)
Department of Surgery, University of Wisconsin Hospital and Clinics, 600 Highland Avenue, 53792-7375 Madison, WI, USA
e-mail: wilke@surgery.wisc.edu

J.G. Steiman, MD
Department of Surgery, University of Wisconsin,
Madison, WI, USA

H. Chen (ed.), *Illustrative Handbook of General Surgery*, 97
DOI 10.1007/978-3-319-24557-7_9,

Introduction

The surgical removal of a benign breast lesion, an unknown breast abnormality or the excision of a breast malignancy has become progressively less invasive over time without negatively impacting the diagnostic or oncologic outcomes. For a mass or area of the breast with an imaging abnormality that is not amenable to image guided biopsy, a surgical biopsy involves removing the area for diagnosis. This procedure is used with less frequency due to the ability for most lesions to be diagnosed via image or palpation guided biopsy. For a known benign lesion the primary procedure utilized is the lumpectomy with indications being growth of a benign mass, size causing discomfort or patient desire for removal. This can be performed with image localization if the lesion is not palpable. For a lesion with malignant potential such as a radial scar or atypical ductal, lobular or papillary changes, a lumpectomy of the area is recommended with image localization. For a breast cancer, the radical mastectomy is now rarely indicated but included the resection of the breast, overlying skin, pectoralis muscles and axillary lymph nodes and had many concomitant morbidities [1]. Subsequent randomized trials demonstrated equivalent results between radical mastectomy and modified radical mastectomy which motivated providers to uncover less invasive means for excision of a cancer [2]. Beginning in the 1970s, multiple randomized trials from the United States and Europe validated that partial mastectomy or breast conservation surgery plus radiation was as effective as total mastectomy [3–5]. The continued evolution of breast cancer operations has led to the use of "oncoplastic" techniques to permit adequate removal of a breast cancer while simultaneously providing surgical techniques to facilitate excellent cosmetic outcomes. Oncoplastic techniques can be as simple as a mastopexy or "lift" type operation that is performed by the oncologic surgeon verses more complex reduction techniques that involve both a plastic and oncologic surgical team [6].

For a patient with a breast malignancy, the decision to undergo breast conservation or a mastectomy is driven by multiple factors which include the tumor to breast size ratio, the expected extension of an in-situ component, genetic susceptibility to breast cancer and the patient's own approach to her cancer based on education from her providers regarding the pros and cons of each surgical approach. Excision of a benign lesion should always involve the most direct approach to the lesion with the least amount of tissue excision which will facilitate complete removal of the abnormality. Excision of a cancer involves more complex planning to ensure that the maximum of amount of tissue is removed to ensure a negative "margin" yet so much is not removed as to cause a significant cosmetic defect and deformity.

Surgical Biopsy/Lumpectomy

There are many benign lesions of the breast as well as many lesions that require excision for diagnosis or to confirm an image guided biopsy accurately diagnosed a lesion of interest. A surgical biopsy or lumpectomy involves removing a lesion with a minimal rim of normal tissue around the lesion. For some suspected benign lesions the "rim" can be very small and almost negligible in the case of the benign fibroadenoma or nonatypical papilloma. If the lesion is one that could not undergo image guided biopsy or is a lesion with potential malignant diagnosis (radial scar, atypical hyperplasia or atypical papilloma) direct excision of the area is recommended with removal of the lesion in total with minimal surrounding breast tissue. Incisional breast biopsy is rarely indicated due to the ability of image guided biopsies to provide a diagnosis.

Lesion Localization

For non-palpable lesions, localization is required. The two most popular techniques utilized for breast lesion localization are the wire or a radioactive iodine-125 seed [7]. In addition, for the surgeon skilled in intraoperative ultrasound, this imaging modality can be used for localization of a non palpable lesion [8]. Either of the seed or wire localization procedures can be done via mammogram, ultrasound or more rarely MRI, whichever will be easier for the patient and permits the most direct access to the breast lesion or lesions of interest. The radioactive seed localization procedure is not available in most breast centers and institutions due to the stringent requirements for a radioactive safety program to prevent loss of a radioactive point source, the seed. Retrospective studies and randomized trials in patients with cancer have shown the two procedures to be equivalent with a slightly lower re-excision rate with seed localized procedures. Prior to the lumpectomy surgery, two-view mammogram (CC and MLO) is necessary to determine the exact location of the lesion and localization wire or seed within the breast and should be available to the surgeon in the operating room. Figure 9.1a, b show an example wire and seed in patients undergoing localization for nonpalpable lesions.

Surgical Procedure

Anesthesia for a breast surgery can involve the use of local anesthetic with sedation, a paravertebral block or general anesthetic. Incision placement for a surgical biopsy or lumpectomy can vary depending on the size and type of lesion to be excised. For a known benign lesion either an incision directly over the lesion or a periareolar incision which facilitates access to the benign lesion can be selected if cosmesis is of importance to the patient and a periareolar incision will not compromise future breast feeding in premenopausal women. For an excisional biopsy of an unknown abnormality the incision with the most direct access to the area is desired. Mammographic or MRI localization may not have facilitated placement of a localization wire directly adjacent to the lesion so the surgeon must evaluate the location of the abnormality and determine the best incision placement without necessarily following the wire through the breast which may lead to an excess of tissue removed. Incision placements are commonly radial in the

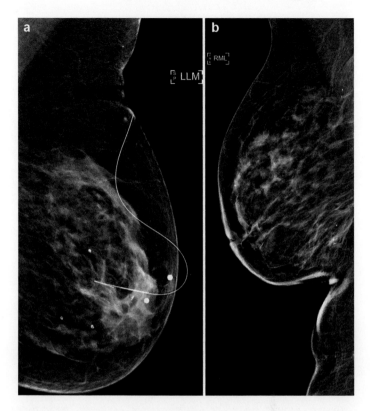

FIGURE 9.1 (**a**) Left breast wire localization prior to lumpectomy. (**b**) Radioactive seed localization of inferior breast lesion

lower breast and periareolar or along Langer's lines in the superior breast but should be selected based on patient breast size, lesion size and best location to avoid a convexity post surgical removal. Excision of a lesion can use electrocautery, knife or scissors depending on surgeon preference. Once removed, the specimen requires orientation in three dimensions, using either suture, clips or ink (Fig. 9.2). Even if known to be benign a breast lesion should be oriented to prevent need for re-excision if an unsuspected cancer is detected. A radiograph of the tissue is then necessary for non-palpable lesions

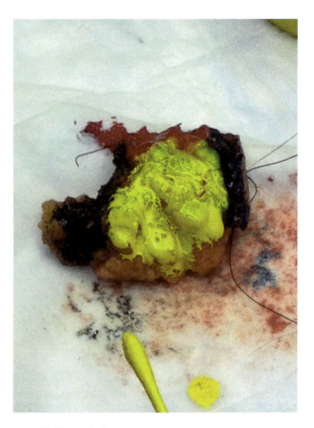

FIGURE 9.2 Inking of a lumpectomy specimen

to ensure inclusion of the area of concern. If a biopsy was performed pre-operatively for the diagnosis, then often a metallic clip will be present and should be confirmed within the specimen as well as the lesion of interest. A 3-0 Vicryl suture should then be used, in an interrupted fashion, to re-approximate the deep dermal layer. A 4-0 Monocryl or non absorbable suture (which will be removed post operatively), in a running fashion, should finally be used for the subcuticular layer. Apply either Steri-Strips or a liquid adhesive to the skin to complete the operation.

Nipple Exploration

For nonlactating patients with bloody nipple discharge or unilateral spontaneous discharge, nipple exploration and duct excision is recommended. The procedure is performed once examination has confirmed the discharge and imaging is negative for abnormality that is amenable to biopsy. The procedure involves use of local or regional anesthesia with incision placement in a periareolar location near the duct with discharge. The patient should be advised to not express the discharge for several days prior to the surgery. The breast tissue is incised up to the posterior ducts and then a lacrimal duct probe placed through the duct of interest. Blunt dissection is performed to the duct and then the duct excised with knife or cautery from the nipple insertion site to 5-7 cm deep into the breast. The lacrimal duct probe is removed once the duct is identified and excision started. The specimen is oriented and then the breast tissue closed with 3-0 Vicryl and skin closed with absorbable or nonabsorbable suture (to be removed 1 week later in clinic). Steri-strips and dressing are then applied.

Partial Mastectomy/Oncoplastic Breast Surgery

For patients undergoing breast conservation surgery for cancer, the localization procedures with wire, seed or ultrasound are similar to those described in Sect. 9.2. The only note of difference is that for patients with several abnormalities (multi-focal disease within one quadrant of the breast) which are felt to be amenable to partial mastectomy several wires may be used for "bracketing" of a lesion. In these and all cases of localization for cancer the surgeon and breast radiologist should discuss the case together to ensure each provider understands the operative plan for the patient. For patients with mulit-centric disease, or cancers in more than 1 quadrant of the breast, currently mastectomy is advised but is undergoing review in a clinical trial to determine if breast conservation is possible for lesions separated by more than 2 cm (Alliance/American College of Surgeons Oncology Group trial Z11102). For multi-focal disease, the operative procedure will likely involve a larger excision than a diagnostic lumpectomy or excision of a benign lesion. Incision placement is frequently over the lesion or periareolar but as more oncoplastic techniques are employed the surgeon may select an incision based on the ability to provide the best internal breast closure post excision [6, 9].

Intraoperatively the surgeon is advised to again label the specimen on three sides or to ink all six sides to ensure the pathologist knows the orientation of the specimen to facilitate accurate assessment of tumor margins. Recent data suggests that the surgeon should consider shave excision of each margin (except anterior if removed from under the skin or posterior if removed off the pectoralis fascia) to reduce the re-excision rate associated with breast conservation surgery. The shave involves the entire margin but is of minimal thickness. The use of this technique has been evaluated in a retrospective fashion as well as a randomized clinical trial and supports a reduced second surgery rate for patients with a breast malignancy [10, 11]. The operative surgeon is not advised to use intraoperative pathology unless they are in a location that has an established frozen section program for breast conservation tissue assessment. Another difference between benign lumpectomy or excisional biopsy and partial mastectomy is the recommendation to place a clip or 2–3 clips in the lumpectomy cavity for radiation localization for cavity boost. There is no level 1 evidence that this improves outcomes but is minimal risk and is therefore recommended. Surgical closure is as described in Sect. 9.2 and consideration should be given for a compressive bra post operatively if a large oncoplastic surgery was performed to facilitate healing and prevention of seroma. For patients requiring a reduction or larger oncoplastic excision with their breast conservation surgery consideration should be given to working collaboratively with a plastic surgeon to ensure the best cosmetic outcome for the patient.

References

1. Halsted WS. I. The results of operations for the cure of cancer of the breast performed at the Johns Hopkins Hospital from June, 1889, to January, 1894. Ann Surg. 1894;20(5):497–555. PMCID: 1493925.
2. Maddox WA, Carpenter Jr JT, Laws HL, Soong SJ, Cloud G, Urist MM, et al. A randomized prospective trial of radical (Halsted) mastectomy versus modified radical mastectomy in 311 breast cancer patients. Ann Surg. 1983;198(2):207–12. PMCID: 1353081.
3. Fisher B, Anderson S, Bryant J, Margolese RG, Deutsch M, Fisher ER, et al. Twenty-year follow-up of a randomized trial comparing total mastectomy, lumpectomy, and lumpectomy plus irradiation for the treatment of invasive breast cancer. N Engl J Med. 2002;347(16):1233–41.
4. Veronesi U, Cascinelli N, Mariani L, Greco M, Saccozzi R, Luini A, et al. Twenty-year follow-up of a randomized study comparing breast-conserving surgery with radical mastectomy for early breast cancer. N Engl J Med. 2002;347(16):1227–32.
5. Morris AD, Morris RD, Wilson JF, White J, Steinberg S, Okunieff P, et al. Breast-conserving therapy vs mastectomy in early-stage breast cancer: a meta-analysis of 10-year survival. Cancer J Sci Am. 1997;3(1):6–12.
6. Clough K, Kaufman GJ, Nos C, et al. Improving breast cancer surgery: a classification and quadrant per quadrant atlas for oncoplastic surgery. Ann Sug Onc. 2010;17:1375–91.
7. Lovrics PJ, Goldsmith CH, Hodgson N, et al. A multi-centered randomized, controlled trial comparing radioguided seed localization to standard wire localization for nonpalpable, invasive and in-situ breast carcinomas. Ann Surg Oncol. 2011;18(12):3407–14.
8. Ngo C, Pollet AG, Laperrelle J, et al. Intraoperative ultrasound localization of nonpalpable breast cancers. Ann Surg Oncol. 2007;14(9):2485–9.
9. Anderson BO, Masetti R, Silverstein MJ. Oncoplastic approaches to partial mastectomy: an overview of volume displacement techniques. Lancet Oncol. 2005;6(3):145–57.
10. Chagpar AB, Killelea BK, Tsangaris TN, et al. A randomized, controlled trial of cavity shave margins in breast cancer. N Engl J Med. 2015;373:503–10.
11. Moo TA, Choi L, Culpepper C, et al. Impact of margin assessment method on positive margin rate and total volume excised. Ann Surg Oncol. 2014;21(1):86–92.

Chapter 10
Mastectomy

Jacquelynn D. Arbuckle and Lee G. Wilke

Abstract   The mastectomy has evolved over the past 50 years into a less "radical" operation which is utilized for removal of a breast cancer as well as prevention of future malignancy. This operation is frequently coupled with implant or autologous reconstructive techniques.

Keywords   Mastectomy • Reconstruction

Introduction

In modern breast practice the surgeon works collaboratively with a multi-disciplinary team of oncologists to ensure the best long term outcome for patients with a breast malignancy. Though the partial mastectomy or breast conservation surgery is the more frequent operation for removal of a breast tumor,

———

J.D. Arbuckle, MD (✉)
Department of Surgery, University of Wisconsin School
of Medicine and Public Health, Madison, WI, USA
e-mail: Arbuckle@surgery.wisc.edu

L.G. Wilke, MD
Department of Surgery, University of Wisconsin Hospital
and Clinics, Madison, WI, USA

H. Chen (ed.), *Illustrative Handbook of General Surgery*,
DOI 10.1007/978-3-319-24557-7_10,
© Springer International Publishing Switzerland 2016

the mastectomy remains a key operative option. This option is undertaken after a shared decision making discussion with the patient about her tumor size, tumor type and desired long term approach to the cancer. In some situations, such as patients with large tumors which are not amenable to neoadjvuant therapy or those with extensive calcifications or multi-centric disease, a mastectomy is the only choice for complete excision of the disease. For some patients with a known genetic mutation or strong family history without known mutation, a mastectomy may be the patient's choice for surgical treatment. For some patients without a family history they may elect mastectomy to avoid future imaging and interventions. It is important for patients to be counseled on the equivalent survival between mastectomy and breast conservation surgery but it is ultimately the patient's decision regarding her operative choice for excision of a breast cancer. There are multiple oncologically safe options for patients and it is surgeon's role to help the patient navigate these options to achieve a desired long term outcome with a good quality of life.

The Radical Halstad mastectomy is an operation of primary historical interest but set an important precedent for the techniques required for removal of the breast, chest muscles and axillary contents. The more extensive operation performed in today's operating room is the Modified Radical Mastectomy (MRM) which removes the breast and axillary contents and occasionally the pectoralis minor muscle. More commonly as less invasive procedures have improved over the past 25 years and clinical trials have validated the use of a more minimalist approach, the simple mastectomy with sentinel node surgery has replaced the MRM [1]. A simple mastectomy is an operation intended to remove all breast tissue and can be performed with or without reconstruction. There are three types of mastectomies: total or simple, skin-sparing and nipple-sparing.

Simple Mastectomy Without Reconstruction

A total/simple mastectomy is performed in settings without immediate reconstruction. Consultation with a plastic surgeon should be offered to all patients undergoing a mastectomy. In some cases the patient may prefer no reconstruction or may elect a delayed reconstruction option based on the need for adjuvant radiation or medical therapy. As previously noted a simple mastectomy can be performed with a sentinel node excision or with axillary dissection which would be labeled a modified radical mastectomy. The type of axillary surgery is dependent on preoperative imaging, preoperative or neoadjvuant therapy and prior biopsy of axillary nodes. Anesthesia for a simple mastectomy can utilize a paravertebral block vs general anesthesia. Increasingly breast surgery can be performed with a paravertebral block with institutional studies revealing decreased post operative pain and nausea with the regional anesthestic approach [2].

Surgical Procedure

A total/simple mastectomy removes as much skin as possible to create flaps that will lie flat against the chest wall (Fig. 10.1). An elliptical incision surrounding the nipple-areolar complex is employed. The most medial point should be lateral to the border of the sternum at the level of the nipple with some surgeons "tailing" the incision towards the xiphoid to prevent a "dog ear" or excess skin in the medial location. The lateral edge should be placed along the chest wall lateral to the breast mound but adjusted superiorly pending the need for axillary surgery or to prevent excess skin this location. The superior and inferior incisions are placed to remove the most amount of skin but to also allow for closure of the wound. Some surgeons utilize a piece of suture to ensure the upper and lower incisions are of similar length.

The skin flaps for all mastectomies should be created between the breast capsule and the skin. A bloodless tissue plane is often identified with adequate retraction which can employ several skin hooks or facelift retractors. Thickness is dependent upon the patient and the amount of adipose overlying the breast tissue. No standard thickness exists, but the tissue remaining should, at a minimum, cover the dermal layer of the skin completely. If inadequate tissue remains,

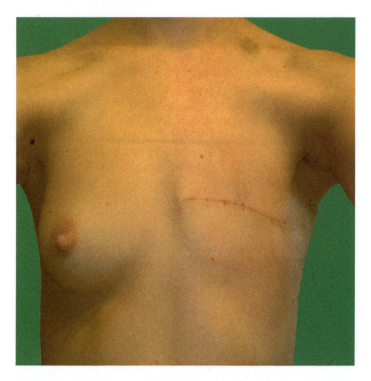

FIGURE 10.1 Simple mastectomy without reconstruction

then there is a risk for skin necrosis. Dissection commonly employs cautery though more recently some surgeons are utilizing the lower energy devices such as ultrasonic or plasma blades. The borders of the dissection include the second rib superiorly, the upper border of the rectus sheath inferiorly, the lateral border of the sternum and the latissimus dorsi muscle laterally [3]. Another option to sharp mastectomy flap dissection is to use tumescent solution for mastectomy flap creation. The solution consists of normal saline, lidocaine and epinephrine. A 20 g spinal needle is used for infiltration in multiple locations once the skin edge is incised with a knife. The solution is injected into the breast/subcutaneous plane and then scissors are used to complete the flaps [4]. The surgeon performing the mastectomy needs to select the approach with which they achieve the lowest skin flap necrosis. Once the breast capsule has been dissected from the skin layer, the tissue should be removed from the pectoralis muscle. The overlying pectoralis fascia should but does not have to be included as well. This dissection is commonly performed in a superior to inferior fashion. The breast tissue should be retracted inferiorly for the duration of the dissection. Care should be taken to avoid entrance into the axilla laterally but should include the entire axillary tail breast contents. The fascia of the serratus anterior muscle should be left intact as well.

After removal of the specimen, the tissue should be oriented with sutures superiorly and laterally. The wound is copiously irrigated with water, and hemostasis is confirmed. The flaps should be examined in a systematic fashion, starting at the 12 o'clock position of the chest and working clockwise. Gently retract the skin and patiently observe for any bleeding. Cautery or a low energy device can be used, pending the thickness of the flaps. Re-examine the pectoralis muscle, along with any ligated vessel, to ensure adequate hemostasis.

A closed drain system should be used within the mastectomy bed. A 10 or 15 French drain is placed beneath the inferior flap with exit laterally. If a sizeable amount of tissue was removed with concern for a potentially large postoperative seroma, a second drain can be placed. The drains can then be sutured to the skin with either a nonabsorbable suture; usually a Nylon. Closure of the wound should then proceed with a 3-0 Vicryl suture, in an interrupted fashion, for the deep dermal layer and then an absorbable or non absorbable suture (removed post operatively) in the subcuticular space. Surgical glue can be used for incisional coverage vs steristrips. A fitted bra or breast binder can be placed with gauze for added support post operatively. There are several companies which have developed post mastectomy bras. The surgeon should select the one that works best for his/her patient population.

Skin and/or Nipple Sparing Simple Mastectomy with Immediate Reconstruction

The primary differences between a simple mastectomy and those which are skin and/or nipple sparing is the incision placement as well as the immediate reconstruction with either an expander/implant or autologous flap. Patient selection for these operations is not standardized but for those desiring nipple preservation, patients usually have tumors which are greater than 2 cm from the nipple or are undergoing prophylactic breast surgery [5]. With negative imaging and pre operative evaluation the rate of finding disease in the nipple areolar complex is low but not negative and therefore this procedure is felt to be oncologically safe for selected patients. The borders of the mastectomy as well the technique of dissection options is the same as noted for the simple mastectomy. The incision placement for a skin sparing mastectomy with nipple/areolar removal is a simple ellipse around the nipple areolar complex (Fig. 10.2). There are several incisions for a skin and nipple

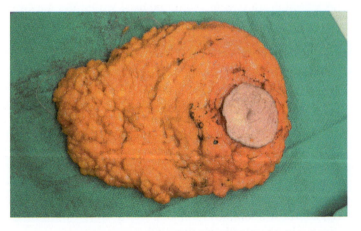

FIGURE 10.2 Skin sparing mastectomy specimen

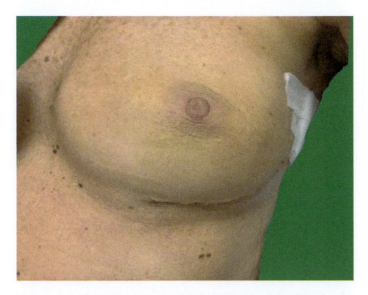

FIGURE 10.3 Nipple sparing mastectomy with implant reconstruction

sparing mastectomy and include those which extend partially around the areola with extensions medially or laterally and those along the inframammary fold. The incision placement is dependent on the patients' breast size and skin envelope and should be discussed with the patient and plastic surgeon prior to surgical intervention (Fig. 10.3). The dissection uses similar techniques but may employ a lighted retractor for better visibility of the skin flaps during the dissection. In addition if the nipple is preserved this area can be dissected with a knife to avoid thermal injury close to the nipple and may include a separate excision of the "button" of tissue beneath the nipple to provide a "margin" evaluation of the mastectomy specimen. Drain placement post mastectomy is dependent upon the type of reconstruction employed and closure is commonly performed by the plastic surgical team.

References

1. Julian TB, Venditti CA, Duggal S. Landmark clinical trials influencing surgical management of non-invasive and invasive breast cancer. Breast J. 2015;21(1):60–6.
2. Schnabel A, Reichl SU, Kranke P, Pogatzki-Zahn EM, Zahn PK. Efficacy and safety of paravertebral blocks in breast surgery: a meta-analysis of randomized controlled trials. Br J Anaesth. 2010;105(6):842–52.
3. Kuerer HM, editor. Kuerer's breast surgical oncology. New York: McGraw-Hill; 2010.
4. Abbott AM, Miller BT, Tuttle TM. Outcomes after tumescence technique versus electrocautery mastectomy. Ann Surg Oncol. 2012;19:2607–11.
5. Maxwell GP, Sorm-Dickerson T, Whitworth P, et al. Advances in nipple-sparing mastectomy: oncological safety and incision selection. Aesthet Surg J. 2011;31:310–9.

Chapter 11
Axillary Procedures for Breast Cancer

Sara E. Holden and Heather B. Neuman

Abstract The status of the axillary lymph nodes in breast cancer patients remains an important predictor of overall survival. The complete axillary node dissection has been largely replaced by the sentinel node mapping surgery in the past 15 years. The indications and techniques for sentinel node surgery have evolved over the past 10 years with resultant decreases in operative morbidity.

Keywords Sentinel node • Axillary dissection • Axillary lymph nodes • Sentinel node mapping • Operative morbidity

S.E. Holden, MD (⊠)
Department of General Surgery, University of Wisconsin Hospital and Clinics, 600 Highland Ave, BX7375
Clinical Science Center, Madison, WI 53792, USA
e-mail: sholden@uwhealth.org

H.B. Neuman, MD, MS
Department of Surgery, University of Wisconsin School of Medicine and Public Health, H4/726 CSC, 600 Highland Ave, Madison, WI 53792-7375, USA
e-mail: Neuman@surgery.wisc.edu

H. Chen (ed.), *Illustrative Handbook of General Surgery*,
DOI 10.1007/978-3-319-24557-7_11,
© Springer International Publishing Switzerland 2016

Introduction

The status of the axillary lymph nodes is the most predictive factor of overall survival in patients with breast cancer [1]. Historically, axillary staging was accomplished by performing a formal axillary lymph node dissection (ALND). However, ALND is now reserved for patients who present with a clinically positive axilla or are found to have pathologically confirmed positive lymph nodes. For the majority of breast cancer patients who present with a clinically negative axilla, a sentinel lymph node (SLN) biopsy is now considered the standard of care [2], offering a low-morbidity staging procedure with reliable identification of axillary metastases (Table 11.1) [3–7, 9].

Axillary Sentinel Lymph Node Surgery

The SLN biopsy is based on the concept that breast cancers will drain to a single node or group of nodes prior to draining to more distal nodes. The status of the SLN can then be used

TABLE 11.1 Associated morbidity of sentinel lymph node biopsy versus axillary lymph node dissection

	Sentinel lymph node biopsy	Axillary lymph node dissection
Infection	1–11 % [3–5]	8–15 % [3, 5]
Seroma	6–7.1 % [4, 5]	14 % [5]
Hematoma	1.4 % [4]	NA
Brachial Plexopathy	0.2 % [4]	0.97 % [5]
Lymphedema (objective)	0–8 % [5–8]	8–16 % [5–9]
Lymphedema (subjective)	2–5 % [3, 5, 10]	13–27 % [3, 5, 10]
Axillary sensations (objective)	9 % [3]	31 % [3]
Axillary sensations (subjective)	1–11 % [3–7, 9]	15–68 % [3, 5–7, 9]

as a marker for the status of the axilla as a whole; if there are no metastases present in the SLN, there should be a low likelihood of additional nodes being positive. Numerous prospective, multi-institutional studies have concluded that surgeons can successfully identify a SLN in >97 % of patients [11, 12]. Additionally, the SLN biopsy accurately reflects the axillary status in 97 % of patients, with a false negative rate of less than 9 % in earlier studies and less than 2–3 % in more modern use of the technique [12]. Based on these results, further axillary surgery can be safely avoided in patients with a negative SLN. Most patients with a clinically negative axilla are candidates for SLN biopsy; however, this technique is contraindicated in patients with inflammatory cancer or those patients unable to receive the mapping agents (use of dye in pregnancy, allergies to tracers or dye).

Operative Technique

Injection of Radiocolloid and Blue Dye

The most common technique when performing a SLN biopsy is to utilize both blue dye and radiotracer for lymphatic mapping. Although either technique alone is reliable when performed by experienced surgeons, the combination may be the most accurate for surgeons early in their SLN learning curve [13]. Injection of the radioactive tracer, typically technetium-99 m (^{99m}Tc) sulfur colloid, should occur within 24 h of surgery and may be followed by lymphoscintigraphy to confirm localization. Injections are most commonly peritumoral or subareolar, with high identification and concordance rates between the two injection sites [14]. In addition, subareolar injection is generally favored for injection of non-palpable tumors and multicentric disease.

Injection of blue dye occurs in a similar fashion as radiocolloid. Either 1 % isosulfan blue (5 cc) or dilute methylene blue (1–2 cc diluted to 5 cc with normal saline) should be injected 5–15 min prior to the procedure in the periareolar or peritumoral location. Methylene blue should not be injected too superficially due to risk of skin or nipple necrosis.

Furthermore, the anesthesiologist should be informed when injection of the blue dye occurs, as this can cause decreased oxygen saturation, mild blue rash or hives (0.4 %), or in rare cases a severe anaphylactic reaction (0.2 %) [12]. Gentle massage is applied to the breast for 3–5 min to facilitate drainage through the lymphatic channels to the nodal basin.

Pre-incision Localization of SLN

The majority of SLN biopsies can be conducted under regional block. If general anesthesia is required, paralytics are typically avoided. The patient should be positioned with the involved arm extended out on an arm board; some prefer to place a roll under the ipsilateral shoulder to elevate the axillary contents into the field. After the blue dye has been injected, the ipsilateral chest and involved axilla are prepped. The hand-held gamma probe is then used to localize the area of maximal radioactive uptake within the axilla, and this spot is marked. For patients undergoing mastectomy, the SLN can be identified through the mastectomy incision. For breast conservation patients, it is helpful to consider what the optimal ALND incision would look like when planning the SLN incision (see ALND section next). A small portion of this ALND incision which overlies the area of greatest radioactivity can then be used for the SLN biopsy. Most commonly, this is an approximately 3 cm incision just inferior to the axillary hairline. If the radiotracer has failed to identify a SLN, the incision should be made at the base of the axillary hairline, just posterior and perpendicular to the pectoralis major.

Incision, Dissection, and Excision

A scalpel is used to make the skin incision, and electrocautery used to dissect down through the subcutaneous tissue and clavipectoral fascia to expose the axillary contents. Utilizing the blue lymphatic channels and gamma probe as a guide, a combination of blunt dissection and electrocautery is used to localize SLNs. All nodes should be harvested that meet the following criteria: the "hottest" (most radioactive) node, nodes with ex vivo counts >10 % of the hottest node, any blue node, any node at the end of a blue lymphatic channel, or suspicious nodes. All lymph nodes removed should have an ex vivo count taken using the gamma probe. Once all SLNs have been excised, a final background count of the axilla should be obtained. If this final count is higher than 10 % of the "hottest" node, a search for additional SLNs should be performed. Dissection should be performed along lymphatic channels and close to the SLNs to minimize damage to surrounding tissues. Although rarely visualized during the SLN biopsy procedure, care should be taken to avoid injury to the thoracodorsal or long thoracic nerve, as the SLN dissection is sometimes quite deep in the axilla.

Intraoperative Pathology

The options for intraoperative pathologic evaluation of a SLN includes frozen section or touch cytology (i.e. stamping the cut SLN pieces onto a glass slide and performing hematoxylin and eosin stain). Intraoperative pathologic evaluation is controversial in patients undergoing partial mastectomy, as not all patients may require a full ALND per the American College of Surgeons Oncology Group (ACOSOG) Z0011 trial [15]. However, if planning a completion axillary dissection in the case of a positive SLN, intraoperative evaluation may allow for completion ALND in a single operation.

Closure

Hemostasis is achieved and the wound is irrigated. The clavipectoral fascia is closed with 3-0 absorbable suture, which may decrease the rate of lymphocele. No drains are necessary.

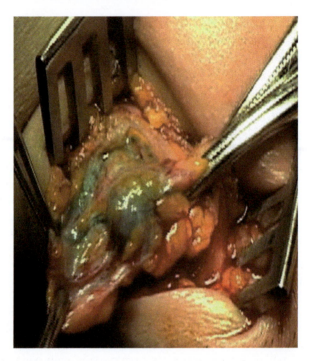

FIGURE 11.1 Identification of a blue sentinel lymph node in the axillary fat

An additional closure in the deep dermal layer is performed. Finally, the skin is closed in a subcuticular fashion with 4-0 absorbable suture, and Steri-Strips or Dermabond are applied (Fig. 11.1).

Axillary Lymph Node Dissection

ALND is currently indicated for the majority of patients with clinically palpable nodes with biopsy-proven metastases, positive SLN, a failed attempt at SLN biopsy, or patients with contraindications to SLN biopsy.

Operative Technique

Positioning

ALND is typically performed under general anesthesia without the use of muscle relaxant to allow for easy identification of the nerves during the dissection; however, it can be performed under regional anesthesia for some patients. The patient should be placed supine with the involved arm extended out to 90° and can be fully prepped into the surgical field by the use of a stockinette. A towel roll may be placed under the ipsilateral hemithorax and shoulder to lift the axillary contents into the surgical field. A single dose of perioperative antibiotic with coverage of skin flora is administered.

Incision, Dissection, Excision, and Closure

The borders of the axilla (lateral border of pectoralis major and medial border of latissimus dorsi) should be marked. A curvilinear incision is then made in an anterior to posterior fashion between the lateral border of the pectoralis major and the medial aspect of the latissimus dorsi, just inferior to the hairline. The skin incision is deepened down to the clavipectoral fascia. The fascia is incised and circumferential skin flaps are made just deep to the fascia to allow room for the dissection; this should extend laterally to the anterior border of the latissimus dorsi muscle, medially to the lateral aspect of the pectoralis muscle, superiorly to the approximate level of the axillary vein, and inferiorly to the fourth or fifth rib. Care should be taken during the lateral dissection to avoid dissecting a flap lateral to the latissimus muscle as this can be cosmetically unsatisfactory. The borders of the axilla are then defined by dissecting medially along the lateral aspect of the pectoralis major muscle and incising the pectoralis major fascia to expose the pectoralis minor muscle; at this point the medial pectoral nerve is identified and spared. The lateral dissection continues along the anterior surface of latissimus dorsi muscle.

The axillary vein can then be identified using one of two approaches. The vein can be identified laterally by following the latissimus dorsi muscle superiorly until its tendinous portion, where it crosses the axillary vein. Medially, the vein can be identified by looking superior and deep to the medial pectoral bundle. The inferior aspect of the vein should then be skeletonized. During this dissection, the thoracodorsal neurovascular bundle should be identified. Multiple venous tributaries may be encountered along the inferior border of the axillary vein; these should be divided with care until the thoracodorsal neurovascular bundle has been clearly identified. The largest of these vessels is the thoracoepigastric vein – a landmark for the thoracodorsal neurovascular bundle, which lies just deep and inferior. To confirm identification of the thoracodorsal neurovascular bundle, the thoracodorsal nerve joining the vascular pedicle should be visualized (usually identified medial to the thoracodorsal vein).

The dissection then continues medially along the vein. The pectoralis minor is dissected free along its lateral aspect to allow medial retraction and access to level II nodes. These nodes are then cleared inferior to the axillary vein and swept down with the specimen. The long thoracic nerve is then visualized coursing along the chest wall. It typically lies relatively deep in the axilla, and approximately 1 cm off of the chest wall. It should remain attached to the chest wall medially with dissection of all lateral tissues off the nerve and included in the specimen.

The fibro-fatty tissue between the thoracodorsal neurovascular bundle and the long thoracic nerve can then be freed. Skeletonization of the thoracodorsal neurovascular bundle is the last step required to clear the axillary contents. Hemostasis is achieved and a closed suction drain is placed in the anterior axillary line. The incision is closed in 1 or 2 layers (depending on the thickness of the subcutaneous flaps) with interrupted deep dermal 3-0 absorbable sutures followed by an absorbable 4-0 continuous subcuticular stitch.

References

1. Fisher B, Bauer M, Wickerham DL, et al. Relation of number of positive axillary nodes to the prognosis of patients with primary breast cancer. An NSABP update. Cancer. 1983;52(9):1551–7.
2. Krag DN, Anderson SJ, Julian TB, et al. Sentinel-lymph-node resection compared with conventional axillary-lymph-node dissection in clinically node-negative patients with breast cancer: overall survival findings from the NSABP B-32 randomised phase 3 trial. Lancet Oncol. 2010;11(10):927–33.
3. Mansel RE, Fallowfield L, Kissin M, et al. Randomized multi-center trial of sentinel node biopsy versus standard axillary treatment in operable breast cancer: the ALMANAC trial. J Natl Cancer Inst. 2006;98(9):599–609.
4. Wilke LG, McCall LM, Posther KE, et al. Surgical complications associated with sentinel lymph node biopsy: results from a prospective international cooperative group trial. Ann Surg Oncol. 2006;13(4):491–500.
5. Lucci A, McCall LM, Beitsch PD, et al. Surgical complications associated with sentinel lymph node dissection (SLND) plus axillary lymph node dissection compared with SLND alone in the American College of Surgeons Oncology Group Trial Z0011. J Clin Oncol. 2007;25(24):3657–63.
6. Ashikaga T, Krag DN, Land SR, et al. Morbidity results from the NSABP B-32 trial comparing sentinel lymph node dissection versus axillary dissection. J Surg Oncol. 2010;102(2):111–8.
7. Veronesi U, Paganelli G, Viale G, et al. A randomized comparison of sentinel-node biopsy with routine axillary dissection in breast cancer. N Engl J Med. 2003;349(6):546–53.
8. McLaughlin SA, Wright MJ, Morris KT, et al. Prevalence of lymphedema in women with breast cancer 5 years after sentinel lymph node biopsy or axillary dissection: objective measurements. J Clin Oncol. 2008;26(32):5213–9.
9. Del Bianco P, Zavagno G, Burelli P, et al. Morbidity comparison of sentinel lymph node biopsy versus conventional axillary lymph node dissection for breast cancer patients: results of the sentinella-GIVOM Italian randomised clinical trial. Eur J Surg Oncol. 2008;34(5):508–13.
10. McLaughlin SA, Wright MJ, Morris KT, et al. Prevalence of lymphedema in women with breast cancer 5 years after sentinel lymph node biopsy or axillary dissection: patient perceptions and precautionary behaviors. J Clin Oncol. 2008;26(32):5220–6.

11. Posther KE, McCall LM, Blumencranz PW, et al. Sentinel node skills verification and surgeon performance: data from a multicenter clinical trial for early-stage breast cancer. Ann Surg. 2005;242(4):593–9; discussion 599–602.
12. Krag DN, Anderson SJ, Julian TB, et al. Technical outcomes of sentinel-lymph-node resection and conventional axillary-lymph-node dissection in patients with clinically node-negative breast cancer: results from the NSABP B-32 randomised phase III trial. Lancet Oncol. 2007;8(10):881–8.
13. Kim T, Giuliano AE, Lyman GH. Lymphatic mapping and sentinel lymph node biopsy in early-stage breast carcinoma: a meta-analysis. Cancer. 2006;106(1):4–16.
14. Rodier JF, Velten M, Wilt M, et al. Prospective multicentric randomized study comparing periareolar and peritumoral injection of radiotracer and blue dye for the detection of sentinel lymph node in breast sparing procedures: FRANSENODE trial. J Clin Oncol. 2007;25(24):3664–9.
15. Giuliano AE, Hunt KK, Ballman KV, et al. Axillary dissection vs no axillary dissection in women with invasive breast cancer and sentinel node metastasis: a randomized clinical trial. JAMA. 2011;305(6):569–75.

Part III
Esophageal and Gastric Surgery

Guilherme M. Campos

Chapter 12
Laparoscopic Antireflux Surgery

Francesco Palazzo, Jad Khoraki, and Guilherme M. Campos

Abstract Gastroesophageal reflux disease (GERD) is a common disease. Established treatment options are lifestyle modifications, medications and laparoscopic anti-reflux surgery (LARS). In this chapter we present the definition of GERD, a basic diagnostic algorithm, indication for LARS and details of the common surgical techniques in use.

F. Palazzo, MD, FACS
Department of Surgery, Thomas Jefferson University,
1100 Walnut Street, 5 Floor, 19107 Philadelphia, PA, USA
e-mail: francesco.palazzo@jefferson.edu

J. Khoraki, MD
Department of Surgery, University of Wisconsin Hospital
and Clinics, Madison, WI, USA

Department of Surgery, University of Wisconsin School
of Medicine and Public Health, 600 Highland Avenue,
K4/730 CSC, 53792-7375 Madison, WI, USA

G.M. Campos, MD, FACS (✉)
Division of Bariatric and Gastrointestinal Surgery, Department of
Surgery, Virginia Commonwealth University, 1200 East Broad Street,
PO Box 980519, Richmond, Virginia 23298, USA
e-mail: guilherme.campos@vcuhealth.org

H. Chen (ed.), *Illustrative Handbook of General Surgery*,   127
DOI 10.1007/978-3-319-24557-7_12,
© Springer International Publishing Switzerland 2016

Keywords Gastroesophageal reflux disease • Esophageal reflux • Hiatal hernia • Esophagus • Fundoplication • Nissen • Laparoscopic surgery

Introduction

The incidence of gastroesophageal reflux disease (GERD) and its related complications (erosive esophagitis, peptic stricture, Barrett's esophagus (BE), and esophageal adenocarcinoma) is increasing worldwide [1]. GERD is the most common admitting diagnosis for Emergency Room visits, with an estimated 7 % of U.S. adults reporting heartburn once a day and 42 % once a month [2–4], with significant impact on quality of life.

GERD is defined as "Symptoms or Mucosal Damage Produced by the Abnormal Reflux of Gastric Contents into the Esophagus" [5]. Most common GERD symptoms are heartburn, regurgitation, and dysphagia but it may also manifest with extraesophageal symptoms like cough, hoarseness, asthma, tooth decay, aspiration pneumonia, among others [6].

While many patients can be managed with lifestyle modifications and acid suppressive medications, surgery is an option to provide long term symptoms relief. Once performed only via laparotomy or thoracotomy, today a laparoscopic approach to Antireflux Surgery (LARS) is considered the gold standard and will be presented in the following sections.

Indications and Preoperative Workup

Patients are considered candidates for LARS after they have objective documentation for the presence of GERD [7, 8]. There are three independent predictors of a successful outcome after LARS [9], they are:

1. GERD symptoms are responsive to acid suppressive therapy,
2. Main symptoms are heartburn and regurgitation ('typical' GERD symptoms), and
3. Patient has abnormal esophageal acid exposure determined by 24-h pH monitoring.

Patients may opt for surgery despite successful medical treatment (due to concerns related to side effects of long term use of medications use, expenses, quality of life) or if they have GERD related complications (peptic stricture or Barrett's Esophagus).

Patients with extraesophageal or atypical GERD symptoms experience, as a group, a lower success rates with LARS, but when GERD is properly documented by objective testing LARS is a therapeutic option [9].

Once a patient is referred for consideration of LARS a thorough preoperative workup needs to be completed in order to: (a) confirm the diagnosis, (b) rule out coexisting conditions (i.e. stricture, diverticulum, ineffective esophageal motility), (c) plan the most appropriate surgical procedure, and (d) set clear expectations for the patient.

Recently a group of experts – the *Esophageal Diagnostic Advisory Panel* – published an evidence and experience-based consensus on the preoperative workup prior to antireflux surgery [10]. In line with most previous recommendations the panel's proposed work up includes the following:

1. Symptomatic evaluation: grading of typical (heartburn, dysphagia, regurgitation) and atypical symptoms (cough, asthma, chest pain, dental erosions, and hoarseness) as well as response to proton pump inhibitors;
2. Barium esophagram: this study, ideally video recorded, provides anatomic description of the esophageal anatomic landmarks such as length and diameter, presence/size/type of hiatal hernia, presence of diverticulum or strictures, and a basic evaluation of esophageal motility;
3. Upper endoscopy: evaluates for mucosal injury and presence/size/type of hiatal hernia;
4. Esophageal Manometry: rules out achalasia and aids in selecting full or partial fundoplication.
5. 24-h pH study (off PPI), ideally Multichannel Intraluminal Impedance (MII)-pH: confirms pathologic reflux. This may be omitted in patients with severe esophagitis or BE on Endoscopy. MII-Ph demonstrates any kind of reflux (acid vs weakly acidic). Critical to the assessment and diagnosis is the <u>association of symptoms with the reflux event</u> (generally within 2 min).

Patients with recurrent symptoms of nausea, vomiting, bloating or retained food on upper endoscopy after overnight fasting should undergo a 4 h gastric emptying study. The presence of gastroparesis should prompt the surgeon and clinician to re-evaluate indication for LARS.

While a Nissen fundoplication (posterior 360° fundoplication) seem currently the most commonly performed fundoplication in the U.S., surgeons must be familiar with the 180° anterior (Dor) and 270° posterior (Toupet) partial fundoplication techniques that may benefit patients with ineffective esophageal motility and also that have been found on recent RCT's to provide equivalent long term results to full fundoplications but with less side effects and need for re-operation [11–13]

Operative Planning, Positioning and Room Setup for Antireflux Surgery

The procedure requires general anesthesia with the patient intubated with a single-lumen endotracheal tube. Adequate muscle relaxation is critical as it improves abdominal wall compliance allowing for better exposure secondary to increased pneumoperitoneum. An orogastric tube is inserted to decompress the stomach.

The patient is placed in a modified lithotomy position with legs on stirrups or, if a split table is available, supine with legs parted. Care must be taken to secure the patient to the bed with all pressure points padded and protected. The procedure will be conducted using a steep reverse Trendelenburg position. It is generally recommended to confirm patient's stability on the table by briefly placing the patient in the proposed position prior to prepping and draping (test flight); this practice minimizes surprises after the laparoscopic procedure has begun.

Pneumatic compression stockings are routinely used for deep vein thrombosis prophylaxis.

The procedure usually requires five (5) trocars. The equipment required is listed in Table 12.1. The surgeon stands between the patient's legs with the assistant on the patient's left side.

TABLE 12.1 Basic instrumentation for Laparoscopic antireflux surgery	
	Hasson 12 mm trocar (1)
	5 mm blunt trocar (3)
	11 mm blunt trocar (1)
	10 mm – 30° scope
	Atraumatic laparoscopic graspers
	Laparoscopic needle holder
	Babcock clamp
	L-shaped hook cautery with suction-irrigation capacity
	Laparoscopic scissors
	Vessel sealing system
	Liver retractor
	Fast clamp or laparoscopic BookWalter retractor
	Penrose drain
	0 and 2-0 SurgiDac sutures
	56 French esophageal bougie
	Laparoscopic clip applier

Technical Steps for Laparoscopic Antireflux Procedure

Placement of Trocars

Five trocars are used for the operation. The initial trocar is placed about 15 cm below the xiphoid process about 1–2 cm to the left of the midline; this port is used for insertion of the scope. The method for first trocar insertion maybe the Hasson technique, direct trocar insertion with or without pneumoperitoneum and will vary depending on patient's specific characteristics and surgeon's preference. The second port (5 mm) is placed at the same level as the Hasson between the left midclavicular and the left anterior axillary line; this is the assistant's port utilized for retraction via Babcock or Penrose drain. The third port (5 mm) is placed at the same level as the previous two ports but in the right mid-clavicular line or the sub-xiphoid location. It is used for inser-tion of the diamond liver retractor, the purpose of which is to lift the lateral segment of the left lobe of the liver and expose the esophagogastric junction. The last two trocars (5 mm on the right of the patients and 11 mm on the left) are placed as high as possible under the costal margin and about 5–6 cm to the right and the left of the midline; these ports are used by the operating surgeon for insertion of graspers, energy devices, and for suturing.

Essential Technical Elements of LARS

There are five key technical steps of LARS:

1. Complete crural dissection with identification and preser-vation of both anterior and posterior vagus nerve and reduction/excision of hiatal hernia sac if present,
2. Circumferential dissection of the esophagus and posterior mediastinum to obtain adequate abdominal esophageal length (3 cm),
3. Crural closure,
4. Mobilization of gastric fundus with division of short gastric vessels, and
5. Fundoplication

The last two steps have been source of long debate in the surgical community and while some authors, based on data from RCTs [14], may recommend against routine division of the short gastric vessels, all agree that a form of fundoplication – partial or complete – is a mandatory final step for a successful antireflux procedure.

Dissection of the Esophageal Hiatus and Esophageal Mobilization

The procedure begins with division of the gastrohepatic ligament above the caudate lobe of the liver, where this ligament usually is very thin, and continues toward the diaphragm until the right crus is identified (Fig. 12.1). In 15 % of patients an accessory or replaced left hepatic artery, branching off the left gastric artery, may run in the gastrohepatic ligament altogether with the always present hepatic branch of the vagus nerve. This should be preserved, but if exposure is compromised and the vessel has a small size (indicative that it may be an accessory not a replaced left hepatic artery) it can generally be divided without consequence. The peritoneum and the phrenoesophageal membrane above the esophagus

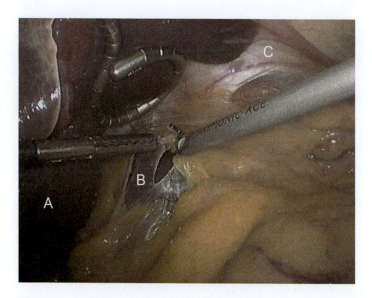

FIGURE 12.1 Division of the gastrohepatic ligament (*A* left lobe of the liver, *B* gastrohepatic ligament, *C* diaphragm)

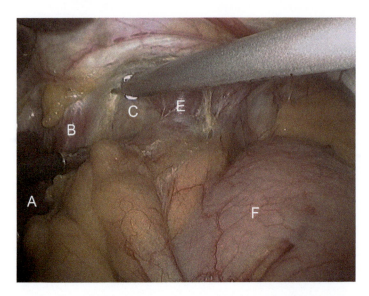

FIGURE 12.2 Opening of the phrenoesophageal membrane and initial dissection into the posterior mediastinum (*A* caudate lobe of the liver, *B* right crus, *C.* areolar tissue of posterior mediastinum, *D* divided phrenoesophageal ligament and fat pad *E* left crus, *F* gastric fundus)

are divided (Fig. 12.2) and the anterior vagus nerve is identified (Fig. 12.3). The Phrenoesophageal fad pad maybe excised and left crus of the diaphragm is exposed (Fig. 12.4).

The right crus is then separated from the right side of the esophagus by sharp and blunt dissection (Fig. 12.5), and the posterior vagus nerve is identified. The right crus is dissected inferiorly toward the junction with the left crus (Fig. 12.6). Care should be taken to leave the peritoneal lining on the right crus in preparation for crural closure.

It is at the beginning of the dissection that care must be taken to identify and excise any potentially present hiatal hernia sac. If present, the sac needs to be reduced in the abdominal cavity and excised in its entirety.

The dissection is continued cranially into the posterior mediastinum to ensure proper mobilization of the distal

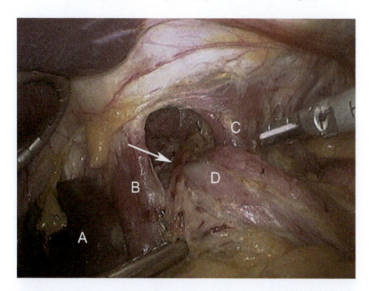

FIGURE 12.3 The anterior vagus nerve (*Arrow*) is identified (*A* caudate lobe of liver, *B* right crus, *C* left crus, *D* esophagus)

esophagus which will then translate into adequate abdominal esophageal length.

Tips and Tricks

To avoid the risk of injuring the inferior vena cava or the left gastric artery at the beginning of the dissection, some surgeons use a different method—the so-called left crus approach. In this approach, the operation begins with identification of the left crus of the diaphragm and division of the peritoneum and the phrenoesophageal membrane overlying it. The next step is division of the short gastric vessels, starting midway along the greater curvature of the stomach and continuing upward to join the area of the previous dissection. When the fundus has been thoroughly mobilized, the peritoneum is divided from the left to the right crus, and the right

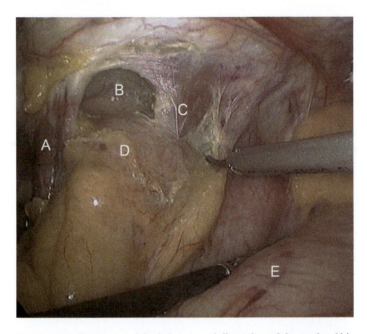

FIGURE 12.4 Exposure of the left crus and dissection of the angle of his (*A*. right crus, *B* posterior mediastinum, *C* left crus, *D* gastroesophageal junction (excised phrenoesophageal fat pad), *E* stomach)

crus is dissected downward to expose the junction of the right and left crura. With this technique, the vena cava is never at risk. In addition, the branches of the anterior vagus nerve and the left gastric artery are less exposed to danger. This technique can be very useful, particularly for management of very large paraesophageal hernias and for re-operative anti-reflux operations.

Mobilization of Greater Curvature with Division of Short Gastric Vessels

If routine Mobilization of Greater curvature with Division of SGV is contemplated, then at this point the vessel sealer of choice is utilized for this part of the procedure. Dissection

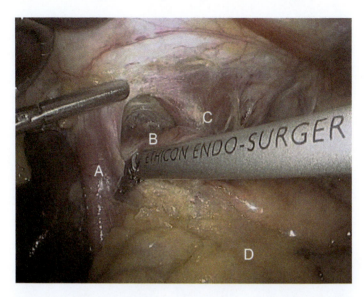

FIGURE 12.5 Dividing the peritoneum in between the right crus and esophagus (*A* right crus, *B* esophagus, *C* left crus, *D* stomach)

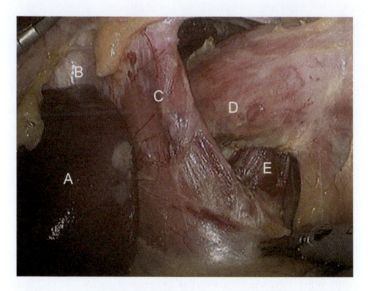

FIGURE 12.6 Dissecting the right crus inferiorly towards the junction with the left crus (*A* caudate lobe of liver, *B* inferior vena cava, *C* right crus, *D* esophagus, *E* left crus)

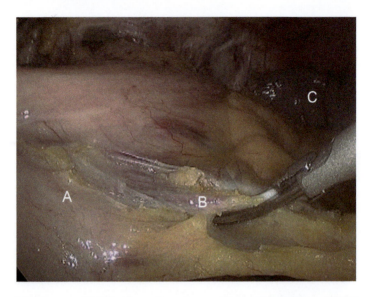

FIGURE 12.7 Mobilization of greater curvature with division of SGV (*A* greater curvature of the stomach, *B* SGV, *C* spleen)

begins at the level of the superior portion of the gastric body (Fig. 12.7) and continues upward until the most proximal short gastric vessel is divided (Figs. 12.8 and 12.9). Importantly, all the attachments of the posterior aspect of the gastric fundus to the left crura and the pancreas should also be divided (Fig. 12.10).

Care must be taken to avoid bleeding, either from the short gastric vessels or from the spleen, and damage to the gastric wall. Placement of endoscopic clips in the more proximal short gastric vessels before dividing it may be used to prevent bleeding.

Creation of a Large Retroesophageal Window

The esophagus is retracted upward with a Babcock clamp applied at the level of the esophagogastric junction. By blunt and sharp dissection, a window is created under the esophagus between the gastric fundus, the esophagus, and the left pillar of the crus. The window is enlarged and a Penrose drain

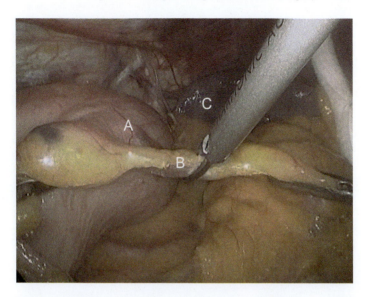

FIGURE 12.8 Mobilization of greater curvature with division of SGV
(*A* greater curvature of the stomach, *B* SGV, *C* spleen)

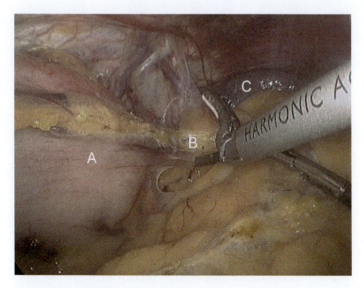

FIGURE 12.9 Mobilization of greater curvature with division of SGV
(*A* greater curvature of the stomach, *B* SGV, *C* spleen)

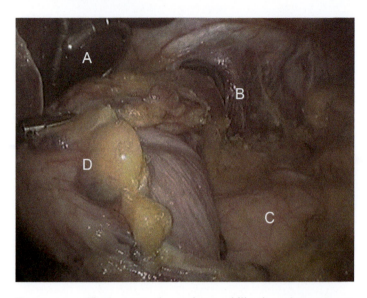

FIGURE 12.10 Final aspect of complete mobilization of greater cur-vature with division of SGV (*A* liver, *B* left crus, *C* pancreas, *D* greater curvature of the stomach)

is passed around the esophagus. This drain is then used for traction instead of the Babcock clamp to reduce the risk of damage to the gastric wall (Fig. 12.11).

During this part of the procedure the surgeon should be aware of a potential common complications such as damage to the pleura and creation of a CO_2 pneumothorax.

A CO_2 pneumothorax is usually caused by dissection done above the pillar of the crus in the mediastinum rather than between the crus and the gastric fundus. This problem can be avoided by properly identifying the pleura and separating it by using blunt dissection.

If the pleura space is entered, the surgeon should immedi-ately notify the anesthesiologist. The anesthesiologist should observe that peak airway pressure has increased (because of a pneumothorax), but this is usually managed without any other intra-operative intervention other than adjusting venti-lation mode and reducing the pneumoperitoneum pressure from 15 mmHg to 8 or 10 mmHg. At the end of the procedure,

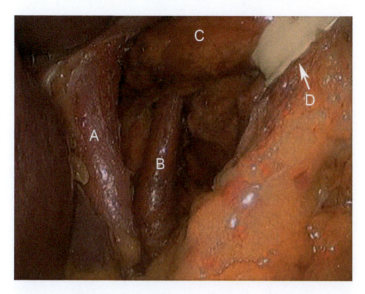

FIGURE 12.11 Final aspect of the creation of the retroesophageal window (*A* right crus, *B* left crus, *C* esophagus, *D* penrose drain around the GE junction)

while deflating the CO_2 pneumoperitoneum, the surgeon should ask the anesthesiologist to provide the patient a few large volume breaths. Due to the easy diffusibility of CO_2, any residual gas in the pleural space is absorbed within 1 h or 2 and chest drainage is not necessary in most cases. Neck and face emphysema related to progression of the pneumomediastinum into the subcutaneous tissue resolves without intervention within a few hours of the end of the procedure. CO_2 pneumothoraces tend to resolve spontaneously, rendering insertion of a chest tube unnecessary.

Crural Closure

The diaphragmatic crura are closed with interrupted 0 nonabsorbable braided sutures. Our preference is to use 0 braided polyester on an Endostitch device (Autosuture, Norwalk, CT); with the sutures tied intracorporeally. This

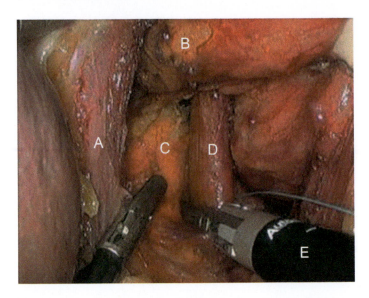

FIGURE 12.12 Closure of the diaphragmatic crura (*A* right crus, *B* esophagus, *C* aorta, *D* left crus, *E* suture device)

device, when used properly, allows for large crura bites while protecting the needle from inadvertently damaging the aorta or IVC (Figs. 12.12 and 12.13). Exposure is provided by retracting the esophagus upward and toward the patient's left with the Penrose drain. The first stitch should be placed just above the junction of the two pillars. We prefer a figure of eight stich configuration. Additional stitches are placed 1 cm apart, and a space of about 1 cm is left between the upper-most stitch and the esophagus (Fig. 12.14).

The bougie is not placed inside the esophagus during this part of the procedure.

If a Nissen 360° fundoplication is planned a 56 French Bougie should be inserted by the anesthesiologist and passed through the esophagogastric junction under laparoscopic vision. A routine Bougie insertion is not necessary when a partial fundoplication is planned. The crura must be snug around the esophagus but not too tight: a closed grasper should slide easily between the esophagus and the crura.

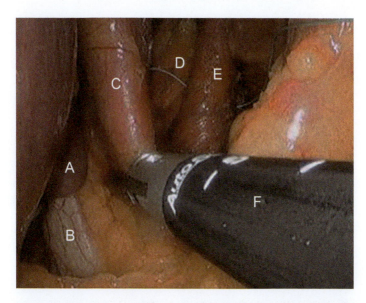

FIGURE 12.13 Closure of the diaphragmatic crura (*A* caudate lobe of the liver, *B* IVC, *C* right crus, *D* aorta, *E* left crus, *F* suture device)

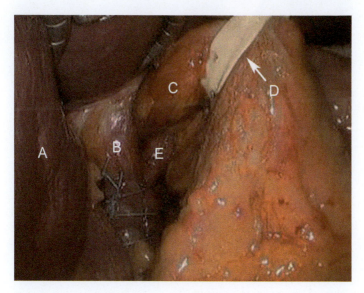

FIGURE 12.14 Crural closure – Final aspect (*A* liver, *B* right crus, *C* esophagus, *D* penrose drain, *E* left crus)

Fundoplication

Laparoscopic Fundoplication

The choice of a posterior complete (360° Nissen) versus posterior partial (270° Toupet) or anterior partial (180° Dor) fundoplication is based on individual patient characteristics and surgeon preferences. In the US, the most commonly used fundoplication is the Nissen fundoplication. However, many centers in Europe and some in North America favor the 270 posterior or 180 anterior partial fundoplications, as they have been associated with smaller rates of post-operative side effect such as gas bloat or dysphagia and need for re-intervention in recent randomized controlled trials [11–13].

Laparoscopic Nissen Fundoplication (Posterior 360° plication)

The posterior and most superior aspect of gastric fundus is gently pulled under the esophagus through the retro-esophageal window with the graspers. The anterior and most superior aspect of the fundus is brought above the esophagus held together. A "shoe-shine" maneuver should be done to ascertain using the appropriate portion of the gastric fundus for the fundoplication. Then, three 2-0 non absorbable braided sutures are used to secure the two ends of the gastric fundus to each other, having them join at a 9 or 10 o'clock position (Fig. 12.15). The middle stitch may incorporate the muscular layer of the esophagus. Two coronal stitches are then placed between the top of the wrap and the esophagus, one on the right and one on the left. Finally, one additional suture is placed between the right side of the wrap and the closed crura. In order to ascertain that at 'floppy' fundoplication was created a grasper can be introduced to elevate the anterior lip of the fundoplication (Fig. 12.16).

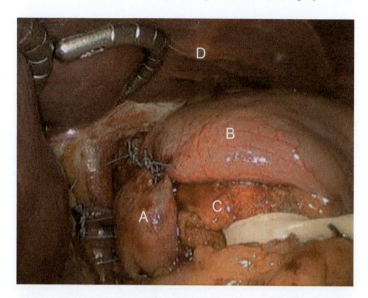

FIGURE 12.15 Nissen fundoplication – Final aspect (*A* posterior lip of the fundoplication, *B* anterior lip of the fundoplication, *C* esophagus, *D* liver)

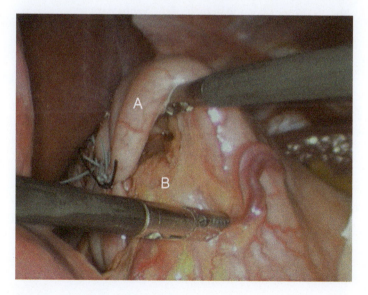

FIGURE 12.16 Nissen fundoplication (*A* anterior lip of the fundoplication, *B* GE junction)

Laparoscopic Toupet Fundoplication (Posterior 270° fundoplication)

The first steps in a Toupet fundoplication are identical to the first steps in a Nissen fundoplication. The wrap, however, differs in that it extends around only 270° of the esophageal circumference. Once the posterior aspect of gastric fundus is delivered under the esophagus, the two sides are not approximated over the esophagus. Instead, 90° of the anterior esophagus is left uncovered, and each of the two sides of the wrap (right and left) is separately affixed to the esophagus with three 2–0 non-absorbable braided sutures, with each stitch including the muscle layer of the esophageal wall. The remaining stitches (i.e., the coronal stitches and the stitch between the right side of the wrap and the closed crura) are identical to those placed in a Nissen fundoplication. One additional stich is place in between the posterior aspect of the gastric fundus and the closed crura (Fig. 12.17). Note that Fig. 12.17 also shows an accessory or replaced left hepatic artery, branching off the left gastric artery, running in the gastrohepatic ligament altogether with the always present hepatic branch of the vagus nerve.

Laparoscopic Dor Fundoplication (Anterior 180° Fundoplication)

The first steps in a Dor fundoplication are identical to the first steps in a Nissen or Toupet fundoplication. The wrap, however, differs in that it extends anteriorly for 180° of the esophageal circumference. It is accomplished by suturing the posterior and most superior aspect of the gastric fundus to the left lateral side of the esophagus with two 2-0 non-absorbable braided sutures, then two stitches from the most superior aspect of the anterior gastric fundus the right lateral side of the esophagus. Three additional stitches are then placed from the anterior aspect of the stomach to the superior aspect of the left crura, right crura and one in between (Fig. 12.18).

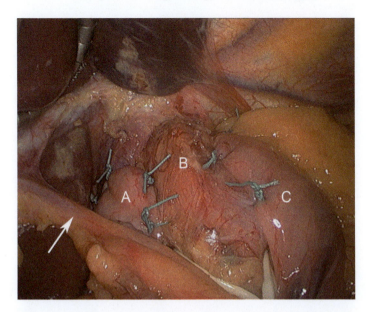

FIGURE 12.17 Toupet fundoplication – Final aspect (*A* posterior lip of the fundoplication, *B* esophagus, *C* anterior lip of the fundoplication, *Arrow* points to a replaced or accessory left hepatic artery running in the gastrohepatic ligament)

Postoperative Care

Patients are generally admitted to a regular floor bed. Narcotic utilization is kept to a minimum by use of long acting local anesthesia at the port sites and NSAIDs. A tight protocol for prevention of postoperative Nausea and Vomiting (PONV) is implemented on all patients. Antiemetics are prescribed as needed during the first 24–48 h. Patients are started on a soft pureed diet on the morning of postoperative day 1 after consulting with a dietician to review appropriate food options. This is continued for about 2 weeks. Patients are usually discharged after 23–48 h.

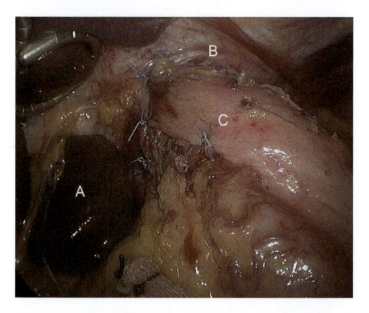

FIGURE 12.18 Dor fundoplication – Final aspect (*A* caudate lobe of the liver, *B* diaphragm, *C* anterior fundoplication)

Perioperative Complications

A feared complication of laparoscopic Nissen fundoplication is esophageal or gastric perforation (0–2.2 %) [15–17], which may result either from traction applied with the Babcock clamp or a grasper to the esophagus or the stomach (particularly when the stomach is pulled under the esophagus) or from inadvertent electrocautery burns during any part of the dissection. A leak will manifest itself during the first 48 h. Peritoneal signs will be noted if the spillage is limited to the abdomen; shortness of breath and a pleural effusion will be noted if spillage also occurs in the chest. The site of the leak should always be confirmed by a contrast study with barium or a water-soluble contrast agent. Optimal management consists of laparotomy and direct repair. If a perforation is detected intra-operatively, it may be closed laparoscopically.

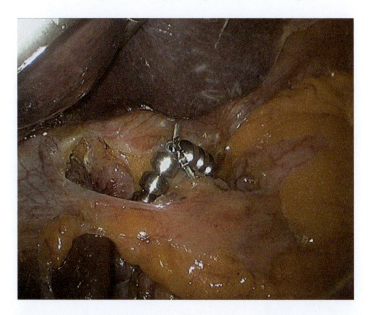

FIGURE 12.19 LINX device placed at gastroesophageal junction

Other known complications in the immediate postoperative period include pneumothorax (0–3.5 %) and Splenic and/or hepatic injury (0–2.2 %) [16–18].

Almost every patient experiences some degree of dysphagia postoperatively. This problem usually resolves after 4–6 weeks, during which period patients receive pain medications in an elixir form and are maintained on a dedicated mechanical soft diet.

Magnetic Augmentation of the LES

In recent years a new tool has been added to the surgical armamentarium for laparoscopic antireflux surgery: a magnetic ring that can be placed at the inferior border of the lower esophageal sphincter to restore the sphincter's competency (LINX Reflux management system, Torax Medical, Shoreview, MN, USA) (Fig. 12.19). The device is designed for patients that do not have large diaphragmatic hiatal hernia defects or advanced mucosal injury such as BE or strictures. As with standard LARS, patients offered LINX should have well documented GERD by 24-h pH monitoring. It is recommended that patients should undergo an esophageal manometry and have documented normal esophageal body motility. The theoretical advantages of the LINX device over a standard fundoplications is that would be easier to perform and associate with fewer side effects; however high quality comparative studies with all fundoplications are still lacking.

The device has been studied prospectively in a group of 100 patients with chronic GERD [19] and results showed that exposure to esophageal acid decreased, reflux symptoms improved, and use of proton-pump inhibitors decreased. Data on the device's safety profile was recently reported for 1000 patients operated worldwide [20]. Intra and perioperative complications occurred in 0.1 % of the patients, with 5.6 % requiring endoscopic dilations, and 3.4 % requiring reoperations (all elective, non-urgent). Erosions occurred in one patient (0.1 %). While more long-term data is still needed; initial results with the LINX device are certainly promising for selected patients.

Final Considerations

LARS has proven to be a safe and effective treatment for chronic GERD in several reports in the short and long term as it pertains to symptoms control and quality of life [21, 22]. Critical elements to a successful procedure are appropriate patient selection and preoperative workup together with surgeon's expertise.

References

1. Boeckxstaens G, El-Serag HB, Smout AJ, Kahrilas PJ. Symptomatic reflux disease: the present, the past and the future. Gut. 2014;63(7):1185–93.
2. Isolauri J, Luostarinen M, Isolauri E, Reinikainen P, Viljakka M, Keyrilainen O. Natural course of gastroesophageal reflux

disease: 17–22 year follow-up of 60 patients. Am J Gastroenterol. 1997;92(1):37–41.

3. Orlando RC. The pathogenesis of gastroesophageal reflux disease: the relationship between epithelial defense, dysmotility, and acid exposure. Am J Gastroenterol. 1997;92(4 Suppl):3S–5. discussion 5S-7S.

4. Peery AF, Dellon ES, Lund J, Crockett SD, McGowan CE, Bulsiewicz WJ, Gangarosa LM, Thiny MT, Stizenberg K, Morgan DR, et al. Burden of gastrointestinal disease in the united states: 2012 update. Gastroenterology. 2012;143(5):1179–87. e1-3.

5. DeVault KR, Castell DO. American college of gastroenterology. Updated guidelines for the diagnosis and treatment of gastroesophageal reflux disease. Am J Gastroenterol. 2005;100(1):190–200.

6. Kahrilas PJ. Clinical practice. gastroesophageal reflux disease. N Engl J Med. 2008;359(16):1700–7.

7. Kahrilas PJ, Shaheen NJ, Vaezi MF, Hiltz SW, Black E, Modlin IM, Johnson SP, Allen J, Brill JV. American Gastroenterological Association. American gastroenterological association medical position statement on the management of gastroesophageal reflux disease. Gastroenterology. 2008;135(4):1383–91. e1-5.

8. Stefanidis D, Hope WW, Kohn GP, Reardon PR, Richardson WS, Fanelli RD. SAGES guidelines committee. Guidelines for surgical treatment of gastroesophageal reflux disease. Surg Endosc. 2010;24(11):2647–69.

9. Campos GM, Peters JH, DeMeester TR, Oberg S, Crookes PF, Tan S, DeMeester SR, Hagen JA, Bremner CG. Multivariate analysis of factors predicting outcome after laparoscopic nissen fundoplication. J Gastrointest Surg. 1999;3(3):292–300.

10. Jobe BA, Richter JE, Hoppo T, Peters JH, Bell R, Dengler WC, DeVault K, Fass R, Gyawali CP, Kahrilas PJ, et al. Preoperative diagnostic workup before antireflux surgery: an evidence and experience-based consensus of the esophageal diagnostic advisory panel. J Am Coll Surg. 2013;217(4):586–97.

11. Broeders JA, Roks DJ, Ahmed Ali U, Draaisma WA, Smout AJ, Hazebroek EJ. Laparoscopic anterior versus posterior fundoplication for gastroesophageal reflux disease: systematic review and meta-analysis of randomized clinical trials. Ann Surg. 2011;254(1):39–47.

12. Broeders JA, Broeders EA, Watson DI, Devitt PG, Holloway RH, Jamieson GG. Objective outcomes 14 years after laparoscopic anterior 180-degree partial versus nissen fundoplication: results from a randomized trial. Ann Surg. 2013;258(2):233–9.

13. Mardani J, Lundell L, Engstrom C. Total or posterior partial fundoplication in the treatment of GERD: results of a randomized trial after 2 decades of follow-up. Ann Surg. 2011;253(5):875–8.
14. Engstrom C, Jamieson GG, Devitt PG, Watson DI. Meta-analysis of two randomized controlled trials to identify long-term symptoms after division of the short gastric vessels during nissen fundoplication. Br J Surg. 2011;98(8):1063–7.
15. Lidor AO, Chang DC, Feinberg RL, Steele KE, Schweitzer MA, Franco MM. Morbidity and mortality associated with antireflux surgery with or without paraesophogeal hernia: a large ACS NSQIP analysis. Surg Endosc. 2011;25(9):3101–8.
16. Colavita PD, Belyansky I, Walters AL, Tsirline VB, Zemlyak AY, Lincourt AE, Heniford BT. Nationwide inpatient sample: have antireflux procedures undergone regionalization? J Gastrointest Surg. 2013;17(1):6–13. discussion p.13.
17. Niebisch S, Fleming FJ, Galey KM, Wilshire CL, Jones CE, Litle VR, Watson TJ, Peters JH. Perioperative risk of laparoscopic fundoplication: safer than previously reported-analysis of the american college of surgeons national surgical quality improvement program 2005 to 2009. J Am Coll Surg. 2012;215(1):61–8. discussion 68–9.
18. Funk LM, Kanji A, Scott Melvin W, Perry KA. Elective antireflux surgery in the US: an analysis of national trends in utilization and inpatient outcomes from 2005 to 2010. Surg Endosc. 2014;28(5):1712–9.
19. Ganz RA, Peters JH, Horgan S, Bemelman WA, Dunst CM, Edmundowicz SA, Lipham JC, Luketich JD, Melvin WS, Oelschlager BK, et al. Esophageal sphincter device for gastroesophageal reflux disease. N Engl J Med. 2013;368(8):719–27.
20. Lipham JC, Taiganides PA, Louie BE, Ganz RA, Demeester TR. Safety analysis of first 1000 patients treated with magnetic sphincter augmentation for gastroesophageal reflux disease. Dis Esophagus. 2014;28(4):305–11.
21. Dallemagne B, Weerts J, Markiewicz S, Dewandre JM, Wahlen C, Monami B, Jehaes C. Clinical results of laparoscopic fundoplication at ten years after surgery. Surg Endosc. 2006;20(1):159–65.
22. Morgenthal CB, Shane MD, Stival A, Gletsu N, Milam G, Swafford V, Hunter JG, Smith CD. The durability of laparoscopic nissen fundoplication: 11-year outcomes. J Gastrointest Surg. 2007;11(6):693–700.

Chapter 13
Laparoscopic Surgery for Para-esophageal Hernias

Clinton T. Morgan, Laura E. Fischer, Jad Khoraki, and Guilherme M. Campos

Abstract   Surgical management of paraesophageal hernias has changed dramatically during the past two decades. Elective laparoscopic paraesophageal hernia repair is now the standard approach to the patient with a symptomatic paraesophageal hernia. The operation is technically challenging and requires numerous intra-operative and peri-operative considerations. Here, we will highlight the key points in the peri-operative and intra-operative management of paraesophageal hernias, emphasizing the operative goals of reduction of the hernia contents, excision of the hernia sac, a tension free repair with complete esophageal mobilization, crural repair, and fundoplication.

C.T. Morgan, MD, PhD • L.E. Fischer, MD, MS • J. Khoraki, MD
Department of Surgery, University of Wisconsin,
University of Wisconsin School of Medicine
and Public Health, Madison, WI, USA

G.M. Campos, MD, FACS (✉)
Division of Bariatric and Gastrointestinal Surgery,
Department of Surgery, Virginia Commonwealth University,
1200 East Broad Street, PO Box 980519,
Richmond, Virginia 23298, USA
e-mail: guilherme.campos@vcuhealth.org

H. Chen (ed.), *Illustrative Handbook of General Surgery*,   153
DOI 10.1007/978-3-319-24557-7_13,
© Springer International Publishing Switzerland 2016

Keywords Hiatus • Paraesophageal • Diaphragm •
Esophagus • Gastric volvulus • Mesh • Fundoplication

Indications

Immediate open repair of all paraesophageal hernias,
irrespective of symptoms, was standard practice for many
years. This pre-emptive approach was based on the surgical
dogma that paraesophageal hernias were at high risk for
life-threatening gastric volvulus and gastric necrosis [1].
However, this practice is no longer recommended, as it is
now known that the annual risk of paraesophageal hernias
progressing to life-threatening gastric volvulus and necrosis is low at approximately 1 % [2]. Therefore, these hernias can be managed on an elective basis when not
incarcerated.

Patients with asymptomatic paraesophageal hernias
identified incidentally can be offered watchful waiting as
a treatment option; though elective repair is an option in
patients with appropriate performance status. Common
presenting symptoms of paraesophageal hernias include
early satiety, gastroesophageal reflux symptoms such as
dysphagia, heartburn or regurgitation; epigastric discomfort, dyspnea, recurrent pneumonia (secondary to chronic
reflux and aspiration), and anemia [3]. Anemia develops
secondary to Cameron's ulcers: linear gastric ulcers that
form as a result of diaphragmatic compression of the
stomach at the hiatus. Notably, this anemia reliably
resolves following surgical treatment of paraesophageal
hernias [4].

Gastric volvulus with incarceration is a rare emergency in
which the stomach can rotate on either the long axis
(organoaxial) or short axis (mesenteroaxial) and become
ischemic [5]. An influential study by Drs. David Skinner and
Ronald Belsey in 1967 reported that 29 % (6 of 21) patients
with documented paraesophageal hernias and minimal symptoms died of gastric strangulation, perforation, or bleeding

[1]. However, subsequent studies have documented a much lower rate of lethal complications [2, 6], thus changing surgical practice to allow elective repair or watchful waiting of asymptomatic patients. Although uncommon, gastric volvulus with incarceration is typically seen in elderly patients and is a true emergency. Typical presenting symptoms include severe chest pain, vomiting, and epigastric distention [5]. If endoscopic decompression is unsuccessful patients should be taken to the operating room emergently for laparoscopic versus open reduction and repair. The urgency of an operation for paraesophageal hernia is a significant predictor of morbidity, especially with respect to pulmonary complications and mortality [7, 8].

Classification

There are four types of hiatal hernias (Fig. 13.1): sliding hiatal hernia (type I), and para-esophageal hernias types II, III and IV. Normally, the phreno-esophageal membrane is attached to the diaphragm and acts as an anchor, maintaining the gastroesophageal junction (GEJ), angle of His, and stomach in position (Fig. 13.1, top left). Sliding hiatal hernias (type 1) are the most common (95 %) and occur when the GEJ and the proximal stomach move above diaphragm. Sliding hernias (Fig. 13.1, top middle) and are repaired only when patients have surgery for recalcitrant gastroesophageal reflux disease [5]. Type II paraesophageal hernias (also referred to as "rolling" or "true" paraesophageal hernias) occur when the gastric fundus moves into the chest alongside a normally positioned GEJ (Fig. 13.1, top right). Type III paraesophageal hernias are characterized by the herniation of both GEJ and the variable portion of the stomach to an intra-thoracic position and account for the majority of the paraesophageal hiatal hernias (Fig. 13.1, bottom left) [5]. Most authors would call a hiatal hernia a Type III paraesophageal hernia when at least 50 % of the stomach is herniated into the chest. Finally, Type IV paraesophageal hernias are defined as the

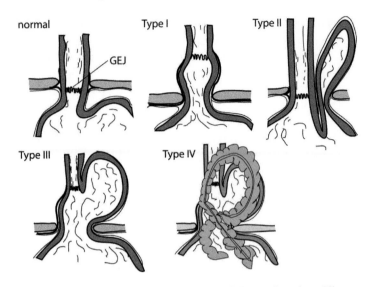

FIGURE 13.1 Types of hiatal hernia (Illustration by Clinton T. Morgan, M.D.)

herniation of other viscera such as colon, small bowel, or others alongside a Type III paraesophageal hernia (Fig. 13.1, bottom right).

Preoperative Preparation

Pre-operative management varies according to patient presentation. For the symptomatic patient seeking surgical intervention, a thorough pre-operative evaluation is recommended. Patients are generally older and often have significant co-morbidities requiring cardiopulmonary evaluation. Patients should undergo a barium esophagram [9] in order to define the anatomy, assess for volvulus, and evaluate for esophageal shortening, esophageal bolus transport and gastric emptying. Figure 13.2 shows a barium esophagram of a patient with a large type III para-esophageal hiatal hernia with all the stomach in the chest and with an organoaxial

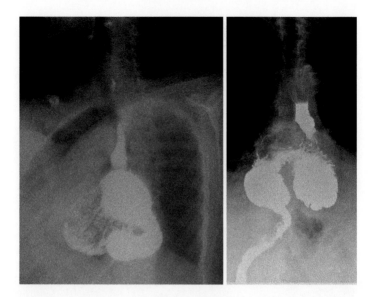

FIGURE 13.2 Barium esophagram showing large type III para-esophageal hiatal hernia with organoaxial volvulus of the intrathoracic stomach

volvulus of the intrathoracic stomach. Upper endoscopy with biopsy is also routinely performed (preferably by the operating surgeon). Esophageal manometry can be attempted to assess esophageal motility to guide the surgeon's operative planning with regard to the type of fundoplication and rule out esophageal motility disorders. High-resolution computed tomography, although not required pre-operatively, can depict the anatomical abnormalities well (Fig. 13.3).

Positioning and Anesthesia

All patients should undergo induction of general anesthesia with endotracheal intubation using techniques to prevent aspiration. The patient should be placed in either the supine

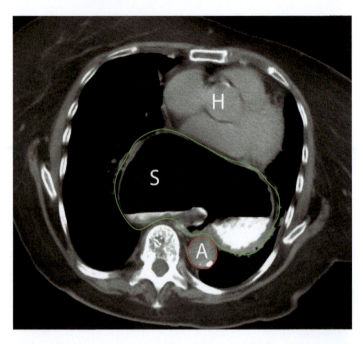

FIGURE 13.3 Computed tomography of the chest showing a paraesopha-geal hernia. A large portion of the stomach *S* green outline, is noted high in the mediastinum, at the level of the heart *H* note the proximity of the posterior aspect of the hernia to the aorta (*A* red outline)

position or on a split-leg table. The arms are secured on padded arm boards at a 90° angle to the body's axis. A footboard is placed and the patient secured to the bed in anticipation of a steep reverse Trendelenburg position during the case. An orogastric or nasogastric Levine tube can be placed as needed to decompress the stomach. Our preference is to introduce the Levine tube after the stomach is reduced and gastro-esophageal junction is under direct visualization. Sequential compression devices should be placed on the lower legs bilaterally and subcutaneous heparin can be administered for deep vein thrombosis prophylaxis. A foley catheter can be considered for close monitoring of urine output if the procedure is emergent or the patient has multiple comorbidities. The skin of the abdomen should be widely prepped after hair has been clipped short using an atraumatic electric clipper [10]. A single dose of antibiotics should be administered within 1 h of incision [11], typically a second-generation cephalosporin.

Operative Approach

Paraesophageal hernias can be repaired using laparoscopic, open trans-abdominal, or trans-thoracic (via a left thoracotomy) approaches. The laparoscopic approach is currently preferred in most centers. The possible benefits of the trans-thoracic approach include direct visualization of the sac and hernia, complete mobilization of the esophagus to the aortic arch and the ease of a relaxing incision on the left hemidiaphragm [3, 9]. Disadvantages include the pain of a thoracotomy, higher risk of peri-operative complications and the extended length of hospital stay [3, 9]. Most centers in the U.S. favor the use of laparoscopic techniques as complication rates seem lower than open approaches and recurrence rates with laparoscopic techniques seem similar to the ones obtained with the trans-thoracic and open abdominal approach [12, 13].

The laparoscopic approach to repair of paraesophageal hernias was first described in 1992 and emphasized crural approximation and fundoplication [14]. Five steps are essential components of a laparoscopic repair of a paraesophageal hernia:

1. reduction of the hernia contents
2. excision of the hernia sac,
3. complete esophageal mobilization,
4. crural repair, and
5. fundoplication [9, 14].

One of the most important aspects of successful paraesophageal hernia repair is to create a tension-free repair. Axial tension can be addressed with mediastinal esophageal mobilization in most cases. Occasionally, a Collis gastroplasty may be necessary. Lateral tension, due to a large diaphragmatic defect, is usually addressed by using appropriate technique for crural closure or an absorbable synthetic or biologic mesh. However, in selected cases relaxing incisions with or without absorbable mesh placement may be beneficial [9, 12, 15]. Only absorbable synthetic or biologic mesh should be used at the hiatus. Non-absorbable meshes should be avoided as they have potential to erode into the esophagus. However, even the use of absorbable synthetic or biologic mesh is controversial since its efficacy in long-term objective recurrence has not been demonstrated [12]. Reduction of early recurrences with biologic mesh placement, however, may be one advantage over primary repair [16].

Laparoscopic repair is associated with less blood loss, fewer intraoperative complications, faster diet advancement, and shorter hospital stays [3, 17]. Unfortunately, the radiographic recurrence rate is still quite high, ranging from 23 to 50 % in selected series [15, 17–20]. However most radiographic recurrence are small recurrences of a small portion of the proximal stomach and the vast majority are asymptomatic, thus of little clinical significance and needing no treatment [18, 20].

Laparoscopic port sites are positioned in a configuration similar to that of a standard Nissen fundoplication. An additional 5 mm port in the left lower quadrant may be beneficial to assist with retraction and dissection. After inspection of the abdominal contents, the left lobe of the liver is retracted cephalad with a self-retaining laparoscopic retractor, exposing the hiatal defect and hernia (Fig. 13.4).

Description of the Laparoscopic Procedure

Reduction of Hernia Contents and Esophageal Hiatus Dissection

It is our preference to start the dissection at the gastrohepatic ligament, which is bluntly grasped and divided with the harmonic scalpel (Fig. 13.5). Care should be taken to identify

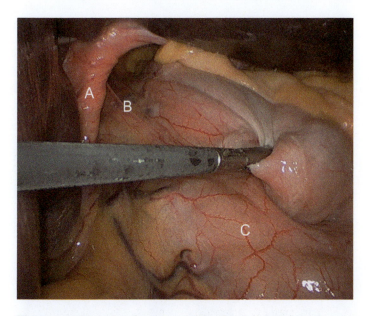

FIGURE 13.4 Reducing the stomach into the abdomen (*A* right crus, *B* preno-esophageal membrane, *C* stomach)

and, if present, preserve a replaced left hepatic artery arising from the left gastric artery and traversing the gastrohepatic ligament. Next, the phrenoesophageal ligament is identified at the right crus. The ligament is grasped with an atraumatic grasper and pulled caudally. It is then divided with the harmonic scalpel, exposing an avascular plane while delivering the hiatal hernia sac medially (Fig. 13.6). Blunt dissection allows development of this avascular plane, which is extended cephalad into the thoracic cavity (Figs. 13.7 and 13.8). The dissection is then extended circumferentially in a clockwise fashion to the left crus. Then, the peritoneal coverage of the right crus is opened and the avascular plane dissected to release the hernia sac in that location (Figs. 13.9, 13.10 and 13.11). Care is taken to identify and avoid entry into the pleura both the right and left side. Figure 13.12 shows the dissection to the base of the right crus and in proximity to

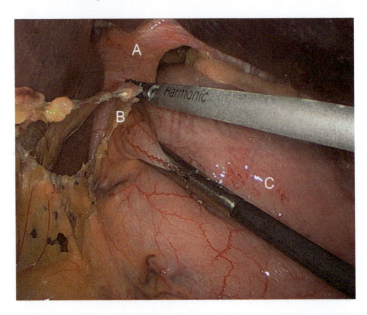

FIGURE 13.5 Division of the gastrohepatic ligament (*A* right crus, *B* gastrohepatic ligament, *C* stomach)

the left gastric vessels. Dissection on the left side is facilitated by reduction of the gastric fundus (Fig. 13.13), opening the gastro-colic ligament, entering the lesser sac, and dividing the short gastric vessels (Figs. 13.14, 13.15, 13.16, 13.17, and 13.18). Some surgeons prefer to start the operation by identifying the left crus (as opposed to the right crus as described above) and then move to the right side. For this portion of the operation, we employ the harmonic scalpel. Clips should be placed on the larger and more proximal short gastric vessels (Fig. 13.17). Division of the short gastric vessels and

FIGURE 13.7 Dissection of the anterior aspect of the hernia sac (*A* hernia sac *B* gastric fundus *C* left crus)

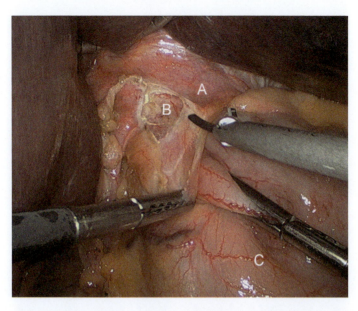

FIGURE 13.6 Division of the phrenoesophageal membrane (*A* phrenoesophageal membrane, *B* hernia sac, *C* stomach)

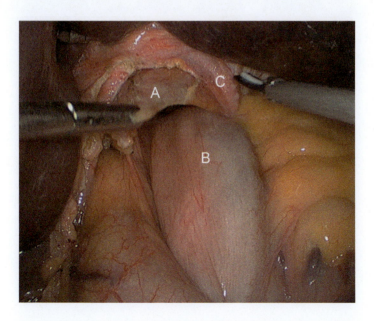

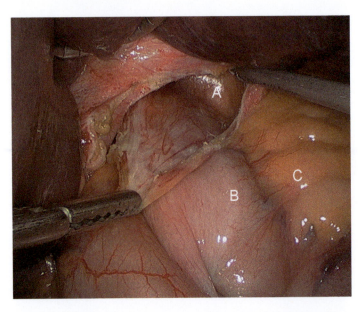

FIGURE 13.8 Opening the hernia sac laterally (*A* areolar tissue inside hernia sac, *B* gastric fundus, *C* gastrosplenic ligament)

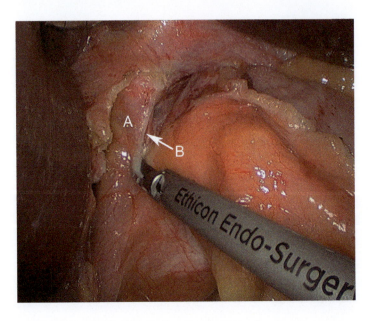

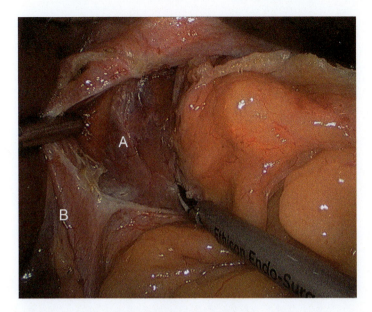

FIGURE 13.10 Dissecting the avascular space in between right crus and the hernia sac (*A* avascular space, *B* right crus)

mobilization of the stomach aids in complete circumferential dissection of the hernia sac (Figs. 13.19 and 13.20) and will facilitate the creation of a proper fundoplication, which is performed later in the operation.

Excision of the Hernia Sac

Once the stomach is reduced and the hernia sac has been opened circumferentially around the crura, the hernia sac dissection is extended further into the mediastinum (Fig. 13.20). Much of this dissection can be accomplished by blunt

FIGURE 13.9 Incising the peritoneal coverage of the right crus (*A* right crus, *B* entering the avascular space to access the hernia sac)

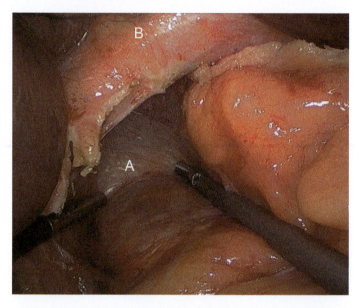

FIGURE 13.11 Dissecting the avascular space in between right crus and the hernia sac (*A* avascular space, *B* right crus)

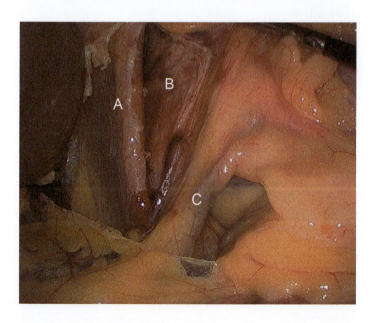

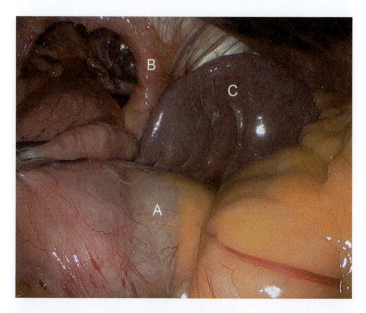

FIGURE 13.13 Exposure of gastroesplenic ligament for dissection (*A* stomach, *B* left crus, *C* spleen)

dissection in the avascular plane. We frequently employ rolled 4 x 4" gauze to aid blunt dissection. Critically, the right and left pleura, inferior vena cava, and aorta must be identified early and protected during the procedure. Complete dissection of the hernia sac is an essential component of the operation [21]. Dissection of the hernia sac proceeds by alternating between the left anterior and right anterior thoracic cavity until the sac has been circumferentially released from its intrathoracic attachments. Placement of a Penrose around the esophagus near the GEJ facilitates alternating the direction of retraction during this dissection. Once the hernia

←─────────────────────────────

FIGURE 13.12 Left gastric vessels (*C*) at the base of the hernia sac dissection (*A* right crus, *B* hernia sac)

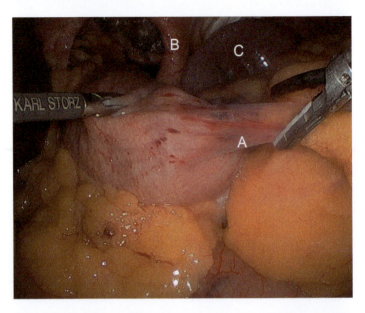

FIGURE 13.14 Division of the short gastric vessels (SGV) for mobilization of the gastric fundus (*A* SGV, *B* left crus, *C* spleen)

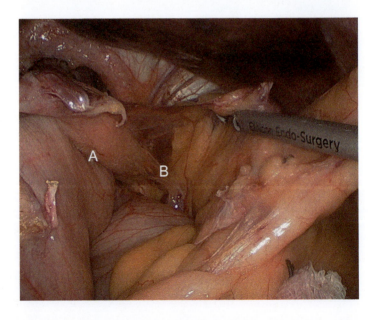

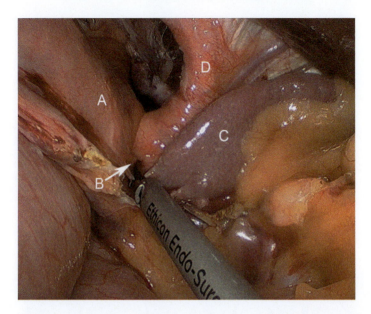

FIGURE 13.16 Division of the short gastric vessels and mobilization of the stomach up to the angle of his (*A* stomach, *B* angle of his, *C* spleen, *D* left crus)

sac is dissected off all intra-thoracic attachments it can be retracted into the abdomen and excised (Fig. 13.21). Care is taken to identify and preserve the anterior and posterior Vagus nerves during the dissection and excision of the sac. The excision of the sac maybe omitted if the presence of the sac would not interfere with the fundoplication. It is our preference to excise the hernia sac as it allows for a clearer identification of the gastroesophageal junction and the distal esophagus.

FIGURE 13.15 Division of the short gastric vessels and mobilization of the stomach (*A* stomach, *B* SGV)

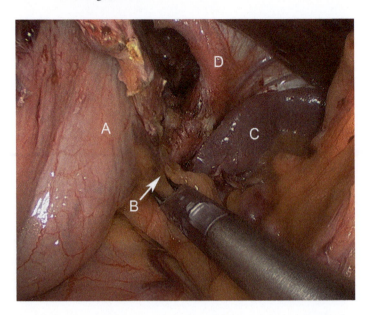

FIGURE 13.17 Applying a clip on a more posterior and superior short gastric vessel (*A* stomach, *B* SGV, *C* spleen, *D* left crus)

Crural Repair

Once the hernia sac has been excised, we turn our attention to repair of the hiatal defect. The right crus and left crus are approximated with sutures (Fig. 13.22). It is our preference to use interrupted zero braided polyester sutures in a figure of eight configuration. The number of sutures place will vary according to the size of the defect. The goal is to close the diaphragmatic defect while allowing only a 1–2 cm space in between the esophagus and the crural closure. If there is excessive lateral tension on the crural approximation, reducing CO_2 insufflation from 15 mmHg to 10 or 12 mmHg may assist in allowing closure without tension.

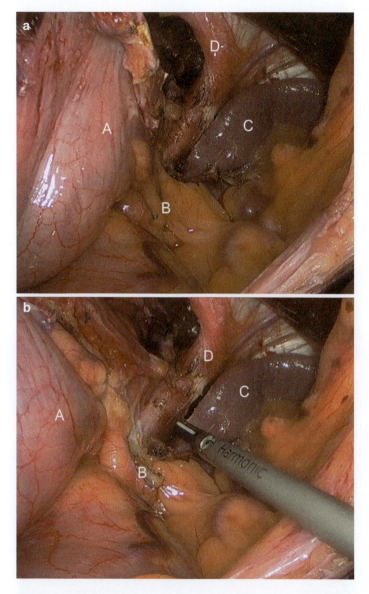

FIGURE 13.18 Completed SGV and stomach greater curvature mobilization (*A* stomach, *B* SGV, *C* spleen, *D* left crus)

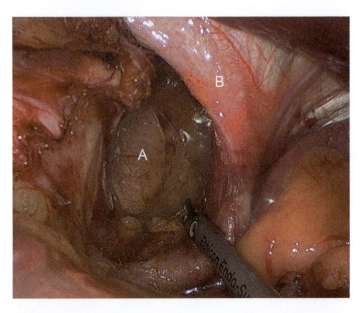

FIGURE 13.19 Left lateral and inferior dissection of the hernia sac (*A* aorta, *B* left crus)

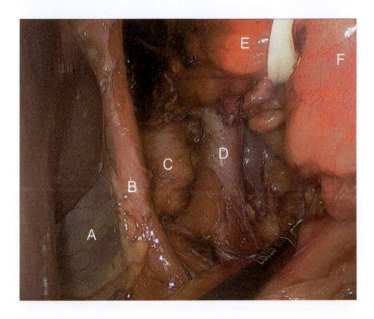

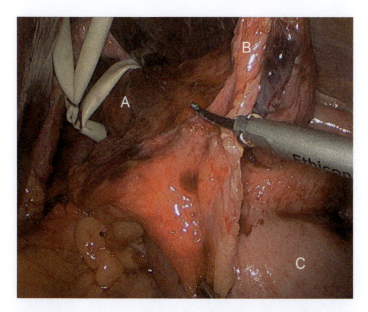

FIGURE 13.21 Excision of the hernia sac (*A* GE junction, *B* hernia sac, *C* stomach)

Absorbable Synthetic and Biological Mesh Placement

The use of mesh to reinforce the crural closure during repair large hiatal hernia has been used in an attempt to reduce the relatively high recurrence rates observed after the repair of these hernias [22]. Radiologic, objective recurrence rates (re-herniation >than 2 cm) have been reported to occur in approximately 40–60 % of patients after laparoscopic repair of paraesophageal hernia [20, 23], however, most patients with noted recurrences report no return of symptoms. Studies

FIGURE 13.20 Final aspect of dissection and retroesophageal window (*A*, *B* right crus, *C* aorta *D* left crus *E* esophagus *F* stomach)

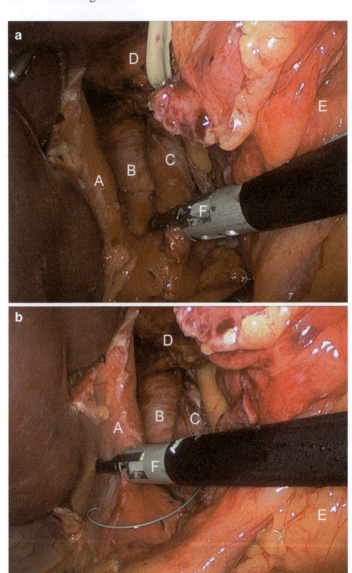

FIGURE 13.22 (**a, b, c, d**) Closure of the crura (*A* right crus, *B* aorta, *C* left crus, *D* esophagus, *E* stomach, *F* suturing device, *G* suture)

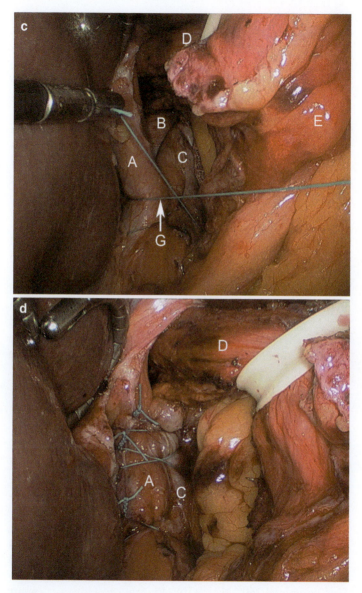

FIGURE 13.22 (continued)

report long-term relief of symptoms in 75–87 % of patients and a 61–91 % satisfaction rate with the result of the procedure [16, 22–24]. The only randomized controlled trial comparing the use of biologic mesh to no mesh with both 6 month and 2 year results suggest that the objective success rate seems to be improved with mesh over non-mesh repair in the short term [16, 25]. However, appropriate long-term follow-up is lacking and objective recurrence tends to increase over time [22, 24, 25]. Notably, the complications from non-absorbable mesh usage can be severe, including esophageal erosion (0.2 %) and extensive hiatal fibrosis (0.5 %) [3, 22, 26]. For these reasons, absorbable mesh is advised [16, 24]. Despite radiographic evidence of recurrence after a large hiatal hernia repair, most patients report enduring and dramatic symptomatic improvement [24, 25].

Despite the lack of level I evidence that the use of mesh reduces recurrence rates, newer biological and absorbable synthetic products that are less expensive are commonly used in practice. We place a U-shaped absorbable mesh around the esophagus at the level of the hiatus. The mesh onlay is placed posteriorly, with the esophagus cupped by the U and the approximated hiatus covered (Fig. 13.23). The mesh may be secured in place with fibrin glue or sutures.

Fundoplication

A gastric fundoplication around the distal esophagus is recommended after the closure of the hiatal defect to prevent de-novo or recurrent GERD symptoms after surgery. Some types of fundoplication also assist in securing the gastric fundus to the esophagus and diaphragm. The choice of a posterior complete (360° Nissen), posterior partial (270° Toupet), or anterior partial (180° Dor) fundoplication is based on individual patient characteristics and surgeon preferences. In the US, the most commonly used fundoplication is the posterior complete 360° Nissen fundoplication. However, many centers in Europe and also in North America favor the

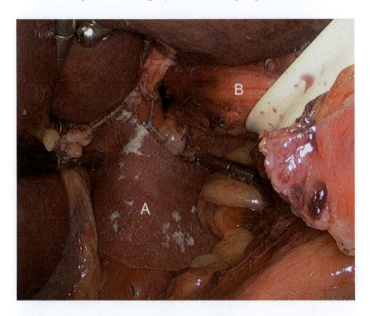

FIGURE 13.23 Absorbable synthetic Mesh (*A* covering the crural repair, *B* esophagus)

Toupet or Dor fundoplications, as they have been associated with lower rates of post-operative side effect such as gas bloat, dysphagia, and need for additional interventions in recent randomized controlled trials [27–29].

We favor a partial fundoplication as most of these patients have reflux as the main presenting symptom, and most have inherent esophageal motility dysfunction related to advanced age or the chronic nature of the partial obstruction caused by the paraesophageal herniation. A completed anterior 180° Dor fundoplication is shown in Fig 13.24. The technical steps for the creation of the Nissen, Toupet and Dor fundoplications can be found in the "Laparoscopic Antireflux Surgery" chapter of this book.

Occasionally, a "short esophagus" may be encountered and such a condition is diagnosed when less than 2.5 cm of intra-abdominal esophageal length is attainable. In these

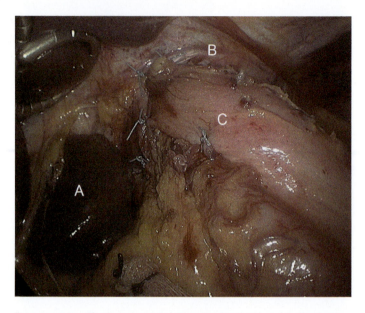

FIGURE 13.24 Final aspect of a Dor fundoplication (*A* diaphragm, *B* fundoplication, *C* caudate lobe of the liver)

cases, a Collis gastroplasty may be performed in conjunction with a fundoplication [3, 30–32]. Finally, the addition of a wedge fundectomy to Collis gastroplasty should be considered when a short esophagus is encountered as this procedure has recently been shown to have a lower prevalence of post-operative dysphagia and esophagitis [33].

Post-operative Care and Complications

Due to extensive mediastinal dissection, subcutaneous emphysema is commonly observed. This is rarely of clinical significance as long as the anesthesiologist has been attentive to the patient's PCO_2 during the procedure. Another relatively common intra-operative complication is a pleural tear. This is usually managed by communication with the anesthesiologist and altering the ventilation mode without the need for any intervention. Other peri-operative complications include atrial fibrillation, bleeding, deep venous thrombosis, and pneumonia, among others. Most patients can begin with a clear liquid meal within the first 24 h of the operation. Patients rapidly advance to a pureed or soft diet and remain on this diet for about 2 weeks. Most patients can be discharged on post-operative day number 1 or 2.

Summary

Elective repair is recommended for patients with symptomatic para-esophageal hiatal hernia that are not acutely incarcerated and laparoscopic repair is the standard of care. We describe the operative approach to achieve the critical goals of paraesophageal hernia repair:

1. reduction of the hernia contents
2. excision of the hernia sac,
3. complete esophageal mobilization,
4. crural repair, and
5. fundoplication

References

1. Skinner DB, Belsey RH. Surgical management of esophageal reflux and hiatus hernia: long-term results with 1,030 patients. J Thorac Cardiovasc Surg. 1967;53(1):33–54.
2. Stylopoulos N, Gazelle GS, Rattner DW. Paraesophageal hernia: operation or observation? Ann Surg. 2002;236(4):492–500.
3. Schieman C, Grondin S. Paraesophageal hernia: clinical presentation, evaluation, and management controversies. Thorac Surg Clin. 2009;19:473–84.
4. Carrott PW, Markar SR, Hong J, Kuppusamy MK, Koehler RP, Low DE. Iron-deficiency anemia is a common presenting issue with giant paraesophageal hernia and resolves following repair. J Gastrointest Surg. 2013;17(5):858–62.
5. Kohn GP, Price RR, DeMeester SR, Zehetner J, Muensterer OJ, Awad Z, Mittal SK, Richardson WS, Stefanidis D, Fanelli

RD. SAGES guidelines committee. Guidelines for the management of hiatal hernia. Surg Endosc. 2013;27(12):4409–28.

6. Allen MS, Trastek VF, Deschamps C, Pairolero PC. Intrathoracic stomach: presentation and results of operation. J Thorac Cardiovasc Surg. 1993;105(2):253–8.

7. Ballian N, Luketich JD, Levy RM, Awais O, Winger D, Weksler B, Landreneau RJ, Nason KS. A clinical prediction rule for perioperative mortality and major morbidity after laparoscopic giant paraesophageal hernia repair. J Thorac Cardiovasc Surg. 2013;145(3):721–9.

8. Poulose BK, Gosen C, Marks JM, Khaitan L, Rosen MJ, Onders RP, Trunzo JA, Ponsky JL. Inpatient mortality analysis of paraesophageal hernia repair in octogenarians. J Gastrointest Surg. 2008;12:1888–92.

9. DeMeester SR. Laparoscopic paraesophageal hernia repair: critical steps and adjunct techniques to minimize recurrence. Surg Laparosc Endosc Percutan Tech. 2013;23:429–35.

10. Tanner J, Norrie P, Melen K. Preoperative hair removal to reduce surgical site infection. Cochrane Database Syst Rev. 2011;11:1–49.

11. Nelson RL, Gladman E, Barbateskovic M. Antimicrobial prophylaxis for colorectal surgery. Cochrane Database Syst Rev. 2014;5:1–262.

12. Zehetner J, DeMeester SR, Ayazi S, Kilday P, Augustin F, Hagen JA, Lipham JC, Sohn HJ, DeMeester TR. Laparoscopic versus open repair of paraesophageal hernia: the second decade. J Am Coll Surg. 2011;212:813–20.

13. Luketich JD, Nason KS, Christie NA, Pennathur A, Jobe BA, Landreneau RJ, Schuchert MJ. Outcomes after a decade of laparoscopic giant paraesophageal hernia repair. J Thorac Cardiovasc Surg. 2010;139(2):395–404.

14. Cuschieri A, Shimi S, Nathanson LK. Laparoscopic reduction, crural repair, and fundoplication of large hiatal hernia. Am J Surg. 1992;163:425–30.

15. Greene CL, DeMeester SR, Zehetner J, Worrell SG, Oh DS, Hagen JA. Diaphragmatic relaxing incisions during laparoscopic paraesophageal hernia repair. Surg Endosc. 2013;27:4532–8.

16. Oelschlager BK, Pellegrini CA, Hunter J, Soper N, Brunt M, Sheppard B, Jobe B, Polissar N, Mitsumori L, Nelson J, Swanstrom L. Biologic prosthesis reduces hernia recurrence after laparoscopic paraesophageal hernia repair: a multicenter, prospective, randomized trial. Ann Surg. 2006;244:481–90.

17. Ferri LE, Feldman LS, Stanbridge D, Mayrand S, Stein L, Fried GM. Should laparoscopic paraesophageal hernia repair be abandoned in favor of the open approach? Surg Endosc. 2005;19:4–8.
18. Furnee EJ, Draaisma WA, Simmermacher RK, Stapper G, Broeders IA. Long-term symptomatic outcome and radiologic assessment of laparoscopic hiatal hernia repair. Am J Surg. 2010;199:695–701.
19. Rathore MA, Andrabi SI, Bhatti MI, Najfi SM, McMurray A. Meta analysis of recurrence after laparoscopic repair of paraesophageal hernia. JSLS. 2007;11:456–60.
20. Hashemi M, Peters JH, DeMeester TR, Huprich JE, Quek M, Hagen JA, Crookes PF, Theisen J, DeMeester SR, Sillin LF, Bremner CG. Laparoscopic repair of large type III hiatal hernia: objective follow-up reveals high recurrence rate. J Am Coll Surg. 2000;190:553–61.
21. Edye M, Salky B, Posner A, Fierer A. Sac excision is essential to adequate laparoscopic repair of paraesophageal hernia. Surg Endosc. 1998;12(10):1259–63.
22. Furnee E, Hazebroek E. Mesh in laparoscopic large hiatal hernia repair: a systematic review of the literature. Surg Endosc. 2013;27:3998–4008.
23. Dallemagne B, Kohnen L, Perretta S, Weerts J, Markiewicz S, Jehaes C. Laparoscopic repair of paraesophageal hernia. Long-term follow-up reveals good clinical outcome despite high radiological recurrence rate. Ann Surg. 2011;253(2):291–6.
24. Jones R, Simorov A, Lomelin D, Tadaki C, Oleynikov D. Long-term outcomes of radiologic recurrence after paraesophageal hernia repair with mesh. Surg Endosc. 2015;29(2):425–30.
25. Oelschlager BK, Pellegrini CA, Hunter J, Brunt ML, Soper N, Sheppard BC, Polissar NL, Neradilek MB, Mitsumori L, Rohrmann CA, Swanstrom L. Biologic prosthesis to prevent recurrence after laparoscopic paraesophageal hernia repair: long-term follow-up from a multicenter, prospective, randomized trial. J Am Coll Surg. 2011;213:461–8.
26. Stadlhuber RJ, Sherif AE, Mittal SK, Fitzgibbons Jr RJ, Michael Brunt L, Hunter JG, Demeester TR, Swanstrom LL, Daniel Smith C, Filipi CJ. Mesh complications after prosthetic reinforcement of hiatal closure: a 28-case series. Surg Endosc. 2009;23(6):1219–26.
27. Broeders JA, Roks DJ, Ahmed Ali U, Draaisma WA, Smout AJ, Hazebroek EJ. Laparoscopic anterior versus posterior fundoplication for gastroesophageal reflux disease: systematic review

and meta-analysis of randomized clinical trials. Ann Surg. 2011; 254(1):39–47.

28. Broeders JA, Broeders EA, Watson DI, Devitt PG, Holloway RH, Jamieson GG. Objective outcomes 14 years after laparoscopic anterior 180-degree partial versus Nissen fundoplication: results from a randomized trial. Ann Surg. 2013;258(2):233–9.

29. Mardani J, Lundell L, Engstrom C. Total or posterior partial fundoplication in the treatment of GERD: results of a randomized trial after 2 decades of follow-up. Ann Surg. 2011; 253:875–8.

30. Darling G, Deschamps C. Technical controversies in fundoplication surgery. Thorac Surg Clin. 2005;15(3):437–44.

31. Horvath KD, Swanstrom LL, Jobe BA. The short esophagus: pathophysiology, incidence, presentation, and treatment in the era of laparoscopic antireflux surgery. Ann Surg. 2000;232: 630–40.

32. Mitiek MO, Andrade RS. Giant hiatal hernia. Ann Thorac Surg. 2010;89:S2168–73.

33. Zehetner J, Demeester SR, Ayazi S, Kilday P, Alicuben ET, Demeester TR. Laparoscopic wedge fundectomy for collis gastroplasty creation in patients with a foreshortened esophagus. Ann Surg. 2014;260(6):1030–3.

Chapter 14
Minimally Invasive Treatment of Esophageal Achalasia

Charlotte Rabl and Guilherme M. Campos

Abstract Achalasia is a rare neurodegenerative disease of the esophagus and the lower esophageal sphincter characterized by the inability of the lower esophageal sphincter to relax and by failure of esophageal body peristalsis, most commonly resulting in dysphagia. Current treatment options are directed at palliation of symptoms. Therapies include pharmacological, endoscopic and surgical therapy. Endoscopic dilation was the first line of therapy until the introduction of minimally invasive surgical techniques in the early 1990s that paved the way for the introduction of laparoscopic myotomy. Laparoscopic Heller myotomy with partial fundoplication performed at an experienced center is currently the first line of therapy because it offers a low complication rate, the most durable symptom relief, and the lowest incidence of postoperative gastro-esophageal reflux.

C. Rabl, MD, FACS
Department of Surgery, Paracelsus Medical University Salzburg, Muellner Hauptstrasse 48, Salzburg 5020, Austria
e-mail: c.rabl@salk.at

G.M. Campos, MD, FACS (✉)
Division of Bariatric and Gastrointestinal Surgery, Department of Surgery, Virginia Commonwealth University, 1200 East Broad Street, PO Box 980519, Richmond, Virginia 23298, USA
e-mail: guilherme.campos@vcuhealth.org

H. Chen (ed.), *Illustrative Handbook of General Surgery*, 183
DOI 10.1007/978-3-319-24557-7_14,
© Springer International Publishing Switzerland 2016

Keywords Esophageal achalasia • Heller myotomy • Laparoscopic surgery • Endoscopic dilation • Review

Introduction

Achalasia is a rare neurodegenerative esophageal disease that primarily involves the myoenteric plexus of the esophagus, lower esophageal sphincter (LES), the vagal trunks and the dorsal vagal nucleus without associated synchronous systemic manifestations [1–3]. The expected annual incidence of achalasia is 1 to 3 per 100.000 persons in the Western world [4]. Most commonly it occurs between the ages of 20 to 40 years although this disease has been reported from infancy through the ninth decade of life. Achalasia seems to affect all races and both genders equally [5]. Although the etiology is unclear, Achalasia is the best described primary esophageal motility disorder and has clear clinical, manometric, radiologic, and pathologic correlates [6–9]. Achalasia is characterized by the inability of the LES to relax in response to swallowing and by absent peristaltic contractions in the esophageal body, leading to dysphagia and other associated symptoms.

The goal of therapy is to promote relief of dysphagia while preventing gastro-esophageal reflux (GER). This can be accomplished by reducing both the resting and swallow-induced residual pressures of the LES, but there is no specific therapy for managing the underlying disease process because the pathogenesis for the impaired esophageal peristalsis and LES relaxation is still unknown. None of the treatment options currently available reestablish normal muscle activity of the esophageal body and LES. Instead, all relieve the functional obstruction caused by the failure of LES to relax upon deglutition.

Because achalasia is rare and the spectrum of disease severity is wide, few randomized controlled clinical trials have properly delineated the best treatment strategy. The safety, effectiveness, and durability of current treatment options, including pharmacologic, endoscopic, and surgical therapy, varied widely. Until the late 1980s, endoscopic dilation was considered first-line therapy but after minimally invasive surgical techniques were introduced toward the end of the last century, expert opinion shifted [10, 11]. Currently, most experts agree that first-line therapy should be laparoscopic myotomy with partial fundoplication, performed by an experienced surgeon, and that endoscopic methods should be reserved as an alternative to surgery for patients who are poor surgical candidates, refuse an operation, and possibly patients for whom surgery fails [12–19].

Evaluation and Diagnosis of Achalasia

The evaluation of every patient with foregut complaints starts in the office with a complete and detailed history and physical examination. The definition and classification of the type, duration and severity of symptoms are essential in determining which diagnostic tests to order. The sum of the objective findings obtained with endoscopic, radiologic and physiologic testing will ultimately establish a best diagnosis and then guide therapy.

Symptoms of Achalasia

Patients with achalasia present to the gastroenterologist within a spectrum of disease severity related to the progressive pathological changes affecting the esophagus, such as grades of esophageal dilation, and associated conditions, such as esophageal diverticulum. The most common presenting symptom of achalasia is dysphagia, which can often become so debilitating that profound weight loss occurs. However, the primary symptom of achalasia in up to 40 % of patients may be regurgitation of undigested food, unexplained chest pain, "heartburn" mimicking reflux, cough, or recurrent pneumonia.

The standard current workup of a patient suspected of having esophageal achalasia consists of upper endoscopy, barium esophagram and esophageal manometry [20].

1. Upper endoscopy: Endoscopy can provide insight into the extent and the severity of the disease. It has to be performed in all patients with suspected achalasia to rule out secondary achalasia or pseudoachalasia (strictures, tumors, neurological disorders, among others). In up to 44 % of cases endoscopy may be normal [3].

   The endoscopist should always provide information on the condition of the esophageal mucosa, presence of mechanical lesions, appearance and location of the squamo-columnar junction, the location of the crural impression upon gastroesophageal junction (GEJ) and presence and size of a hiatal hernia. Endoscopy also allows direct sampling of abnormal tissue from the esophagus, GEJ and gastric epithelium.

2. Barium esophagram: The combination of peristaltic failure and non-relaxation of the sphincter causes a functional stasis of ingested material in the esophagus, resulting in dilatation of the atonic esophageal body. Roentgenographic studies will reveal a dilated esophagus with a tapering, beak-like narrowing of the distal end (classic "bird's beak" deformity (Fig. 14.1). There is usually an air fluid level in the esophagus that reflects the degree of resistance imposed by the non-relaxing sphincter and build up of residual food and fluid above the LES. Transit of barium through the LES is slow. As the disease progresses, the esophagus may become massively dilated and subsequently tortuous (megaesophagus or a sigmoid esophagus). In patients with advanced disease the roentgenographic study can show a corkscrew deformity of the esophagus and diverticulum formation.

3. Esophageal manometry: Esophageal manometry is the best method to characterize the motility of the upper esophageal sphincter, esophageal body and the LES, and is currently considered the gold standard method for the diagnosis of achalasia. Nowadays, esophageal manometry catheters have been equipped with high resolution capacity

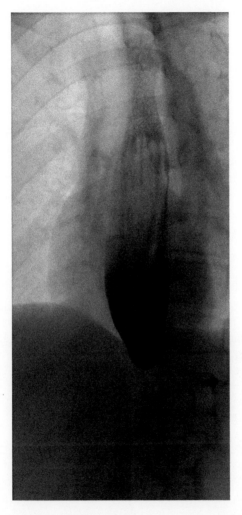

FIGURE 14.1 Barium Swallow Study in a patient with achalasia showing a mildly dilated esophagus and the classic "bird's beak" deformity at the gastro-esophageal junction

and impedance sensors to further correlate esophageal motor function with the bolus clearance capacity. The classic motility pattern includes two requirements: the loss of progressive peristalsis in the body of the esophagus, and failure of complete LES relaxation in response to deglutition [20]. As peristalsis is absent, the contractions recorded at different esophageal levels are simultaneous and usually of low amplitude (Fig. 14.2). Other features that can be seen include elevation of intraluminal esophageal pressure and hypertension of the LES (50 % of the patients) [21]. A subgroup of patients with otherwise typical features consistent with classic achalasia show higher amplitude, active simultaneous contractions of their esophageal body; this manometric pattern has been termed vigorous achalasia [22] and may be manifested as frequently atypical chest pain episodes as by progressive dysphagia.

Treatment of Achalasia

Different treatment options for achalasia are available. Several factors should be taken into consideration when determining the appropriate therapy including patient's age, overall medical condition and the patient's expectations for symptom relief. Treatment options consist of pharmacologic therapy, endoscopic therapy, and surgical therapy.

Pharmacologic Therapy

The goal of pharmacological therapy is to lower the resting LES pressure. Because drug absorption can be impaired due to the poor esophageal emptying, sublingual medications are preferred. Sublingual calcium channel blockers (nifedipine)

FIGURE 14.2 High resolution manometry (**a, c**) with impedance measurement (**b, d**) in a patient with normal esophageal peristalsis and LES relaxation (**a, b**) and in a patient with achalasia (**c, d**). (**a**) Shows a normal peristalsis and LES. (**b**) Shows appropriate clearance of the swallowed bolus. (**c**) Shows absent peristalsis at swallow with no LES relaxation. (**d**) Shows no clearance of the swallowed bolus

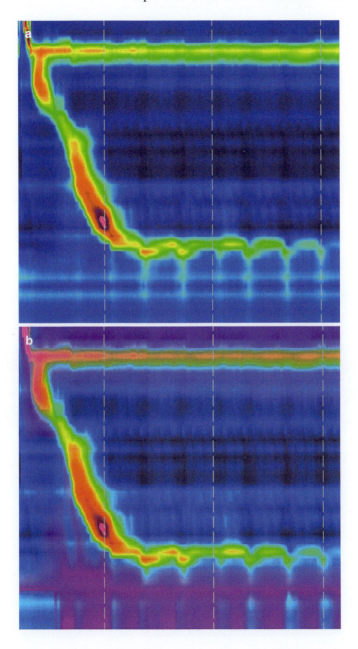

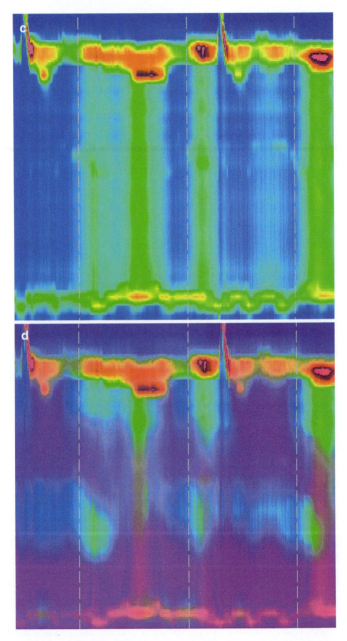

FIGURE 14.2 (continued)

and sublingual isorbide dinitrates (nitrates) are the two most common medications used [23, 24]. Less commonly used medications include anticholinergics, beta-blockers, beta-adrenergic agonists, nitroglycerine, and theophylline [25–28].

Improvement of symptoms is reported in 61 % of patients after use of nifedipine and 70 % of patients after use of nitrates [11]. Manometry showed a transient decrease in LES pressure in 46 % of patients, which was better after nitrate use than after nifedipine use. The time to maximum effect was better after nitrates than after nifedipine (25 vs 9 min), but the duration of effect was longer for nifedipine (40 vs 30 min). The short clinical response and common presence of side effects such as headache, dizziness, tachycardia, hypotension, nausea, and ankle edema were limiting problems with pharmacological therapy. It should be considered only for patients who decline or are considered too frail for endoscopic or surgical treatment options.

Endoscopic Therapy

Endoscopic treatments are directed at relieving the obstruction caused by the LES. Standard endoscopic techniques include endoscopic botulinum toxin injection (EBTI) and endoscopic dilation (ED) of the LES. Recently, a novel totally endoscopic esophagomyotomy technique (peroral endoscopic myotomy, POEM) has been introduced in which the endoscope is advanced into an esophageal submucosa tunnel to then divide the inner circular layers of the LES. Currently, no high quality evidence and enough follow up data exist to recommend POEM as a standard therapeutic option for Achalasia, but there are ongoing clinical research trials [29].

Endoscopic Botulinum Toxin Injection (EBTI)

EBTI decreases tonic and swallow-induced LES pressure by inhibiting acetylcholine release from the inhibitory cholinergic presynaptic nerve innervating the LES [30]. EBTI relieves symptoms in 79 % of patients surveyed up to 1 month after treatment, but the symptom relief declines to 70 % at 3 months, 53 % at 6 months, and 41 % after 12 months [1]. Therefore, almost half (47 %) of the patients undergoing EBTI required repeat injection [1]. Relief of dysphagia was found to be better if a second injection was planned at a 1-month interval after the first, but again, symptoms returned in 66 % of patients at 2 years [31]. Primary failure of EBTI can also be due to antibody formation that causes resistance to the acetylcholine injection in 26 % of patients [32–34]. In addition EBTI leads to fibrosis of the mucosa and muscle layers that could make a myotomy, during a future surgical therapy, more challenging [35, 36].

Endoscopic Dilation (ED)

ED attempts to produce a controlled division of the esophageal muscle while leaving the mucosa intact. The current method of choice for dilation is a controlled pneumatic dilation [11]. A balloon is placed across the LES under direct endoscopic or fluoroscopic visualization. The balloon is inflated for 1–3 min, to a pressure of 300 mmHg (10– 12 psi). To obtain an acceptable therapeutic effect, dilation to a diameter of at least 3.0 up to 4.0 cm must be performed; with the 3.0 cm size being preferred as it has a lower perforation rate [37]. Symptom relief seems to dependent on dilator size, the amount of pressure applied and duration of dilation. ED is a relatively safe procedure and the most serious complication of the currently used methods of ED is perforation of the esophagus, which was seen in 1.6 % of patients in a review of 1,065 patients [1]. A systematic review and meta-analysis showed that symptom relief after ED was obtained in 85 % of patients at 1 month and declined with time to 68 % at 12 months and 58 % at 1.5 years [1]. The need for further procedures after ED was 25 % in this review. In addition to dysphagia recurrence, patients undergoing ED can experience the onset of GER [11].

In summary, ED is consistently more durable than EBTI, but after ED, symptoms recur in 42 % of patients over the time and about 30 % of all of the patients treated with ED require further therapy. In a multicenter randomized controlled study [37] clinical outcomes 1 and 2 years after ED were comparable to laparoscopic Heller myotomy with Dor fundoplication. However, patients with ED needed 2 initial dilations with an interval of 1–3 weeks. During the 2 years follow up 4 % did not had a clinical response to initial dilation and additional 27 % had recurrent symptoms with the need for further dilations. Twenty-nine % of the patients with repeated dilations needed an operation. Prior to any surgical intervention, knowledge of the patient's history of previous endoscopic therapies at the GEJ is important to the surgeon because some experts propose that ED and EBTI lead to fibrosis of the mucosa and muscular layers of the esophagus. Less predictable symptom relief has been reported in patients who have been previously treated with endoscopic therapy [36, 38], which could be due to the greater technical difficulty of doing the operation in these patients.

Peroral Endoscopic Myotomy (POEM)

With this new endoscopic technique (that requires general anesthesia), an esophageal submucosal tunnel through a small opening of the mucosa about 13 cm proximal to the GEJ is created to access the LES and perform a myotomy of the inner circular esophageal muscle LES fibres [29, 39, 40]. Published studies showed good short-term results after POEM with dysphagia remission>80 % at 12 months [39, 41, 42]. However long-term follow up results are still lacking. Furthermore, results from randomized-controlled trials comparing POEM with other endoscopic techniques or laparoscopic myotomy are not available until now. One major problem after POEM seems to be GER, which has been reported to be up to 46 % [43], because an antireflux procedure cannot be performed simultaneously [29].

Surgical Therapy

The first successful surgical myotomy of the lower esophagus and LES was reported in 1913, by the German surgeon Ernest Heller [44]. His original technique used anterior and posterior myotomies extending for 8 cm or more along the distal esophagus and GEJ through a left thoracoabdominal approach. In 1918, the Dutch surgeon Zaaijer [45] described a modification of Heller's original technique to a single, anterior cardiomyotomy that has remained the myotomy of choice until now. Both the transabdominal and transthoracic approach have been used to perform a myotomy since. During the end of the last century there was shift from open surgery in the chest and abdomen towards thoracoscopic and laparoscopic surgery. The first laparoscopic Heller myotomy was described by Shimi et al. in 1991 [46]. Thoracoscopic myotomy is more technically challenging and associated with a lower symptom relief but a higher incidence of postoperative GER, making the laparoscopic operation the preferred approach performed at most experienced centers [1, 11]. Laparoscopic myotomy of the LES has proven over the time to be the approach that consistently produces the most durable symptom relief [1, 47].

Some authors have debated the need to perform an antireflux procedure (ARP) after the myotomy [48–50]. A 2009 systematic review and meta-analysis [1] evaluated the development of postoperative GER and found that adding an ARP after laparoscopic myotomy dramatically decreased the incidence of GER symptoms from 31 % down to 9 % (OR 4.3; 95 % CI 1.9–9.7; P=0.001) without altering the resolution of dysphagia (90 % vs 90 %; OR 1.6; 95 % CI 0.74–3.3; P=0.23). When measured by 24-h pH monitoring, the incidence of GER after laparoscopic myotomy without fundoplication was 42 % vs 15 % after laparoscopic myotomy with fundoplication (OR 4.2; 95 % CI 1.5–12.8; P=0.01). The addition of an ARP seems crucial for satisfactory outcome in the treatment of achalasia, and the addition of a fundoplication does not increase morbidity [11, 51].

Laparoscopic Heller Myotomy

Positioning of the patient and Anesthesia

After general anesthesia is induced, the patient is positioned in modified lithotomy and the operating table in reverse Trendelenburg. The patient should be secured to the operating table and all extremities should be padded. The surgeon stands in between the legs of the patient, the first assistant stands on the left side of the patient, and a static retractor (or a second assistant) holds the camera on the right side of the table. In addition to the standard laparoscopic equipment, we also suggest using two graspers with soft grab, scissors, hook cautery, a needle holder, a babcock clamp, a 30° scope, and a 5-mm ultrasonic Harmonic scalpel (Ethicon Endosurgery, Cincinnati OH).

Port Placement

The operation begins with trocar placement similar to that for any laparoscopic operation taking place at the GEJ [47]. Pneumoperitoneum is established to 12 mmHg. Five laparoscopic ports are utilized (three 5 mm and two 10–12 mm). The camera is placed above the umbilicus, one third of the distance to the xiphoid process. In most patients, placement of the camera in the umbilicus will not allow adequate visualization of the hiatal structures once dissected. Two lateral retracting ports are placed in the right and left anterior axillary lines respectively. The port utilized for the liver retractor can be placed at the surgeon's preference in the sub-xiphoid location or in the right mid abdomen (mid-clavicular line), at or slightly below the camera port. A second retraction port is placed at the level of the umbilicus, in the left anterior axillary line. The surgeons right and left handed trocars are placed in the right and left midclavicular lines, 2–3 inches below the costal margin. Placing the operating trocars on either side of the midline allows triangulation between the camera and the two instruments, avoiding the difficulty associated with the instruments being in direct line with the camera. The falciform ligament hangs low in many patients and provides a barrier around which the left-handed instrument must be manipulated.

Initial Exposure and Dissection

Initial retraction is accomplished with exposure of the esophageal hiatus. A 5 or 10 mm retractor is placed into the sub-xiphoid or right anterior axillary port, and positioned to hold the left lateral segments of the liver towards the anterior abdominal wall. Trauma to the liver should be meticulously avoided, because subsequent bleeding will obscure the field. Mobilization of the left lateral segments by division of the triangular ligament is not necessary. A Babcock clamp is placed into the left anterior axillary port and the stomach retracted toward the patients left foot. This maneuver exposes the esophageal hiatus. An atraumatic clamp should be used, and care taken not to grasp the stomach too vigorously, as gastric perforations can occur. Dissection is typically performed with electrocautery or an ultrasonic dissector. The gastrohepatic ligament is incised to identify and expose the right pillar of the crus. If a replaced left hepatic artery is encountered, it should be preserved. To plan for the extent of the myotomy, the phrenoesophageal membrane is divided and blunt dissection is used to expose the anterior aspect of the abdominal esophagus and the distal portion of the intra-thoracic esophagus. This dissection is started by incising just medial to the right crus and dissecting clockwise in a usually avascular plane in between the diaphragm and the esophagus. The anterior vagus nerve should be identified and protected, when possible, to allow the planned myotomy to be performed underneath it (Fig. 14.3).

Most specialized centers in the United States choose to add a partial fundoplication after the esophageal myotomy is completed to prevent postoperative GER. Technical details of the construction of an anterior or posterior fundoplication (antireflux procedures) are described below. We routinely perform an anterior (Dor) fundoplication; however, some authors advocate a posterior (Toupet) fundoplication [6, 52, 53]. Anterior fundoplication does not require circumferential esophageal dissection thus allowing for a more limited dissection that leaves the natural adhesions between the posterior esophagus and the hiatus intact, which provides an anchor to help keep the GEJ in the proper anatomic location. If a posterior fundoplication is chosen, the posterior surface of the esophagus and esophageal hiatus must be dissected. In a rare case where a large concomitant hiatal hernia is identified a posterior dissection has to be performed always, so that the

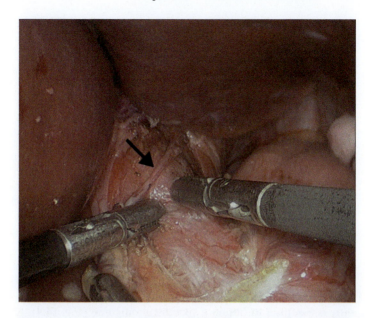

FIGURE 14.3 Dissection of the phrenoesophageal membrane and the right and left pillar of the crus to expose the anterior aspect of the abdominal esophagus and the distal portion of the intrathoracic esophagus. The anterior vagus nerve (*arrow*) should be identified and preserved. Two graspers are used to start the myotomy just above the GEJ (Reprinted with permission from Roll et al. [11])

hernia can be reduced into the abdominal cavity and the crura can be repaired properly.

Mediastinal mobilization of the esophagus should continue until approximately 6 cm of anterior esophagus is accessible for the myotomy. The anterior fat pad covering the GEJ may be removed to facilitate the myotomy and to better identify the GEJ.

Heller Myotomy

After exposure of the distal esophagus and the GEJ, a myotomy is performed to extend proximally for 6 cm above the GEJ onto the esophagus and distally across the gastroesophageal junction for 3 cm onto the stomach, making the total length of the myotomy about 9 cm. A 48 or 52 French bougie may be placed through the patient's mouth and through the GEJ into the stomach to help identify the dissection plane and provide tactile feedback during the dissection. The myotomy is started by separating the external longitudinal esophageal muscle fibers on the anterior distal esophagus above the GEJ (Fig. 14.3). This may be done with scissors, a hook, or by tearing the fibers apart using two graspers. There may be bleeding from small vessels, but this is easily controlled with gentle pressure. Excessive use of electrocautery to control bleeding must be avoided at all times, especially if the dissection has traversed the esophageal circular muscle fibers or adhesions and scarring from previous endoscopic treatment are present. The transection of the circular esophageal muscle fibers and the identification of the blood vessels of the submucosa lead to the recognition of the correct dissection plane. Extension of the myotomy from the GEJ onto 3 cm of the proximal anterior stomach to perform a complete myotomy is essential to obtain a successful outcome (Fig. 14.4). A gastric extension that is too short is one important cause of failure of the myotomy to relieve dysphagia. However, most mucosal perforations occur during the extension of the myotomy from the GEJ onto the stomach, because the identification and separation of the muscle layers from the gastric mucosa is more difficult, where the muscularis becomes thinner and more firmly attached to the submucosa. The surgeon should inspect the myotomy area to identify inadvertent mucosal perforations. If a mucosal perforation is detected it must be closed with absorbable interrupted sutures. After completion of the myotomy, a diagnostic upper endoscopy should be performed to ensure that the myotomy is complete, and to insufflate the stomach with the mucosa under water to evaluate for air bubbles indicating a mucosal perforation.

Antireflux Procedure (Fundoplication)

After the myotomy is completed, an antireflux procedure is performed to prevent postoperative GER by recreating the His angle and keeping the GEJ inside the abdominal cavity.

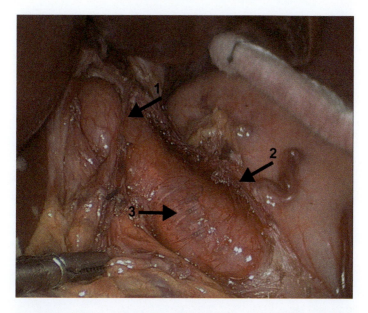

FIGURE 14.4 The myotomy is performed to extend proximally for 6 cm above the GEJ onto the esophagus and distally across the GEJ for 3 cm onto the stomach, making the total length of the myotomy about 9 cm. *Arrow* 1: anterior vagus nerve, *arrow* 2: left edge of the myotomy, *arrow* 3: exposed esophageal submucosa (Reprinted with permission from Roll et al. [11])

A 360° Nissen fundoplication has been used in selected series [51, 54, 55], however, a Nissen fundoplication may hinder esophageal clearance, resulting in progressive postoperative dilatation of the aperistaltic esophagus and recurrent dysphagia. Although a few centers with significant experience in esophageal surgery still advocate a Nissen fundoplication after myotomy [55], most do not recommend it due to reported reoperation rates as high as 29 % [11]. Two partial fundoplications have been used with equipoise, a posterior fundoplication (Toupet fundoplication) and an anterior fundoplication (Dor fundoplication). The theoretical advantages of the Toupet fundoplication are that due to its anatomical configuration, it keeps the edges of the myotomy pulled apart, thus preventing scarring and recurrent dysphagia, and that it can be performed just after the lower esophagus has been pulled downward and straightened, thus improving passage through the cardia and again minimizing postoperative dysphagia [56]. The drawbacks of the Toupet fundoplication are the need for circumferential dissection of the GEJ and the possibility that diverticula may develop at the site of the myotomy years after surgery because the fundoplication does not cover the myotomy site [57]. Proponents of the Dor fundoplication argue that the procedure is faster because the posterior esophageal attachments may be left in place [56]. Another advantage is that a properly constructed Dor fundoplication can prevent post-operative reapproximation of the myotomy [58]. Furthermore, covering the myotomy with the fundoplication may seal inadvertent mucosal injury and prevent future development of diverticulae at the site of the myotomy.

Dor Fundoplication

The creation of the fundoplication begins with a complete mobilization of the fundus of the stomach, including division of the short gastric vessels all the way to the His angle. This can be accomplished by using a 5-mm ultrasonic Harmonic scalpel (Ethicon Endosurgery, Cincinnati, OH) and allows the proper creation of the anterior 180° Dor fundoplication. Two vertical rows of sutures secure the gastric fundus to the left and right edges of the myotomy to create the fundoplication. The first row is on the left and consists of about four stitches. Initially, the inferior edge of the left side of the esophageal myotomy is sutured to the medial gastric fundus. Then, a stitch is placed from a superior portion of the gastric fundus to the left diaphragmatic crus and then the left side of the myotomy about 2 to 3 cm cephalad of the first suture (Fig. 14.5). Two to 3 cm cephalad to the previous suture, a suture secures the left side of the myotomy to the gastric fundus without incorporating the crus. Attention to the geometric arrangement of the fundus produced during this step is important because the reconstructions of the His angle, in addition to having an intra-abdominal GEJ, are what provide

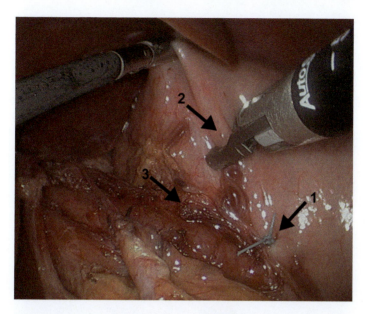

FIGURE 14.5 Creation of the Dor fundoplication. The first stitch sutures the inferior edge of the left side of the esophageal myotomy to the medial gastric fundus (*arrow* 1). The second stitch is placed from a superior portion of the gastric fundus (*arrow* 2) to the left diaphragmatic crus (not shown) and then the left side of the myotomy (*arrow* 3) about 2 to 3 cm above the first suture (Reprinted with permission from Roll et al. [11])

the major antireflux barriers. An additional suture, again on the left and cephalad to the last, my be placed and brings the fundus to the left edge of the myotomy, this time just below the myotomy apex. A suture line is then created down the right edge of the myotomy. The first suture secures the superior right edge of the myotomy to a bite of gastric fundus. The suture line is continued caudally down the right myotomy edge. The second suture incorporates the right diaphragmatic crus to the fundus and the myotomy edge. Two final sutures on the right side bring the fundus to the inferior edge of the myotomy, and the exposed mucosal surface should now be completely covered by the fundus at this point. One or two

202 C. Rabl and G.M. Campos

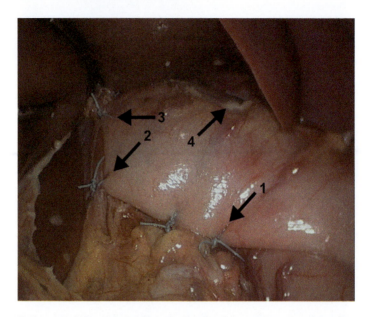

FIGURE 14.6 Completed Dor fundoplication. *Arrows* 1 and 2 point to the suture line that anchors the fundoplication to the right edge of the myotomy. *Arrow* 2 incorporates the fundus, the right crus to the right edge of the myotomy. *Arrow* 3 shows the suture that secures the fundoplication to the diaphragm. *Arrow* 4 points to the divided short gastric vessels (Reprinted with permission from Roll et al. [11])

sutures should then be placed to secure the superior aspect of the fundus to the anterior esophageal hiatus to prevent anterior herniation of the fundoplication into the chest (Fig. 14.6).

Toupet Fundoplication

When planning to perform a Toupet fundoplication a complete circumferential dissection of the esophagus with creation of a posterior window has to be done in advance. After mobilization of the greater curvature with division of the short gastric vessels the posterior part of the gastric fundus is passed behind the esophagus to the right and is fixed with 3 sutures to the right crus. The wrap is then fixed to the anterior wall of the esophagus including the edges of the myotomy by 3 sutures on both sides to form a posterior wrap of about 270°.

Finishing the Operation

The operation field is explored for residual bleeding. The liver retractor and ports are removed under direct vision to evaluate for bleeding. Then, all port sites are infiltrated under direct vision with bupivacaine as local anesthetic. The fascia of the 10 mm ports is closed with an Endoclose device to avoid hernias. The patient's abdomen is deflated and all incisions are closed.

Treatment of Advanced Stages of Achalasia

Treatment of advanced stages of achalasia is controversial when the esophagus has dilated severely and its course in the chest becomes sigmoidal. Some authors have proposed that the gross pathology of the esophagus is so advanced that it will not respond to myotomy and fundoplication and therefore requires esophageal resection. However, recent studies suggest that these patients may have good outcomes after myotomy and fundoplication, although studies with long-term follow-up are still lacking [59, 60]. Esophagectomy may need to be contemplated in selected cases.

Post-operative Care

Oral intake can be initiated immediately postoperative in most patients. We start with clear liquids on the operation day and rapidly increase to a pureed and then soft diet, which should be continued for 2–3 weeks. Most patients are discharged on postoperative day 1.

Complications

Selecting the proper treatment for a given patient requires analysis of the rates of complications of all of the treatment options. With pneumatic balloon dilation, currently the accepted standard, the perforation rate is 1.6 % [1]. Systematic review of the results of 3,086 patients who had laparoscopic myotomy found that complications were reported in 6 % and death in 0.1 % [1]. Intraoperative perforation of the esophageal or gastric mucosa was reported in about 7 % [1]. Most of those injuries were repaired during the index operation, and only 0.7 % experienced symptoms from perforation postoperatively. When overall complication rates reported after laparoscopic myotomy are compared with ED, differences are possibly related to an innate more invasive nature of the laparoscopic surgery, but differences in baseline patient characteristics and severity of the disease likely have an impact on the results of each method reported. A 2001 decision analysis for the treatment of achalasia evaluated four strategies for the initial management of achalasia: (1) laparoscopic Heller myotomy and partial fundoplication, (2) pneumatic dilatation, (3) botulinum toxin injection, and (4) thoracoscopic Heller myotomy [61]. According to the analysis, laparoscopic myotomy with fundoplication was the proper first treatment strategy unless the patient's risk of operative mortality was higher than 0.7 %.

Persistent postoperative dysphagia after laparoscopic myotomy with fundoplication can be the result of the following technical factors: (1) the myotomy is too short distally, (2) the myotomy is too short proximally, or (3) the fundoplication has been constructed incorrectly. Some patients may develop recurrent dysphagia after a symptom-free interval. This type of failure may be due to GER and the development of peptic stricture, healing, and fibrosis of the distal portion of the myotomy [11].

References

1. Campos GM, Vittinghoff E, Rabl C, et al. Endoscopic and surgical treatments for achalasia: a systematic review and meta-analysis. Ann Surg. 2009;249(1):45–57.

2. Nguyen NQ, Holloway RH. Recent developments in esophageal motor disorders. Curr Opin Gastroenterol. 2005;21(4):478–84.

3. Howard PJ, Maher L, Pryde A, Cameron EW, Heading RC. Five year prospective study of the incidence, clinical features, and diagnosis of achalasia in Edinburgh. Gut. 1992;33(8):1011–5.

4. Ruffato A, Mattioli S, Lugaresi ML, D'Ovidio F, Antonacci F, Di Simone MP. Long-term results after Heller-Dor operation for oesophageal achalasia. Eur J Cardiothorac Surg. 2006;29(6):914–9.

5. O'Neill OM, Johnston BT, Coleman HG. Achalasia: a review of clinical diagnosis, epidemiology, treatment and outcomes. World J Gastroenterol. 2013;19(35):5806–12.

6. Balaji NS, Peters JH. Minimally invasive surgery for esophageal motility disorders. Surg Clin North Am. 2002;82(4):763–82.

7. Kraichely RE, Farrugia G. Achalasia: physiology and etiopathogenesis. Dis Esophagus. 2006;19(4):213–23.

8. Gockel I, Bohl JR, Junginger T. Achalasia: new insights in pathogenesis. Am J Gastroenterol. 2006;101(1):202–3.

9. Dogan I, Mittal RK. Esophageal motor disorders: recent advances. Curr Opin Gastroenterol. 2006;22(4):417–22.

10. Bennett JR, Hendrix TR. Treatment of achalasia with pneumatic dilatation. Mod Treat. 1970;7(6):1217–28.

11. Roll GR, Rabl C, Ciovica R, Peeva S, Campos GM. A controversy that has been tough to swallow: is the treatment of achalasia now digested? J Gastrointest Surg. 2010;14 Suppl 1:S33–45.

12. Bonatti H, Hinder RA, Klocker J, et al. Long-term results of laparoscopic Heller myotomy with partial fundoplication for the treatment of achalasia. Am J Surg. 2005;190(6):874–8.

13. Rosemurgy A, Villadolid D, Thometz D, et al. Laparoscopic Heller myotomy provides durable relief from achalasia and salvages failures after botox or dilation. Ann Surg. 2005;241(5): 725–33; discussion 33–5.

14. Frantzides CT, Moore RE, Carlson MA, et al. Minimally invasive surgery for achalasia: a 10-year experience. J Gastrointest Surg. 2004;8(1):18–23.

15. Zaninotto G, Costantini M, Molena D, et al. Treatment of esophageal achalasia with laparoscopic Heller myotomy and Dor partial anterior fundoplication: prospective evaluation of 100 consecutive patients. J Gastrointest Surg. 2000;4(3):282–9.

16. Oelschlager BK, Chang L, Pellegrini CA. Improved outcome after extended gastric myotomy for achalasia. Arch Surg. 2003;138(5):490–5; discussion 5–7.

17. Patti MG, Fisichella PM, Perretta S, et al. Impact of minimally invasive surgery on the treatment of esophageal achalasia: a

decade of change. J Am Coll Surg. 2003;196(5):698–703; discussion –5.

18. Deb S, Deschamps C, Allen MS, et al. Laparoscopic esophageal myotomy for achalasia: factors affecting functional results. Ann Thorac Surg. 2005;80(4):1191–4; discussion 4–5.

19. Ackroyd R, Watson DI, Devitt PG, Jamieson GG. Laparoscopic cardiomyotomy and anterior partial fundoplication for achalasia. Surg Endosc. 2001;15(7):683–6.

20. Boeckxstaens GE, Zaninotto G, Richter JE. Achalasia. Lancet. 2014;383(9911):83–93.

21. Pandolfino JE, Kahrilas PJ. AGA technical review on the clinical use of esophageal manometry. Gastroenterology. 2005;128(1): 209–24.

22. Camacho-Lobato L, Katz PO, Eveland J, Vela M, Castell DO. Vigorous achalasia: original description requires minor change. J Clin Gastroenterol. 2001;33(5):375–7.

23. Hoogerwerf WA, Pasricha PJ. Pharmacologic therapy in treating achalasia. Gastrointest Endosc Clin N Am. 2001;11(2): 311–24, vii.

24. Wen ZH, Gardener E, Wang YP. Nitrates for achalasia. Cochrane Database Syst Rev. 2004;1, CD002299.

25. Wong RK, Maydonovitch C, Garcia JE, Johnson LF, Castell DO. The effect of terbutaline sulfate, nitroglycerin, and aminophylline on lower esophageal sphincter pressure and radionuclide esophageal emptying in patients with achalasia. J Clin Gastroenterol. 1987;9(4):386–9.

26. DiMarino Jr AJ, Cohen S. Effect of an oral beta2-adrenergic agonist on lower esophageal sphincter pressure in normals and in patients with achalasia. Dig Dis Sci. 1982;27(12):1063–6.

27. Marzio L, Grossi L, DeLaurentiis MF, Cennamo L, Lapenna D, Cuccurullo F. Effect of cimetropium bromide on esophageal motility and transit in patients affected by primary achalasia. Dig Dis Sci. 1994;39(7):1389–94.

28. Penagini R, Bartesaghi B, Negri G, Bianchi PA. Effect of loperamide on lower oesophageal sphincter pressure in idiopathic achalasia. Scand J Gastroenterol. 1994;29(12):1057–60.

29. Torres-Villalobos G, Martin-Del-Campo LA. Surgical treatment for achalasia of the esophagus: laparoscopic heller myotomy. Gastroenterol Res Pract. 2013;2013:708327.

30. Roberts KE, Duffy AJ, Bell RL. Controversies in the treatment of gastroesophageal reflux and achalasia. World J Gastroenterol. 2006;12(20):3155–61.

31. Annese V, Bassotti G, Coccia G, et al. A multicentre randomised study of intrasphincteric botulinum toxin in patients with oesophageal achalasia. GISMAD Achalasia Study Group Gut. 2000;46(5):597–600.
32. Pasricha PJ, Rai R, Ravich WJ, Hendrix TR, Kalloo AN. Botulinum toxin for achalasia: long-term outcome and predictors of response. Gastroenterology. 1996;110(5):1410–5.
33. Fishman VM, Parkman HP, Schiano TD, et al. Symptomatic improvement in achalasia after botulinum toxin injection of the lower esophageal sphincter. Am J Gastroenterol. 1996;91(9):1724–30.
34. Annese V, Basciani M, Perri F, et al. Controlled trial of botulinum toxin injection versus placebo and pneumatic dilation in achalasia. Gastroenterology. 1996;111(6):1418–24.
35. Morino M, Rebecchi F, Festa V, Garrone C. Preoperative pneumatic dilatation represents a risk factor for laparoscopic Heller myotomy. Surg Endosc. 1997;11(4):359–61.
36. Portale G, Costantini M, Rizzetto C, et al. Long-term outcome of laparoscopic Heller-Dor surgery for esophageal achalasia: possible detrimental role of previous endoscopic treatment. J Gastrointest Surg. 2005;9(9):1332–9.
37. Boeckxstaens GE, Annese V, des Varannes SB, et al. Pneumatic dilation versus laparoscopic Heller's myotomy for idiopathic achalasia. N Engl J Med. 2011;364(19):1807–16.
38. Smith CD, Stival A, Howell DL, Swafford V. Endoscopic therapy for achalasia before Heller myotomy results in worse outcomes than heller myotomy alone. Ann Surg. 2006;243(5):579–84; discussion 84–6.
39. Chuah SK, Chiu CH, Tai WC, et al. Current status in the treatment options for esophageal achalasia. World J Gastroenterol. 2013;19(33):5421–9.
40. Bello B, Herbella FA, Patti MG. Evolution of the minimally invasive treatment of esophageal achalasia. World J Surg. 2011;35(7):1442–6.
41. Von Renteln D, Fuchs KH, Fockens P, et al. Peroral endoscopic myotomy for the treatment of achalasia: an international prospective multicenter study. Gastroenterology. 2013;145(2), e1–3.
42. Inoue H, Minami H, Kobayashi Y, et al. Peroral endoscopic myotomy (POEM) for esophageal achalasia. Endoscopy. 2010;42(4):265–71.
43. Swanstrom LL, Kurian A, Dunst CM, Sharata A, Bhayani N, Rieder E. Long-term outcomes of an endoscopic myotomy for achalasia: the POEM procedure. Ann Surg. 2012;256(4):659–67.

44. Heller E. Extramukose Cardiaplastik beim chronischen Cardiospasmus mit Dilatation des Osophagus. Mitt Grenzgeb Med Chir. 1914;27:141–9.
45. Zaaijer JH. Cardiospasm in the aged. Ann Surg. 1923;77(5): 615–7.
46. Shimi S, Nathanson LK, Cuschieri A. Laparoscopic cardiomyotomy for achalasia. J R Coll Surg Edinb. 1991;36(3):152–4.
47. Campos G, Ciovica R, Takata M. Laparoscopic myotomie. Oper Tech Gen Surg. 2006;8:161–9.
48. Lyass S, Thoman D, Steiner JP, Phillips E. Current status of an antireflux procedure in laparoscopic Heller myotomy. Surg Endosc. 2003;17(4):554–8.
49. Avtan L, Avci C, Guvenc H, Igci A, Ozmen V. Laparoscopic myotomy for oesophageal achalasia–adding an antireflux procedure is not always necessary. Int J Clin Pract. 2005;59(1):35–8.
50. Ramacciato G, D'Angelo FA, Aurello P, et al. Laparoscopic Heller myotomy with or without partial fundoplication: a matter of debate. World J Gastroenterol. 2005;11(10):1558–61.
51. Rebecchi F, Giaccone C, Farinella E, Campaci R, Morino M. Randomized controlled trial of laparoscopic Heller myotomy plus Dor fundoplication versus Nissen fundoplication for achalasia: long-term results. Ann Surg. 2008;248(6):1023–30.
52. Clemente G. The choice of fundoplication after myotomy for achalasia. Arch Surg. 2006;141(6):612, author reply –3.
53. Iqbal A, Haider M, Desai K, et al. Technique and follow-up of minimally invasive Heller myotomy for achalasia. Surg Endosc. 2006;20(3):394–401.
54. Topart P, Deschamps C, Taillefer R, Duranceau A. Long-term effect of total fundoplication on the myotomized esophagus. Ann Thorac Surg. 1992;54(6):1046–51; discussion 51–2.
55. Falkenback D, Johansson J, Oberg S, et al. Heller's esophagomyotomy with or without a 360 degrees floppy Nissen fundoplication for achalasia. Long-term results from a prospective randomized study. Dis Esophagus. 2003;16(4):284–90.
56. Perrone JM, Frisella MM, Desai KM, Soper NJ. Results of laparoscopic Heller-Toupet operation for achalasia. Surg Endosc. 2004;18(11):1565–71.
57. Dobashi Y, Goseki N, Inutake Y, Kawano T, Endou M, Nemoto T. Giant epiphrenic diverticulum with achalasia occurring 20 years after Heller's operation. J Gastroenterol. 1996;31(6):844–7.
58. Raiser F, Perdikis G, Hinder RA, et al. Heller myotomy via minimal-access surgery. An evaluation of antireflux procedures. Arch Surg. 1996;131(6):593–7; discussion 7–8.

59. Mineo TC, Pompeo E. Long-term outcome of Heller myotomy in achalasic sigmoid esophagus. J Thorac Cardiovasc Surg. 2004;128(3):402–7.
60. Sweet MP, Nipomnick I, Gasper WJ, et al. The outcome of laparoscopic Heller myotomy for achalasia is not influenced by the degree of esophageal dilatation. J Gastrointest Surg. 2008;12(1):159–65.
61. Urbach DR, Hansen PD, Khajanchee YS, Swanstrom LL. A decision analysis of the optimal initial approach to achalasia: laparoscopic Heller myotomy with partial fundoplication, thoracoscopic Heller myotomy, pneumatic dilatation, or botulinum toxin injection. J Gastrointest Surg. 2001;5(2):192–205.

Chapter 15
Bariatric Surgery

**Alain Elian, Charlotte Rabl, Jad Khoraki,
and Guilherme M. Campos**

Abstract Obesity is defined as a body mass index (BMI: weight in kilograms divided by height in meters squared) > 30 kg/m^2. Patients qualify for bariatric surgery with a BMI of 35 kg/m^2 or greater with associated obesity-related comorbid conditions or with a BMI of 40 kg/m^2 or greater. Obesity is associated with increasing rates of a large number of comorbid conditions including type 2 diabetes, obstructive sleep apnea, hypertension, as well as

A. Elian, MD • J. Khoraki, MD
Department of Surgery, University of Wisconsin,
University of Wisconsin School of Medicine and Public Health,
600 Highland Avenue, K4/730 CSC, Madison,
WI 53792-7375, USA

C. Rabl, MD, FACS
Department of Surgery, Paracelsus Medical University,
Salzburg, Austria

G.M. Campos, MD, FACS (✉)
Division of Bariatric and Gastrointestinal Surgery,
Department of Surgery, Virginia Commonwealth University,
1200 East Broad Street, PO Box 980519 Richmond,
Virginia 23298, USA
e-mail: guilherme.campos@vcuhealth.org

H. Chen (ed.), *Illustrative Handbook of General Surgery*,
DOI 10.1007/978-3-319-24557-7_15,
© Springer International Publishing Switzerland 2016

a variety of malignancies including breast, endometrial, and prostate cancer, among others. The current and most commonly used surgical techniques to treat morbid obesity includes procedures designed to restrict gastric capacity (restrictive procedures) such as sleeve gastrectomy and adjustable gastric banding and procedures that combine reducing gastric capacity to different degrees of diversion of food bolus contact with the duodenum and the small bowel (malabsorptive component), such as Roux-en-Y gastric bypass and biliopancreatic diversion with or without duodenal switch (BPD and BPD-DS). The introduction of laparoscopic techniques has led to appreciable decreases in perioperative morbidity while maintaining excellent long-term outcomes. Bariatric surgery provides major and sustained weight loss in most patients, while it improves, cures, or markedly lowers incidence rates of obesity-associated diseases and reduces overall mortality. This chapter describes in detail the two most common bariatric surgical techniques currently in use in the United States: the laparoscopic Roux-en-Y gastric bypass and the laparoscopic sleeve gastrectomy.

Keywords   Obesity • Comorbid conditions • Type 2 diabetes • Apnea • Hypertension • Gastric capacity • Restrictive procedures • Sleeve gastrectomy • Adjustable gastric banding • Malabsorptive component • Biliopancreatic diversion • Roux-en-Y gastric bypass

Introduction

Over the past 40 years there has been a dramatic increase in the rates of obesity in the United States and worldwide and nowadays obesity affects 500 million people worldwide [1]. According to the Center for Diseases Control and Prevention, approximately 35.7 % of US adults and 17 % of children and adolescents ages 2–19 years are obese (body mass index,

TABLE 15.1 Categories of weight

Category	BMI (kg/m^2)
Underweight	<18.5
Normal weight	18.5–24.9
Overweight	25–29.9
Obesity class 1	30–34.9
Obesity class 2	35–39.9
Extreme (severe) obesity class 3	≥40

weight in kilograms divided by height in meters squared; BMI>30 kg/m^2) [2]. In 2005, obesity was responsible for approximately 216,000 deaths in the United States, making it the third most common cause of preventable death behind smoking and hypertension [3]. Additionally, the World Health Organization estimates that the cost of obesity care accounts for 2–7 % of total health care costs worldwide [4]. In the United States, the medical cost of obesity in 2008 was estimated at \$147 billion dollars and is likely to be higher today [5].

Obesity is currently defined as BMI >30 kg/m^2, whereas a BMI>40 kg/m^2 is categorized as extreme (severe) obesity (Table 15.1). Though BMI is the most common marker used to determine obesity, it does have significant limitations. BMI reflects both fat and lean body mass and does not identify the distribution of body fat and/or metabolic active adiposity [6]. In other words, BMI will overestimate obesity in people with a high percentage of lean body mass or muscle mass, such as bodybuilders or athletes. Similarly, BMI will underestimate obesity in patients with a lower percentage of lean body mass such as individuals who have complications of their obesity at lower levels of BMI with preferential fat accumulation in the abdominal region. Other measures of obesity, which are more specific for intra-abdominal adiposity, such as the waist circumference, waist-hip ratio, waist-height ratio and imaging studies, will likely play a significant role in the diagnosis, stratification and classification of obesity in the near future [7].

Obesity is a multifactorial disease with important societal and public health implications. Although the fundamental mechanism is an imbalance between caloric intake and energy expenditure, there is physiologic, biochemical and genetic evidence that obesity and severe obesity are not simple disorders of willpower. In addition, several factors have contributed to the observed increasing rates of obesity over the last 40 years: major changes in the availability, composition, preservation methods and cost of available food products in the United States and worldwide, urbanization, and other changes in modern life style. Important examples are the increase in consumption of sugar, high-fructose corn syrup, fats, and consumption of grain-fed over grass-fed livestock meats during recent decades [8, 9]. Other factors that add to the complexity of the matter include the United States government-policy on farm subsidies, the marketplace involving food manufacturers, revenues from beverage and processed foods, among many others. The low cost of government-subsidized commodities like corn and soybeans, make sugars and fats some of the cheapest food substances to produce. At the same time, prices for fruits and vegetables, grown with relatively little government support, have risen nearly 40 % in the past 20 years [10].

Obesity is associated with severe metabolic disorders, poor quality of life and decrease in life span [11]. While the association between obesity and type II diabetes, hypertension, hypercholesterolemia, and obstructive sleep apnea are well established, many other medical, psychiatric, and oncologic disorders are closely associated with obesity (Table 15.2). The comorbidities associated with obesity can have a massive impact on the overall health and psychological well-being of patients. Most of these comorbidities will correct to some degree with weight loss [12, 13].

While societal changes and treatment strategies aimed at prevention of obesity are essential to stem the rising rates of obesity, treatment for the millions of individuals with established obesity and severe obesity are essential. For individuals with severe obesity, non-surgical treatment modalities have high rates of failure and bariatric surgery should be offered as a therapeutic option. Bariatric surgery is currently

TABLE 15.2 Obesity associated co-morbidities

Cardiovascular	Hypercholesterolemia Hypertension Cardiomyopathy
Pulmonary	Obstructive sleep apnea Obesity hypoventilation syndrome Pickwickian syndrome Asthma
Gastrointestinal	Non-alcoholic steatohepatitis Cholelithiasis Gastroesophageal reflux disease
Endocrine	Type II diabetes mellitus
Orthopedic	Knee arthropathy Low back pain Weight bearing joint pain
Psychologic	Depression Anxiety
Genitourinary	Stress incontinence Polycystic ovarian syndrome Infertility Gestational diabetes Poor maternal and fetal outcomes
Oncologic	Endometrial cancer Breast cancer Prostate cancer Colorectal cancer Esophageal cancer Hepatocellular carcinoma Ovarian cancer

the most effective treatment for severe obesity and has been shown to be cost-effective at approximately $18,000.00 per Quality Adjusted Life Year (QALY) [14]. When the operation is carried out in high-volume centers by expert surgeons, it is associated with a low risk of peri-operative and long-term complications [15], major and sustained weight loss in most patients [16], improvements in or cure of obesity associated

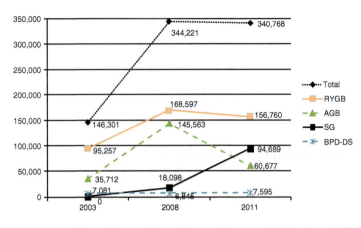

FIGURE 15.1 Trends in numbers of procedures worldwide from 2003 to 2008 to 2011 (Adapted from Buchwald and Oien [1]). *RYGB* Roux-en-Y gastric bypass, *AGB* adjustable gastric band, *SG* sleeve gastrectomy, *BPD-DS* biliopancreatic bypass-duodenal switch

diseases including type 2 diabetes [17], a better quality of life [18] and increased life expectancy resulting from fewer cardiovascular and cancer- related deaths [19, 20].

Historically, there were a number of surgical procedures performed for the treatment of obesity. Many of these procedures, like jejunoileal bypass, were associated with high rates of long-term complications and treatment failure and are thus no longer performed. Others, such as silicone ring gastroplasty, horizontal gastric bypass and vertical banded gastroplasty are seldom performed nowadays. They have fallen out of favor due to high rates of weight recidivism and/or the development of more standardized procedures that can be done using minimally invasive techniques. In the early 1990s roughly only 20,000 bariatric procedures were performed annually in the United States [21]. This number increased to approximately 180,000 by 2006 and continues to climb slowly [21]. A worldwide survey [1] shows that the total global number of bariatric procedures increased from 146,301 in 2003 to 340,768 in 2011 (Fig. 15.1). Many factors have led to this dramatic increase in the utilization of bariatric surgery in the

United States, and include the introduction of laparoscopic minimally invasive techniques, the increasing rates of obesity, the recognition of obesity as a health hazard, the poor outcomes with behavioral and medical management of obesity and the reproducible good outcomes with bariatric surgery in high volume centers [22]. However, weight loss results vary significantly with the different surgical techniques in practice, and the mechanisms promoting weight loss after bariatric surgery are still under scrutiny.

Nowadays, two of the most common performed procedures for the treatment of obesity worldwide are Roux-en-Y gastric bypass (RYGB) and sleeve gastrectomy (SG). A review of the techniques and outcomes of these procedures will be described in this chapter.

Indications for Bariatric Surgery

A decision favoring operative treatment must consider the potential benefits and risks of general anesthesia and an abdominal operation. Assessment of a patient's readiness for operation is a clinical judgment that should be made by a surgeon experienced in the operative management of obese patients in conjunction with other health allied professionals with expertise in the evaluation and management of obesity, such as a mental health care professional and a dietician.

In 1991, the National Institutes of Health (NIH) convened a panel of experts from a variety of specialties to review what were then the current data on the treatment of obesity in order to define a patient population that would most benefit from bariatric surgery. The NIH consensus criteria stated that in order to qualify for surgery, patients must have a BMI >40 kg/m^2 or a BMI of 35–39.9 kg/m^2 with specific obesity-associated comorbid conditions such as severe sleep apnea, type 2 diabetes mellitus (T2DM), or hypertension [23]. They also recommended that patients must be well-informed, self-motivated and of acceptable operative risk. Additionally, they must have failed previous non-surgical treatment options, which include integrated diet, exercise, behavioral modification and psychological support [23]. These criteria were adopted by the Centers for Medicare and Medicaid Services and eventually by most private insurance companies, and they remain to date the accepted indications for operative treatment.

Age alone is no longer a contraindication to operative treatment if a patient has comorbidities that would benefit from sustained weight reduction. Bariatric surgery in adolescents is still considered experimental, and should be done only in specialized medical centers under the supervision of an Institutional Review Board.

While outcomes following bariatric surgery are superior to all other forms of obesity treatment, bariatric procedures may fail over the long term if there is no significant patient motivation to change lifestyle. In addition, it is recommended that bariatric surgical programs should include a multi-disciplinary team for patient evaluation and a structured pathway for pre- and post-operative counseling and medical evaluation. Team members should include bariatric surgeons, health pyschologists, nutritionists, and exercise physiologists. Patients should be advised and agree (1) to comply with lifestyle changes; (2) adhere to nutritional supplement prescriptions; (3) comply with eating behavior modifications; and (4) participate in long-term monitoring and follow-up evaluation.

Laparoscopic Roux-en-Y Gastric Bypass (RYGB)

RYGB was initially described by Drs. Mason and Ito at the University of Iowa in 1969 [24]. Many individuals contributed to the introduction and standardization of laparoscopic minimally invasive techniques. Noteworthy was the work of Dr. Allan Wittgrove with the publication of the first series of laparoscopic RYGB for morbid obesity in 1994 [25]. Since then, most bariatric procedures have been performed utilizing minimally invasive techniques with similar weight loss and resolution of obesity associated disease outcomes [18], but significant decreases in morbidity compared to open bariatric procedures [15].

RYGB combines restriction caused by a small gastric pouch with several other physiologic changes caused by the Roux-en-Y anatomy, because RYGB prevents contact of the food bolus with most of the stomach and the duodenum while allowing for early delivery to the proximal jejunum. Caloric restriction with RYGB leads to negative energy balance and different degrees of weight loss and decreases in total fat and lean body mass and fat in the liver, visceral, and peripheral tissues [12, 26]. These changes are also associated with a decrease in hepatic glucose production and an increase in insulin sensitivity in the liver, muscle, and adipose tissue [27]. RYGB is also known to promote postprandial changes in many gastrointestinal (e.g., ghrelin, glucagon-like-peptide 1, glucose-dependent insulinotropic polypeptide, peptide YY) and pancreatic (insulin, glucagon, pancreatic polypeptide) hormone levels [27–29]. These hormones affect gastric emptying, glucose regulatory mechanisms, central nervous system hunger, and satiety mechanisms [30] in addition to changes in diet induced thermogenesis [31], bile acid metabolism [32] and gut microbiota composition [33]. It has been recently suggested that persons undergoing RYGB may also have increases in weight-adjusted resting energy expenditure after substantial weight loss has occurred [34, 35], a factor that might support the sustained weight loss after RYGB.

Operative Technique of Laparoscopic RYGB

Positioning and Anesthesia

Patients undergoing laparoscopic RYGB are at high risk for deep venous thromboembolism (DVT) and pulmonary embolism. DVT prophylaxis with subcutaneous heparin (unfractionated or low molecular weight heparin) 30 min prior to the induction of anesthesia should be the standard in all cases. Lower extremity sequential compression devices should also be on and operational prior to induction. Proper patient positioning on an appropriate table is critical to avoid injuries. Bariatric patients may be at higher risk for brachial plexus injuries, especially with prolonged cases. Arms should be padded and carefully secured. Arms should be flexed anteriorly when out at the sides on wedges to prevent brachial plexus stretch. Steep reverse Trendelenburg during certain phases of laparoscopic RYGB can be extremely helpful for exposure and the use of a foot board minimizes the chance of a patient sliding off the table. An anesthesia team that is experienced and comfortable intubating extremely obese patients with difficult airways using a variety of techniques is critical. We routinely administer a dexmedetomidine infusion (Precedex, Hospira, Lake Forest, IL) beginning 30 min before the anticipated completion of the procedure and in the recovery room. Dexmedetomidine is an alpha-2 receptor agonist with sedative and analgesic sparing properties. We have found that patients who receive this infusion require less narcotic pain medication for pain control after surgery and are discharged to home sooner following laparoscopic gastric bypass [36].

Description of Procedure

The technique for laparoscopic RYGB varies from center to center. The most common variations relate to the position of the alimentary limb (Roux-limb) and the technique used to create the gastrojejunostomy. The alimentary limb can be placed anterior to both the colon and the gastric remnant (antecolic), posterior to the colon and anterior to the gastric remnant (retrocolic-antegastric), or posterior to both (retrocolic-retrogastric). Most centers in the US now prefer the antecolic approach; however a retrocolic route maybe needed in selected patients to allow for the gastrojejunostomy to be done without tension. Using the retrocolic approach routinely is an option, but that approach creates an additional space for an internal hernia and has been associated with increased risk of internal hernias [37]. The gastrojejunostomy is most often constructed using surgical staplers (either circular staplers or linear staplers) or using hand-sewn techniques with sutures. There are advantages and disadvantages to each technique, and experienced surgical teams can

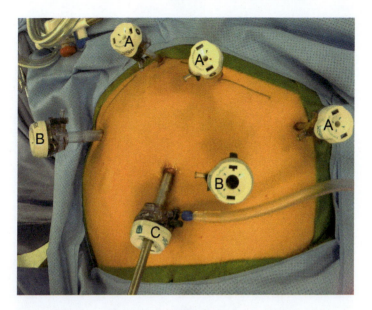

FIGURE 15.2 Ports placement for laparoscopic gastric bypass (*A* 5 mm trocar, *B* 12 mm trocar, *C* 11 mm trocar)

achieve good and safe outcomes in a timely manner with all of these methods. Our standard technique involves the antecolic alimentary limb and a circular stapler gastrojejunostomy. For the circular stapler gastrojejunostomy the stapler anvil maybe 21 or 25 mm and passed either using a transgastric or trans-oral technique.

1. Port placement

We employ a six port technique for laparoscopic RYGB. Initial abdominal access is usually obtained using a direct trocar insertion technique without pneumoperitoneum using 10-mm optical viewing trocar and a 0° scope in the left paramedian supra-umbilical location [38]. A 12 mm port is placed in the right flank. Additional 5 mm ports are then placed in the subxiphoid area, left upper quadrant and left flank. A third 12 mm port is then placed in the left lower quadrant and that incision will also be used to insert the

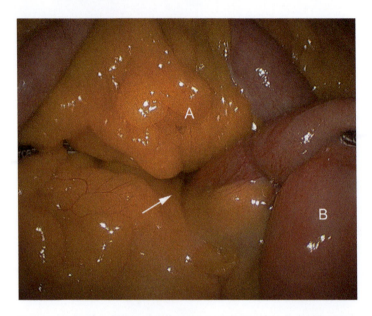

FIGURE 15.3 Identifying the ligament of Treitz (*Arrow*), (*A* transverse mesocolon, *B* jejunum)

circular stapler (Fig. 15.2). The first assistant stands on the patient's left side and holds the camera with his/her left hand and assists through the left lateral port with his/her right hand. The surgeon stands on the patient's right side.

2. Creation of the Alimentary limb and Jejuno-jejunostomy

We routinely create the alimentary limb and jejuno-jejunostomy as the initial step. The omentum is reflected cephalad and tucked in the upper abdomen and the transverse colon elevated. After elevating the transverse mesocolon, the ligament of Treitz is identified at the base of the transverse mesocolon (Fig. 15.3). The ligament of Treitz is clearly identified and the bowel is run for about 50 cm to find a jejunal loop that can reach the upper abdomen without tension. The jejunum is then transected using an endoscopic linear cutting stapler using 2.5 mm height staplers (Fig. 15.4). The mesentery between the bilio-pancreatic and alimentary

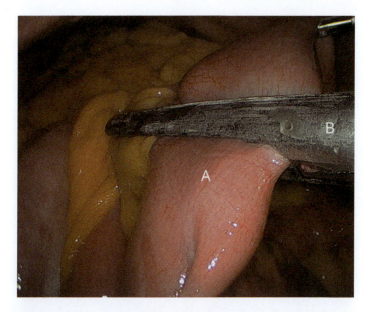

FIGURE 15.4 Transecting the jejunum using an endoscopic linear cutting stapler (*A* jejunum, *B* endo GIA stapler)

limb is then divided for about 2 cm with an ultrasonic dissector. In rare cases, a more complete division of the mesentery is needed. The alimentary limb is marked with two clips to facilitate later the identification when creating the jejuno-jejunostomy and prevent a Roux-en-"O" error (mistakenly connecting the alimentary limb back to itself). The best length of the alimentary limb is still a matter of debate; we choose the alimentary limb length based on the patient's BMI: 100 cm for a BMI < 50 kg/m^2 and 150 cm for a BMI $\geq$ 50 kg/m^2 [39]. Importantly, the alimentary limb should be moved and placed to the left of the bilio-pancreatic limb and angle of Treitz (Fig. 15.5). The jejuno-jejunostomy is then created by connecting the biliopancreatic limb to the 100 or 150 cm location of the alimentary limb. Enterotomies are created in each segment with the ultrasonic shears (Fig. 15.6). The enterotomy in the bilio-pancraetic limb is done at the top of the cut staple line and the enterotomy in the alimentary

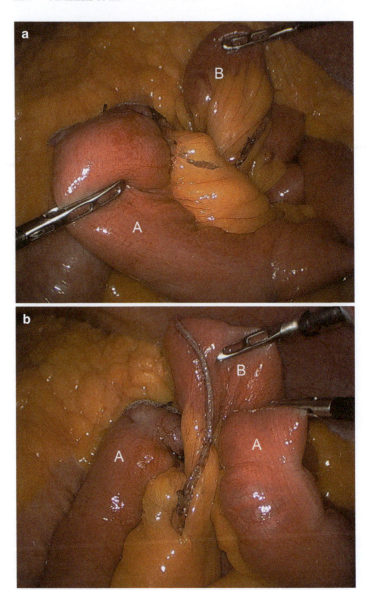

FIGURE 15.5 Placing the alimentary limb (*A*) to the left of the bilio-pancreatic limb (*B*)

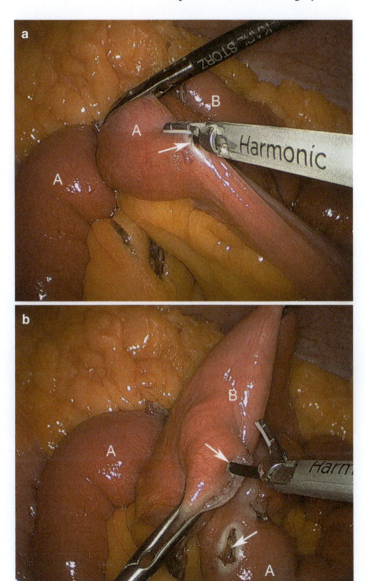

FIGURE 15.6 Creating enterotomies (*Arrows*) in the alimentary limb (*A*) and bilio-pancreatic limb (*B*)

limb should be done in the left lateral side of the small bowel mid-way between the mesentery and the anti-mesenteric border to prevent narrowing the lumen when closing the common enterotomy (Fig. 15.6). An endoscopic linear cutting stapler of 60 mm length with 2.5 mm height staples is inserted down each lumen and fired, creating a side-to-side functional end-to-end jejunojejunostomy (Figs. 15.7 and 15.8). The staple lines are inspected for hemostasis. The opening in the bowel is closed with an additional load of the endoscopic linear cutting stapler with 3.5 mm height staples, taking care not to compromise the caliber of the lumen of the jejunojeju-nostomy (Fig. 15.9). An anti-kinking stitch is placed to prevent obstruction at the jejunojejunostomy (Fig. 15.10). The mesenteric defect is then closed with a running locking 2–0 braided polyester suture from the anastomosis to the base of the mesentery (Fig. 15.11).

Closing Peterson's space (between the mesentery of the alimentary limb and the transverse colon when the antecolic technique is used) is advocated by many. We split the omentum up the middle from the mid transverse colon using ultrasonic shears (Fig. 15.12). The alimentary limb is brought anterior to the mid-transverse colon and into the proximal abdomen between the leaves of the omentum. At this point, attention is turned to creating the gastric pouch.

3. Creation of the Gastric Pouch

The patient is positioned in steep reverse Trendelenburg at this time to facilitate exposure of the proximal stomach. A liver retractor is inserted through a subxiphoid 5 mm incision and secured with a mechanical arm retractor to lift the left lobe of the liver anteriorly. We start by dissecting the gastroesophageal junction fat pad off the left crus of the diaphragm at the angle of His. This makes later visualization of the proximal stomach during gastric pouch creation a bit easier. We then dissect between the proximal lesser curve gastric wall and the lesser curve neurovascular bundle and into the lesser sac (Figs. 15.13 and 15.14). This location is typically between the fat pad and the visible first lesser curve

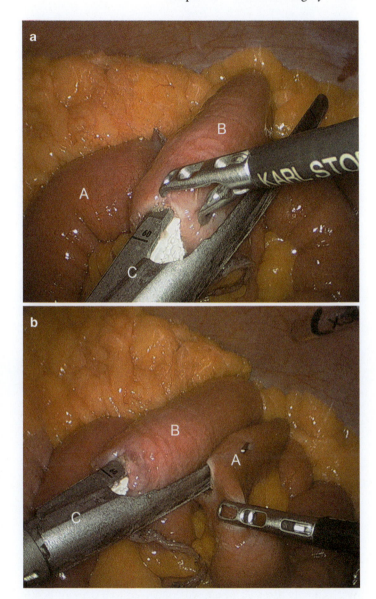

FIGURE 15.7 Placing the bilio-pancreatic limb (*B*) and the alimentary limb (*A*) in the linear stapler (*C*)

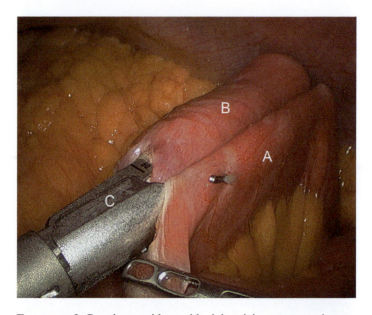

FIGURE 15.8 Creating a side-to-side jejunojejunostomy using an endoscopic linear cutting stapler (*A* alimentary limb, *B* bilio-pancreatic limb, *C* endo GIA Stapler)

vessel on the anterior proximal stomach (about 5 cm distal from the estimated location of the gastroesophageal junction). A 3.5 mm height, 60 mm linear stapler is initially fired to divide the stomach in a right-to-left horizontal plane (Fig. 15.15). Next, two or three 3.5 mm height, 60 mm linear staplers are used to create a 30 ml gastric pouch divided at the level of the angle of His (Fig. 15.16). Specific care is always taken not to leave redundant gastric fundus on the side of the gastric pouch.

4. Creation of the Gastrojejunostomy

We prefer the trans-oral placement of the anvil and with the anvil delivered through the cut staple line of the gastric pouch. We routinely use a 21 mm anvil connected to a 3.5 mm height stapler. However, a 21 mm circular stapler (as opposed to a 25 mm circular stapler) should only be used when the trans-oral

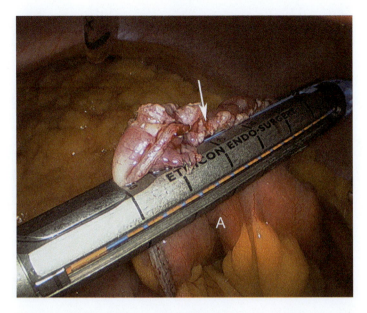

FIGURE 15.9 Closing the opening of the entero-enterostomy (*Arrow*) using an endoscopic linear cutting stapler

technique is used [40]. The transgastric 21 mm stapler technique has been associated with higher stricture rate in ours and others experience [41]. The gastrojejunal anastomosis technique includes passing the 21 mm anvil (OrVil™, Autosuture, Norwalk, CT, USA) trans-orally and through a small opening in the stapled gastric pouch (Fig. 15.17). The OrVil™ 21 mm device is a pre-packaged commercially available device (OrVil™, Autosuture, Norwalk, CT, USA). It combines the anvil head, secured in the tilted position, mounted on a 90-cm long polyvinyl chloride (PVC) delivery tube and secured to the tube with a suture. The PVC delivery tube is inserted through the patient's mouth, delivered through a small opening in the stapled gastric pouch and pulled from left lower quadrant port sites to assist bringing the anvil shaft into the gastric pouch staple line. A critical step of the procedure is then passing the tilted anvil head attached to the delivery tube through the posterior pharynx into the esophagus. We recommend that the anesthesiologist and an

230   A. Elian et al.

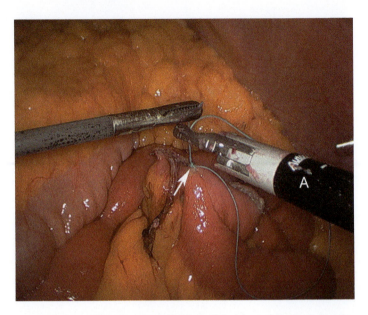

FIGURE 15.10 Placing an anti-kinking stich (*Arrow*) at the jejunojejunostomy

assistant are present for this portion of the procedure. The anvil
head should be generously lubricated, and its convex side
directed and maintained towards the hard palate. Once the anvil
enters the posterior pharynx, elevating the mandible, similar to
a Jaw thrust maneuver, and briefly deflating the balloon of the
double-lumen endotracheal tube, facilitates the anvil passage
into the esophagus. Once the anvil shaft has been exteriorized
through the gastric staple line, the suture that holds it to the
delivery tube is cut and the tube is disconnected from the anvil
while holding the anvil in place (Fig. 15.18). The anastomosis is
completed by joining the anvil to the end-to-end circular stapler
(EEA XL 25 mm with 3.5 mm staples, Autosuture, Norwalk, CT,
USA) inserted into the small bowel (Figs. 15.19, 15.20 and 15.21).
Then, the EEA stapler and anvil were removed, the anastomosis
inspected and the small bowel opening closed using an additional
firing of a 2.5 mm linear stapler (United States Surgical
Corporation, Norwalk, CT, USA) (Fig. 15.22).

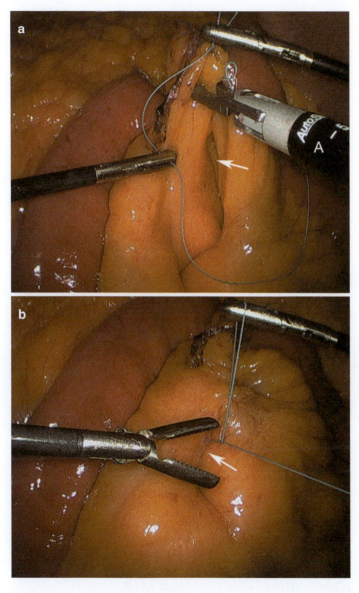

FIGURE 15.11 Closing the mesenteric defect (*Arrow*) using suturing device (*A*)

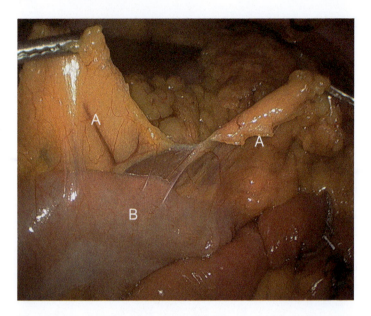

FIGURE 15.12 Dividing the omentum (*A*) in the middle of the transverse colon (*B*)

We routinely place two 2-0 absorbable sutures at the corners of the anastomosis (Fig. 15.23). The use of absorbable rather than permanent sutures at the gastrojejunostomy may help to minimize the incidence of marginal ulcers [42].

A leak test is performed by passing an orogastric tube into the alimentary limb and injecting oxygen at a flow rate of 1 L while the jejunum is pinched distal to the gastrojejunostomy. If air bubbles are identified, the leak should be repaired immediately.

We do not routinely place drains. Final aspect of the gastrojejunostomy is shown (Fig. 15.24). All ports are removed under direct visualization to ensure that there is no abdominal wall bleeding and fascial defects are closed.

Results After Laparoscopic RYGB

The safety profile of RYGB has been confirmed by multiple case series and large administrative database studies [43–45]

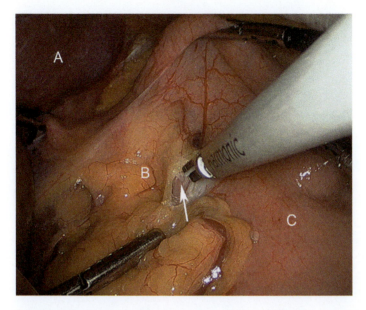

FIGURE 15.13 Dissecting into the lesser sac (*Arrow*) (*A* liver, *B* gastrohepatic ligament, *C* stomach)

and by the results of a prospective, multicenter, observational study of 4,340 consecutive patients at 10 clinical sites in the U.S [15]. Severe complication and mortality rates were low overall (4.1 % and 0.3 %). The study also showed that complications and mortality were significantly lower in patients who had a laparoscopic as opposed to an open RYGB: complication and mortality rates laparoscopic, 4.8 % and 0.2 %; open, 7.8 % and 2.1 %, p < 0.01. Similar data from a randomized controlled trial support the notion that laparoscopic RYGB is associated with fewer overall complications than open RYGB [18].

A series of 608 patients with RYGB who were followed for 14 years was reported in 1995, with 98 % of the patients included in the analysis [46]. The percentage of excess weight loss was 70, 58, 55 and 49 % at 2, 5, 10 and 14 years, respectively. The improvement in comorbidities with this sustained weight reduction included a reduction in the number of patients with hypertension from 58 % to 14 %, while T2DM

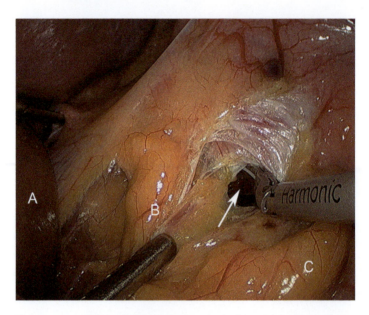

FIGURE 15.14 Dissecting into the lesser sac (*Arrow*) (*A* liver, *B* gastrohepatic ligament, *C* Stomach)

remitted in 83 %. The development of new cases (incidence rates) of T2DM was also reduced; only 1 % of patients who had impaired glucose tolerance preoperatively progressed to T2DM in the postoperative period. It was estimated that 21–38 % of these patients would have become diabetic without sustained weight reduction.

The largest report to-date to evaluate long-term remission and relapse of T2DM after RYGB is a multisite study of 4,434 adults [47]. Postoperative remission and relapse of T2DM followed strict criteria: *Complete remission* was defined as the combination of discontinuing hypoglycemic medication and fasting glucose values <100 mg/dL and/or HbA1c levels <6.0 % occurring more than 90 days after the last prescription. *Relapse of T2DM* was defined as one or more of the following: restarting T2DM medication, one or more HbA1c measures ≥7 %; and/or one or more fasting glucose measures ≥126 mg/dL. Overall, 68.2 % of all

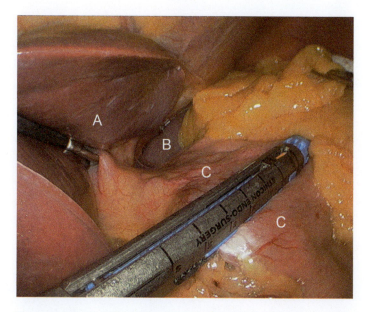

FIGURE 15.15 Creating the gastric pouch with a linear cutting stapler (*A* liver, *B* spleen, *C* stomach)

patients experienced an initial complete diabetes remission within 5 years after surgery and the median duration of remission was 8.3 years. Among those who initially remitted, 35.1 % relapsed within 5 years. Significant predictors of complete remission and relapse were poor preoperative glycemic control, insulin use, and longer duration of diabetes.

Much interest and research is underway to define precisely and understand the mechanisms of diabetes remission and relapse, the optimal timing of operation in effecting a durable remission, and the relationship between remission duration and incident microvascular and macrovascular events. Nevertheless it is clear that bariatric surgery is currently the only available weapon that is capable of providing reliable and enduring rates of T2DM remission.

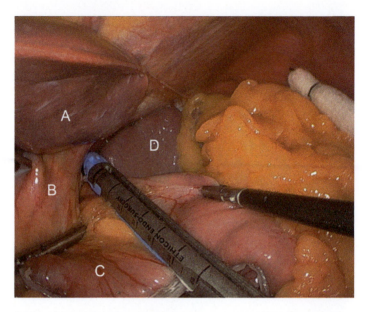

FIGURE 15.16 Creating a gastric pouch by dividing the proximal stomach at the level of angle of His (*A* liver, *B* left crus of diaphragm, *C* gastric pouch, *D* spleen)

Laparoscopic Sleeve Gastrectomy (SG)

Sleeve Gastrectomy (SG) was initially performed in 1988 by Hess and Hess [48] as the gastric restrictive portion of the biliopancreatic diversion with duodenal switch (BPD-DS) [49]. In late 1980, a few centers in the U.S. and in Europe [50–52] started using SG as the first of a two-step procedure to decrease operative time and reduce complication and mortality rate with BPD-DS in the super obese patient. The results after SG in regards of weight loss and resolution of comorbidities were comparable to RYGB [49, 53] and many patients did not need the second step (the BDP-DS part). Therefore, SG was increasingly considered as a sole bariatric procedure and in 2010 the American Society for Metabolic and Bariatric Surgery (ASMBS) recommended SG as an

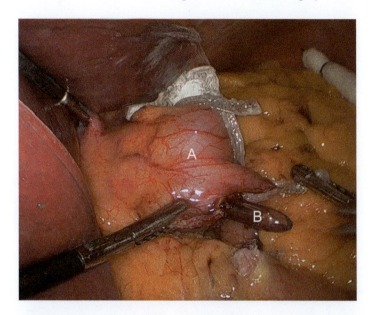

FIGURE 15.17 Passing the delivery tube of the stapler anvil through a small opening in the gastric pouch staple line (*A* gastric pouch, *B* delivery tube)

approved bariatric operation [54]. In 2008 worldwide 18,098 SG were performed and this number increased to 94,689 in 2011, making the SG second most performed bariatric procedure [1] (Fig. 15.1).

SG promotes weight loss by several mechanisms. SG is considered as a purely restrictive procedure with reduction in food intake and early satiety, which results in weight loss [55]. In contrast to other traditional restrictive procedures like adjustable gastric banding, where a tiny gastric pouch of about 15 cc is created, in SG the volume of the remaining stomach is up to 150–200 cc. However, in SG the gastric fundus, the major food storage compartment and upper part of the body of the stomach, including the gastric pacemaker, are removed [56]. Additional, it seems that after SG the gastric emptying is accelerated with an increased small bowel transit time, which leads to decreased nutrient absorption [56]. Another metabolic

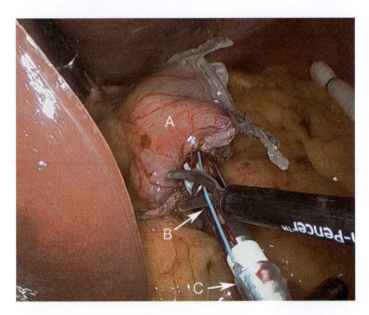

FIGURE 15.18 Cutting the suture to disconnect the delivery tube from the anvil (*A* gastric pouch, *B* anvil shaft, *C* delivery tube)

effect after SG is the reduction in ghrelin [57]. Ghrelin is an orexigenic hormone, which induces preprandial hunger and meal initiation. Ghrelin blocks insulin secretion, stimulates secretion of insulin antagonists growth hormone and adreno-corticotropic hormone, suppresses production of the insulin sensitizing hormone adiponectin and blocks hepatic insulin signaling [55]. Ghrelin is mainly secreted in the gastric fundus [55]. Reduction in Ghrelin-levels, which was found after SG, would have an antidiabetic effect and might be one explanation for the improvement in T2DM, which was seen after SG. Another metabolic effect might be stimulated levels of hindgut hormones [58]. Higher concentrations of undigested food in the terminal ileum might cause stimulation of L-cells with higher concentrations of glucagon-like peptide 1 and peptide YY. Both hormones have an anti-diabetic effect through enhancing glucose dependent insulin secretion, suppressing glucagon secretion and increasing insulin sensitivity [55, 59].

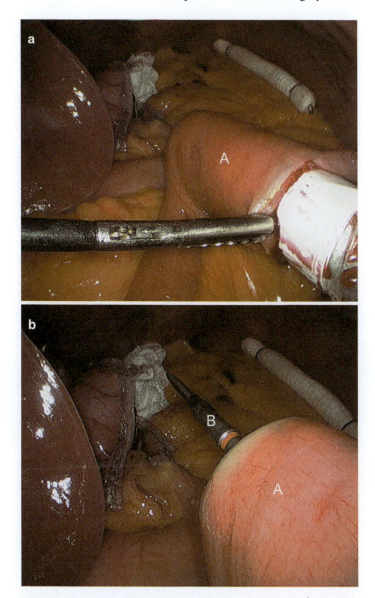

FIGURE 15.19 Placing the jejunum into the circular stapler (*A* jejunum, *B* circular stapler pin)

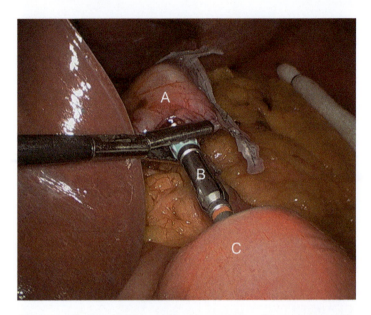

FIGURE 15.20 The circular stapler is engaged to the anvil (*A* gastric pouch, *B* anvil shaft, *C* jejunum)

Current relative contra-indications for SG are patients with Barrett's esophagus, gastro-esophageal reflux disease with esophageal mucosal injury such as erosive esophagitis, strictures, and ulcers, achalasia, large hiatal or paraesophageal hernias, diabetic gastroparesis, and active Crohn's disease. Due to its relative simplicity compared to RYGB and much better results compared to adjustable gastric banding, the utilization of SG has increased markedly both in the US and worldwide [1, 60].

Operative Technique of Laparoscopic Sleeve Gastrectomy

The laparoscopic technique for SG was first described by Ren et al. [61]. Access to the peritoneal cavity is similar to the one described for laparoscopic RYGB. Trocar placement

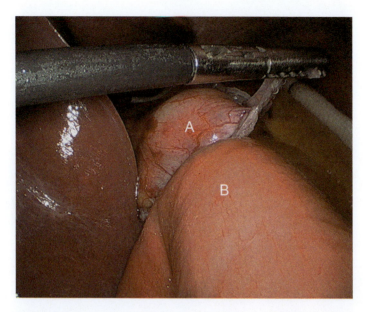

FIGURE 15.21 Closing the EEA circular stapler to create the anastomosis (*A* gastric pouch, *B* jejunum)

varies significantly from center and surgeons. We used 5 trocars, a 12 mm in the right flank, three 5 mm, one in the subxiphoid area, one in the left upper quadrant and one in the left flank, and another 12 mm in the left lower quadrant (Fig. 15.25). The patient is placed in reverse Trendelenburg and the left lobe of the liver is retracted. The stomach is inspected and adequately decompressed through an orogastric tube. Gastric mobilization is started by dividing the gastrocolic ligament about 5 cm proximal to the pylorus (Fig. 15.26) and by dividing it in between the stomach and the right gastroepiploic arcade (Fig. 15.27). This is done with a harmonic scalpel all the way to the Angle of His (Fig. 15.28) and exposing the left crus of the diaphragmatic crura. Larger short gastric vessels maybe clipped (Fig. 15.29). Care must be taken to avoid bleeding or injury to the spleen. We routinely use a 40 French bougie to assure adequate sizing of the sleeve; however this is not standardized and varies from

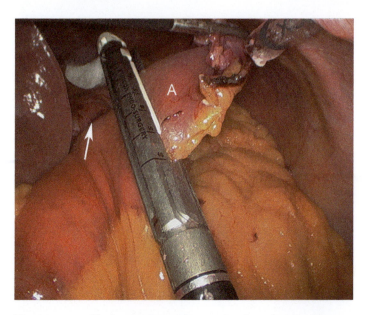

FIGURE 15.22 Closing and excising excess bowel (*A*) using an endoscopic linear cutting stapler (*Arrow* pointing to the gastrojejunostomy)

center to center. The stapling of the stomach is started at 5 cm proximal to the pylorus (Fig. 15.30) and taken superiorly toward the left crus. The initial staple firing should have 4.4 mm height staplers (Fig. 15.31). The use of staple line reinforcement strips is optional. Subsequent firings are done with 4.1 mm height staplers (Fig. 15.32), transitioning to 3.5 mm height staplers in the proximal gastric body and fundus (Fig. 15.33).

The specimen stomach is placed in the LUQ. The staple line is inspected for bleeding. The sizing bougie is removed and a leak test is done using an oro-gastric tubing connected to 1 l flow of oxygen. The resected stomach (Fig. 15.34) is removed through the 12 mm port. The staple line is sewn back to the divided gastrocolic ligament (Figs. 15.35 and 15.36). All ports are removed under direct visualization to ensure that there is no abdominal wall bleeding. The fascia is

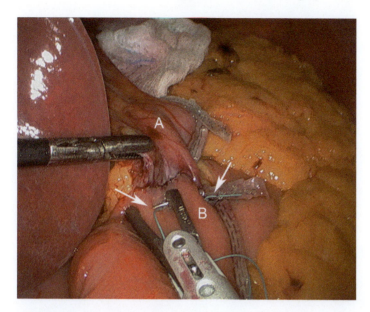

FIGURE 15.23 Placing 2 stiches at the corners of the anastomosis (*Arrows*), (*A* gastric pouch, *B* jejunum)

closed at all trocars over 10 mm. Local anesthesia is infiltrated and the skin edges approximated using subcuticular 4-0 monocryl suture. Sterile dressings are applied.

Comparative Effectiveness of RYGB and Sleeve Gastrectomy

Two large studies compared the results of RYGB, SG and also laparoscopic adjustable gastric banding (AGB) operations.

One study, from the American College of Surgeons-Bariatric Surgery Center Network accreditation program, reported outcomes in 28,616 patients [62]. Weight loss, measured as reduction in BMI, and resolution or improvement in T2DM were significantly better for RYGB (reduction in BMI: 15/resolution in T2DM: 83 %) than for SG (reduction

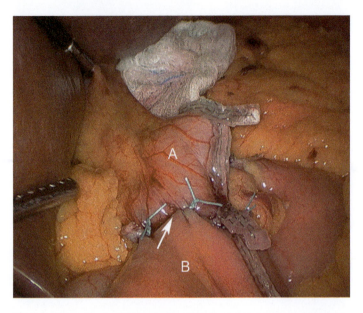

FIGURE 15.24 Gastrojejunostomy – Final aspect (*Arrow*), (*A* gastric pouch, *B* jejunum)

in BMI: 12/resolution in T2DM: 55 %) and AGB (reduction in BMI: 7/resolution in T2DM: 44 %). AGB had the lowest rate of peri-operative complications and SG had a lower reoperation/intervention rate compared to RYGB, though RYGB and SG procedures had similar risk-adjusted morbidity and readmission rates.

The other study came from the Michigan Bariatric Surgery Collaborative Group [63], in which 2,949 SG patients were matched with equal numbers of RYGB and AGB patients on 23 baseline characteristics. Outcomes studied were perioperative 30 day complications, weight loss, quality of life, and comorbidity remission at 1, 2, and 3 years after operation. Overall complication rates in SG patients (6.3 %) were significantly lower than for RYGB (10.0 %, $p < 0.0001$) but higher than for AGB (2.4 %, $p < 0.0001$). An interesting finding was that serious complication rates were similar for SG (2.4 %) and RYGB (2.5 %, $p = 0.7$) but higher than for AGB

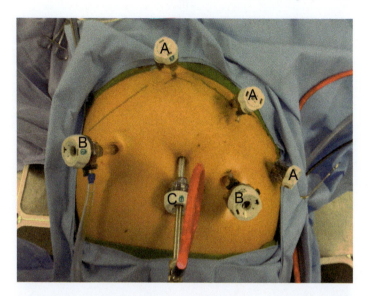

FIGURE 15.25 Port placement for laparoscopic sleeve gastrectomy (*A* 5 mm trocar, *B* 12 mm trocar, *C* 11 mm trocar)

(1.0 %, $p < 0.0001$). Excess body weight loss (EBWL) at 1 year was lower for SG compared to RYGB (EBWL: SG, 60 % vs RYGB, 69 %, $p < 0.0001$), but was 77 % higher for SG than for AGB (EBWL for AGB was only 34 %, $p < 0.0001$). Remission of obesity-associated diseases was similarly closer in between SG and RYGB and superior to AGB.

Lastly, a prospective randomized trial compared SG to RYGB and best medical therapy [64]. It studied 150 patients with a BMI greater than 30 and with T2DM. RYGB had better weight loss than SG at 1 year (BMI reduction: RYGB, 10 vs. SG, 9, $p = 0.03$), but similar rates of T2DM remission (RYGB: 42 % vs. SG: 39 %, $p = 0.59$).

Due to the preservation of the pyloric sphincter, continuing duodenal contact with food bolus and absence of mesenteric defects, SG is not associated with rare complications seen long-term with RYGB, such as marginal ulcers and internal hernias. SG is also an attractive alternative for patients who may be candidates for organ transplant since it

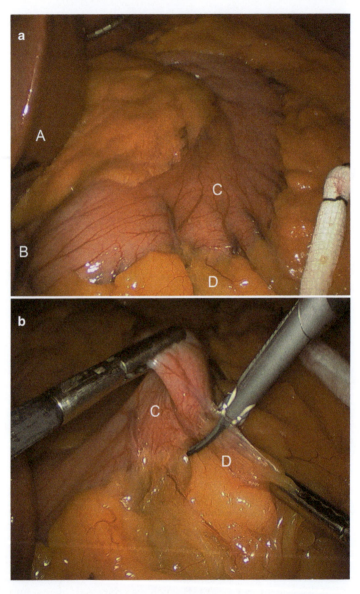

FIGURE 15.26 Dividing the gastrocolic ligament and mobilization of the stomach (*A* liver, *B* pylorus, *C* stomach, *D* gastrocolic ligament)

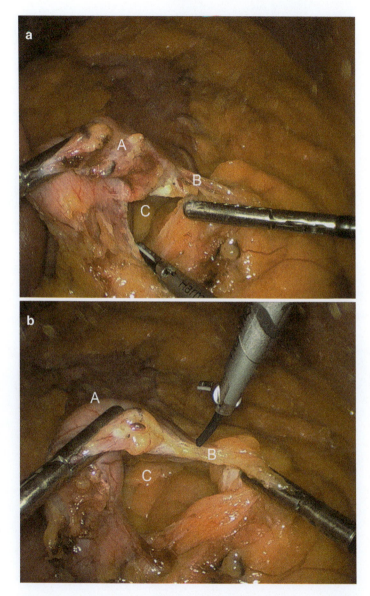

FIGURE 15.27 Division of the gastrocolic ligament and right gastroepiploic arcade (*A* stomach, *B* right gastroepiploic arcade, *C* lesser sac)

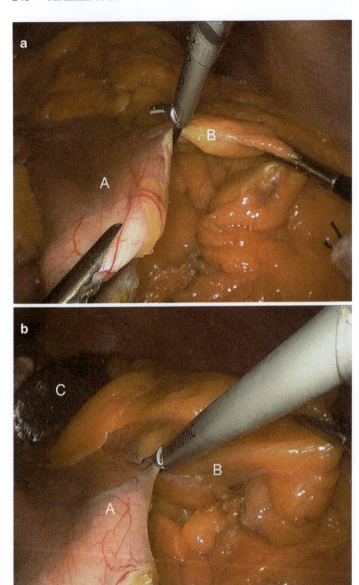

FIGURE 15.28 Division of the gastrocolic ligament and right gastro-epiploic arcade all the way to the angle of HIS (*A* stomach, *B* right gastroepiploic arcade, *C* spleen)

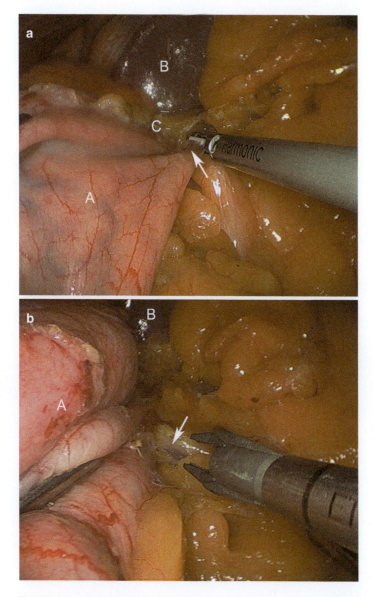

FIGURE 15.29 Dividing the short gastric vessels (*Arrow*), (*A* stomach, *B* spleen, *C* angle of His)

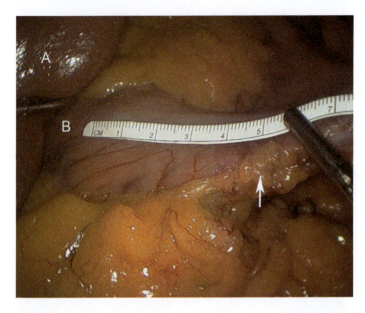

FIGURE 15.30 The *arrow* points to the starting point of stomach transection (*A* liver, *B* pylorus)

preserves normal alimentation pathway for absorption of oral medications [65]. SG is an irreversible procedure, whereas RYGB and AGB can be reversed.

The decision-making process to choose the optimal procedure for a specific patient is complex and should take into account all individual characteristics such as age, obesity-associated diseases, performance status and body habitus. Patients' preferences should be also taken into consideration, but a genuine effort should always be made to inform patients of the known expected benefits and risks of the available operative procedures, including the accepted literature as well as the individual surgeon and center experience.

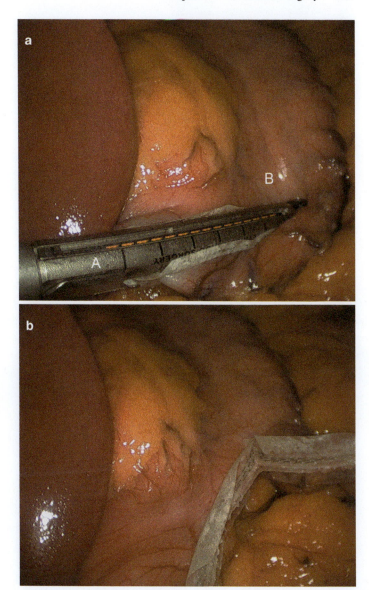

FIGURE 15.31 The initial staple firing using a linear cutting stapler (*A* GIA stapler with 4.4 mm height staplers, *B* stomach)

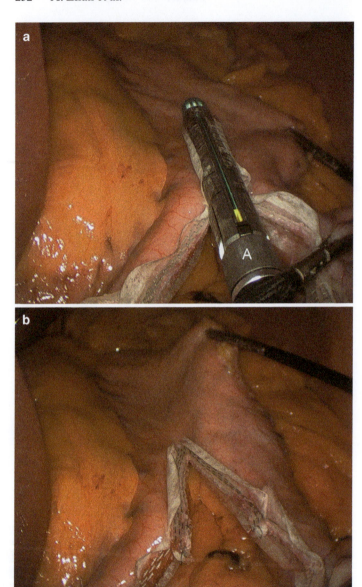

FIGURE 15.32 Stapling of the stomach body with 4.1 mm height staplers (*A*)

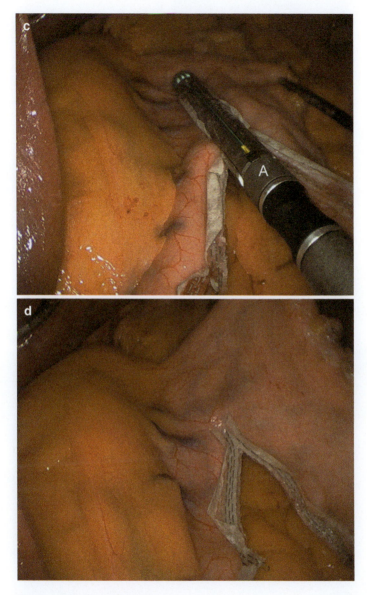

Figure 15.32 (continued)

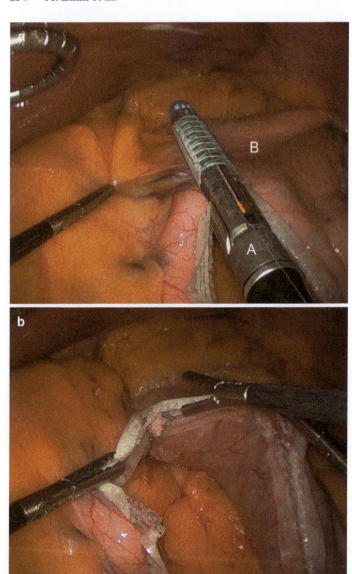

FIGURE 15.33 Stapling of the fundus of the stomach with 3.5 mm height staplers (*A*), (*B* fundus, *C* spleen)

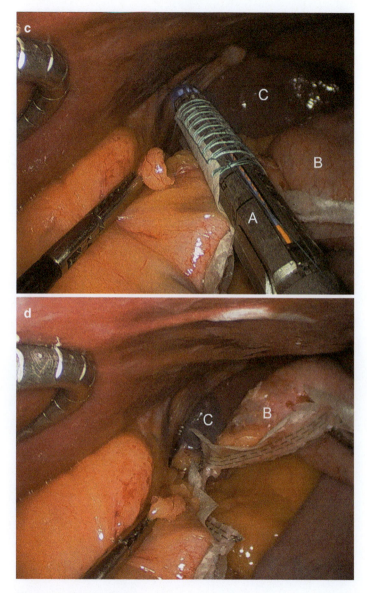

FIGURE 15.33 (continued)

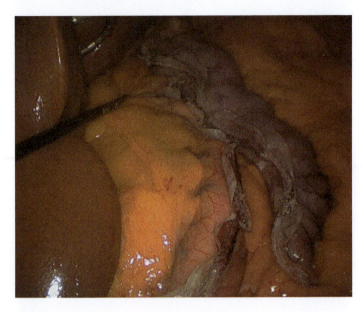

Figure 15.34 Sleeve gastrectomy – final aspect

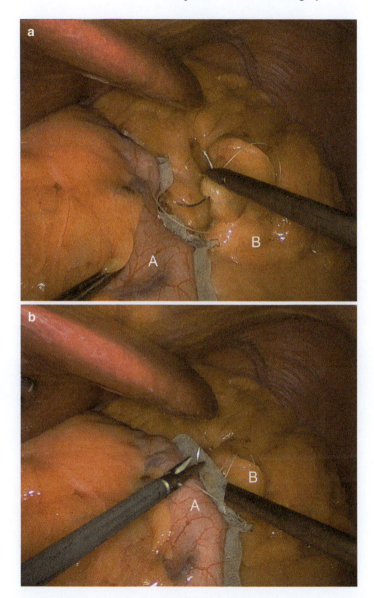

FIGURE 15.35 Securing the divided gastrocolic omentum to the lateral side of the Sleeve. (*A* stomach, *B* omentum)

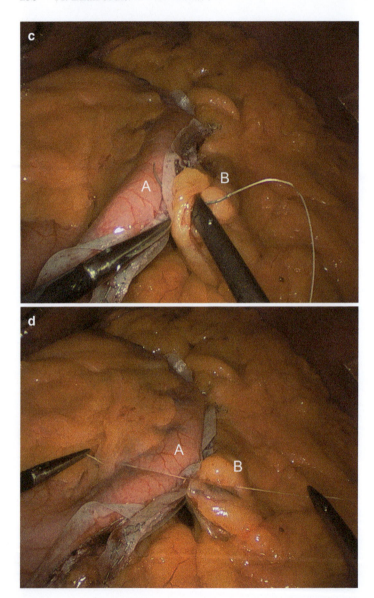

Figure 15.35 (continued)

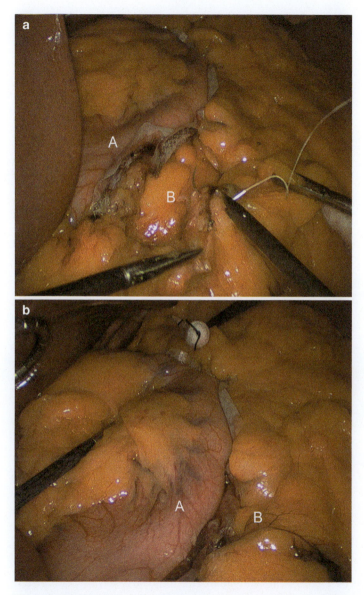

FIGURE 15.36 Securing the divided gastrocolic omentum to the lateral side of the Sleeve and final aspect of the operation. (*A* stomach, *B* omentum)

References

1. Buchwald H, Oien DM. Metabolic/bariatric surgery worldwide 2011. Obes Surg. 2013;23(4):427–36.
2. CDC Adult Obesity Facts and Childhood Obesity Facts. http://www.cdc.gov/obesity/data/facts.html.
3. Danaei G, Ding EL, Mozaffarian D, Taylor B, Rehm J, Murray CJ, et al. The preventable causes of death in the United States: comparative risk assessment of dietary, lifestyle, and metabolic risk factors. PLoS Med. 2009;6(4), e1000058.
4. World Health Organization. Obesity: preventing and managing the global epidemic. Contract No: Geneva (Switzerland). 2000.
5. Finkelstein EA, Trogdon JG, Cohen JW, Dietz W. Annual medical spending attributable to obesity: payer-and service-specific estimates. Health Aff (Millwood). 2009;28(5):w822–31.
6. Reis JP, Macera CA, Aranta MR, Lindsay SP, Marshall SJ, Wingard DL. Comparison of overall obesity and body fat distribution in predicting risk of mortality. Obesity (Silver Spring). 2009;17(6):1232–9.
7. Pischon T, Boeing H, Hoffmann K, Bergmann M, Schulze MB, Overvad K, et al. General and abdominal adiposity and risk of death in Europe. N Engl J Med. 2008;359(20):2105–20.
8. Sievenpiper JL, de Souza RJ, Jenkins DJ. Sugar: fruit fructose is still healthy. Nature. 2012;482(7386):470.
9. Block G. Foods contributing to energy intake in the US: data from NHANES III and NHANES 1999–2000. J Food Compos Anal. 2004;17(3–4):439–47.
10. Putnam J, Allshouse J, Kantor LS. U.S. per capita food supply trends: more calories, refined carbohydrates, and fats. Food Rev. 2002;25(3):2–14.
11. Buchwald H, Avidor Y, Braunwald E, Jensen MD, Pories W, Fahrbach K, et al. Bariatric surgery: a systematic review and meta-analysis. JAMA. 2004;292(14):1724–37.
12. Rabl C, Campos GM. The impact of bariatric surgery on nonalcoholic steatohepatitis. Semin Liver Dis. 2012;32(1):80–91.
13. National Institutes of Health. Clinical guidelines on the identification, evaluation, and treatment of overweight and obesity in adults – the evidence report. Obes Res. 1998;6 Suppl 2:51S–209.
14. Picot J, Jones J, Colquitt JL, Gospodarevskaya E, Loveman E, Baxter L, et al. The clinical effectiveness and cost-effectiveness of bariatric (weight loss) surgery for obesity: a systematic

review and economic evaluation. Health Technol Assess. 2009;13(41):1–190, 215–357, iii–iv.

15. Flum DR, Belle SH, King WC, Wahed AS, Berk P, Chapman W, et al. Perioperative safety in the longitudinal assessment of bariatric surgery. N Engl J Med. 2009;361(5):445–54.

16. Sjostrom L. Review of the key results from the Swedish Obese Subjects (SOS) trial – a prospective controlled intervention study of bariatric surgery. J Intern Med. 2013;273(3):219–34.

17. Buchwald H, Estok R, Fahrbach K, Banel D, Jensen MD, Pories WJ, et al. Weight and type 2 diabetes after bariatric surgery: systematic review and meta-analysis. Am J Med. 2009;122(3):248–56, e5.

18. Nguyen NT, Goldman C, Rosenquist CJ, Arango A, Cole CJ, Lee SJ, et al. Laparoscopic versus open gastric bypass: a randomized study of outcomes, quality of life, and costs. Ann Surg. 2001;234(3):279–89; discussion 89–91.

19. Sjostrom L, Narbro K, Sjostrom CD, Karason K, Larsson B, Wedel H, et al. Effects of bariatric surgery on mortality in Swedish obese subjects. N Engl J Med. 2007;357(8):741–52.

20. Adams TD, Gress RE, Smith SC, Halverson RC, Simper SC, Rosamond WD, et al. Long-term mortality after gastric bypass surgery. N Engl J Med. 2007;357(8):753–61.

21. Kohn GP, Galanko JA, Overby DW, Farrell TM. Recent trends in bariatric surgery case volume in the United States. Surgery. 2009;146(2):375–80.

22. Steinbrook R. Surgery for severe obesity. N Engl J Med. 2004;350(11):1075–9.

23. NIH conference. Gastrointestinal surgery for severe obesity. Consensus development conference panel. Ann Intern Med. 1991;115(12):956–61.

24. Mason EE, Ito C. Gastric bypass. Ann Surg. 1969;170(3):329–39.

25. Wittgrove AC, Clark GW, Tremblay LJ. Laparoscopic gastric bypass, Roux-en-Y: preliminary report of five cases. Obes Surg. 1994;4(4):353–7.

26. Del Genio F, Del Genio G, De Sio I, Marra M, Alfonsi L, Finelli C, et al. Noninvasive evaluation of abdominal fat and liver changes following progressive weight loss in severely obese patients treated with laparoscopic gastric bypass. Obes Surg. 2009;19(12):1664–71.

27. Dirksen C, Jorgensen NB, Bojsen-Moller KN, Jacobsen SH, Hansen DL, Worm D, et al. Mechanisms of improved glycaemic control after Roux-en-Y gastric bypass. Diabetologia. 2012;55(7):1890–901.

28. Campos GM, Rabl C, Havel PJ, Rao M, Schwarz JM, Schambelan M, et al. Changes in post-prandial glucose and pancreatic hormones, and steady-state insulin and free fatty acids after gastric bypass surgery. Surg Obes Relat Dis. 2014;10(1):1–8.

29. Campos GM, Rabl C, Peeva S, Ciovica R, Rao M, Schwarz JM, et al. Improvement in peripheral glucose uptake after gastric bypass surgery is observed only after substantial weight loss has occurred and correlates with the magnitude of weight lost. J Gastrointest Surg. 2010;14(1):15–23.

30. Ashrafian H, le Roux CW. Metabolic surgery and gut hormones – a review of bariatric entero-humoral modulation. Physiol Behav. 2009;97(5):620–31.

31. Faria SL, Faria OP, Cardeal Mde A, de Gouvea HR, Buffington C. Diet-induced thermogenesis and respiratory quotient after Roux-en-Y gastric bypass. Surg Obes Relat Dis. 2012;8(6):797–802.

32. Ashrafian H, Athanasiou T, Li JV, Bueter M, Ahmed K, Nagpal K, et al. Diabetes resolution and hyperinsulinaemia after metabolic Roux-en-Y gastric bypass. Obes Rev. 2011;12(5):e257–72.

33. Ley RE, Turnbaugh PJ, Klein S, Gordon JI. Microbial ecology: human gut microbes associated with obesity. Nature. 2006; 444(7122):1022–3.

34. Faria SL, Faria OP, Buffington C, de Almeida Cardeal M, Rodrigues de Gouvea H. Energy expenditure before and after Roux-en-Y gastric bypass. Obes Surg. 2012;22(9):1450–5.

35. Rabl C, Rao MN, Schwarz JM, Mulligan K, Campos GM. Thermogenic changes after gastric bypass, adjustable gastric banding or diet alone. Surgery. 2014;156(4):806–13.

36. Dholakia C, Beverstein G, Garren M, Nemergut C, Boncyk J, Gould JC. The impact of perioperative dexmedetomidine infusion on postoperative narcotic use and duration of stay after laparoscopic bariatric surgery. J Gastrointest Surg. 2007;11(11):1556–9.

37. Escalona A, Devaud N, Perez G, Crovari F, Boza C, Viviani P, et al. Antecolic versus retrocolic alimentary limb in laparoscopic Roux-en-Y gastric bypass: a comparative study. Surg Obes Relat Dis. 2007;3(4):423–7.

38. Rabl C, Palazzo F, Aoki H, Campos GM. Initial laparoscopic access using an optical trocar without pneumoperitoneum is safe and effective in the morbidly obese. Surg Innov. 2008;15(2):126–31.

39. Ciovica R, Takata M, Vittinghoff E, Lin F, Posselt AM, Rabl C, et al. The impact of roux limb length on weight loss after gastric bypass. Obes Surg. 2008;18(1):5–10.

40. Rondan A, Nijhawan S, Majid S, Martinez T, Wittgrove AC. Low anastomotic stricture rate after Roux-en-Y gastric bypass using a 21-mm circular stapling device. Obes Surg. 2012;22(9):1491–5.

41. Takata MC, Ciovica R, Cello JP, Posselt AM, Rogers SJ, Campos GM. Predictors, treatment, and outcomes of gastrojejunostomy stricture after gastric bypass for morbid obesity. Obes Surg. 2007;17(7):878–84.

42. Sacks BC, Mattar SG, Qureshi FG, Eid GM, Collins JL, Barinas-Mitchell EJ, et al. Incidence of marginal ulcers and the use of absorbable anastomotic sutures in laparoscopic Roux-en-Y gastric bypass. Surg Obes Relat Dis. 2006;2(1):11–6.

43. Gould JC, Kent KC, Wan Y, Rajamanickam V, Leverson G, Campos GM. Perioperative safety and volume: outcomes relationships in bariatric surgery: a study of 32,000 patients. J Am Coll Surg. 2011;213(6):771–7.

44. Campos GM, Ciovica R, Rogers SJ, Posselt AM, Vittinghoff E, Takata M, et al. Spectrum and risk factors of complications after gastric bypass. Arch Surg. 2007;142(10):969–75; discussion 76.

45. Podnos YD, Jimenez JC, Wilson SE, Stevens CM, Nguyen NT. Complications after laparoscopic gastric bypass: a review of 3464 cases. Arch Surg. 2003;138(9):957–61.

46. Pories WJ, Swanson MS, MacDonald KG, Long SB, Morris PG, Brown BM, et al. Who would have thought it? An operation proves to be the most effective therapy for adult-onset diabetes mellitus. Ann Surg. 1995;222(3):339–50; discussion 50–2.

47. Arterburn DE, Bogart A, Sherwood NE, Sidney S, Coleman KJ, Haneuse S, et al. A multisite study of long-term remission and relapse of type 2 diabetes mellitus following gastric bypass. Obes Surg. 2013;23(1):93–102.

48. Hess DS, Hess DW. Biliopancreatic diversion with a duodenal switch. Obes Surg. 1998;8(3):267–82.

49. Soricelli E, Casella G, Di Rocco G, Redler A, Basso N. Longitudinal sleeve gastrectomy: current perspective. Open Access Surg. 2014;7:35–46.

50. Almogy G, Crookes PF, Anthone GJ. Longitudinal gastrectomy as a treatment for the high-risk super-obese patient. Obes Surg. 2004;14(4):492–7.

51. Baltasar A, Serra C, Perez N, Bou R, Bengochea M, Ferri L. Laparoscopic sleeve gastrectomy: a multi-purpose bariatric operation. Obes Surg. 2005;15(8):1124–8.

52. Gagner M, Gumbs AA, Milone L, Yung E, Goldenberg L, Pomp A. Laparoscopic sleeve gastrectomy for the super-super-obese (body mass index >60 kg/m(2)). Surg Today. 2008;38(5):399–403.

53. Boza C, Gamboa C, Salinas J, Achurra P, Vega A, Perez G. Laparoscopic Roux-en-Y gastric bypass versus laparoscopic sleeve gastrectomy: a case–control study and 3 years of follow-up. Surg Obes Relat Dis. 2012;8(3):243–9.

54. Updated position statement on sleeve gastrectomy as a bariatric procedure. Surg Obes Relat Dis. 2010;6(1):1–5.
55. Hoogerboord M, Wiebe S, Klassen D, Ransom T, Lawlor D, Ellsmere J. Laparoscopic sleeve gastrectomy: perioperative outcomes, weight loss and impact on type 2 diabetes mellitus over 2 years. Can J Surg. 2014;57(2):101–5.
56. Melissas J, Koukouraki S, Askoxylakis J, Stathaki M, Daskalakis M, Perisinakis K, et al. Sleeve gastrectomy: a restrictive procedure? Obes Surg. 2007;17(1):57–62.
57. Lee WJ, Chen CY, Chong K, Lee YC, Chen SC, Lee SD. Changes in postprandial gut hormones after metabolic surgery: a comparison of gastric bypass and sleeve gastrectomy. Surg Obes Relat Dis. 2011;7(6):683–90.
58. Thaler JP, Cummings DE. Minireview: Hormonal and metabolic mechanisms of diabetes remission after gastrointestinal surgery. Endocrinology. 2009;150(6):2518–25.
59. Drucker DJ. The role of gut hormones in glucose homeostasis. J Clin Invest. 2007;117(1):24–32.
60. Nguyen NT, Nguyen B, Gebhart A, Hohmann S. Changes in the makeup of bariatric surgery: a national increase in use of laparoscopic sleeve gastrectomy. J Am Coll Surg. 2013;216(2):252–7.
61. Ren CJ, Patterson E, Gagner M. Early results of laparoscopic biliopancreatic diversion with duodenal switch: a case series of 40 consecutive patients. Obes Surg. 2000;10(6):514–23; discussion 24.
62. Hutter MM, Schirmer BD, Jones DB, Ko CY, Cohen ME, Merkow RP, et al. First report from the American College of Surgeons Bariatric Surgery Center Network: laparoscopic sleeve gastrectomy has morbidity and effectiveness positioned between the band and the bypass. Ann Surg. 2011;254(3):410–20; discussion 20–2.
63. Carlin AM, Zeni TM, English WJ, Hawasli AA, Genaw JA, Krause KR, et al. The comparative effectiveness of sleeve gastrectomy, gastric bypass, and adjustable gastric banding procedures for the treatment of morbid obesity. Ann Surg. 2013;257(5):791–7.
64. Schauer PR, Kashyap SR, Wolski K, Brethauer SA, Kirwan JP, Pothier CE, et al. Bariatric surgery versus intensive medical therapy in obese patients with diabetes. N Engl J Med. 2012;366(17):1567–76.
65. Takata MC, Campos GM, Ciovica R, Rabl C, Rogers SJ, Cello JP, et al. Laparoscopic bariatric surgery improves candidacy in morbidly obese patients awaiting transplantation. Surg Obes Relat Dis. 2008;4(2):159–64; discussion 64–5.

Chapter 16
Esophagectomy

Ryan A. Macke and Guilherme M. Campos

Abstract   Resection of the esophagus and proximal stomach followed by reconstruction to reestablish gastrointestinal continuity with a gastric pull-up or other conduit is a complex, multi-step operation that requires considerable attention to detail. An understanding of the surgical anatomy of the esophagus as it courses through the neck, chest, and abdomen is critical, as well as knowledge of the functional changes that occur with this radical change in anatomy.

Esophagectomy is still associated with significant risk of morbidity and mortality, with postoperative morbidity rates of 30–60 % reported in large case series from high volume centers. A technically sound operation, as well as attentive postoperative care and patient education are crucial in order to minimize the risk of post-esophagectomy complications. In

R.A. Macke, MD (✉)
Section of Thoracic Surgery, Division of Cardiothoracic Surgery,
Department of Surgery, University of Wisconsin,
University of Wisconsin School of Medicine and Public Health,
Madison, WI, USA
e-mail: MACKE@surgery.wisc.edu

G.M. Campos, MD, FACS
Division of Bariatric and Gastrointestinal Surgery, Department of
Surgery, Virginia Commonwealth University, 1200 East Broad Street,
PO Box 980519, Richmond, Virginia 23298, USA
e-mail: guilherme.campos@vcuhealth.org

H. Chen (ed.), *Illustrative Handbook of General Surgery*,   265
DOI 10.1007/978-3-319-24557-7_16,
© Springer International Publishing Switzerland 2016

this Chapter we present indications for esophageal resection, standards in pre-operative evaluation and describe common surgical techniques and specific complications.

Keywords Esophagectomy • Esophageal cancer • Complications • Esophageal adenocarcinoma • Ivor Lewis esophagectomy

Introduction

Esophagectomy is considered by many to be one of the most complex and technically challenging gastrointestinal operations performed today. Resection of the esophagus and proximal stomach followed by reconstruction to reestablish gastrointestinal continuity with a gastric pull-up or other conduit (colon or jejunal interposition) is a complex, multi-step operation that requires considerable attention to detail. An understanding of the surgical anatomy of the esophagus as it courses through the neck, chest, and abdomen is critical, as well as knowledge of the functional changes that occur with this radical change in anatomy.

Esophagectomy is associated with significant risk of morbidity and mortality. In 1941, Ochsner and Debakey reported a staggering mortality rate of 72 % in one of the earliest, large series of esophageal resections [1]. Fortunately, with improvements in surgical and anesthetic technique, patient selection, nutritional support, and critical care, mortality rates have declined significantly. A review of 46,692 esophagectomies performed between 1980 and 1988 reported a decrease in mortality to 13 % [2]. A hospital volume relationship has also been established, with mortality rates reported as high as 23.1 % in "low-volume" centers and as low as 8.1 % in "high-volume" centers [3]. More recently, in 2009 an analysis of 2,315 esophagectomies registered in the Society of Thoracic Surgeons' General Thoracic Database reported a mortality rate of 2.7 % for patients treated primarily at tertiary referral centers [4]. Minimally invasive approaches to esophagectomy have been developed in hopes of further improving outcomes. Luketich and colleagues reported a mortality rate of only 0.9 % in a series of 1,011 patients selected for laparoscopic and thoracoscopic esophagectomy [5].

Postoperative morbidity rates of 30–60 % have been reported following esophagectomy [6]. The most common major complications are pulmonary in nature, occurring in approximately 20–40 % of patients, including pneumonia, empyema, and respiratory failure [6]. Anastomotic leaks occur in roughly 10–20 % of cases, with varying degrees of severity and resulting morbidity [6, 7]. Other less common major complications include pulmonary embolism, myocardial infarction, chylothorax, vocal cord palsy, gastric outlet obstruction and gastric conduit ischemic complications. Common minor complications include supraventricular arrhythmias and wound infections. Anastomotic strictures, delayed gastric emptying, and dumping syndrome are complications that occur in the late postoperative period. A technically sound operation, as well as attentive postoperative care and patient education are crucial in order to minimize the risk of post-esophagectomy complications.

Indications

Esophagectomy is most commonly performed for the treatment of esophageal cancer. Invasive adenocarcinoma and squamous cell carcinoma of the middle and distal esophagus without evidence of metastatic disease are standard indications for esophageal resection. Patients with evidence of locoregional nodal metastases, tumors invading the muscularis propria (T2), and tumors invading into the periesophageal adventitia (T3) are typically offered neoadjuvant chemoradiation therapy prior to resection. Tumors invading surrounding structures (T4) that can be completely resected, such as those invading the diaphragm, may also be considered for resection following neoadjuvant therapy. Barrett's esophagus with high-grade dysplasia (HGD) was previously considered an indication for esophagectomy, as many older series reported presence of invasive cancer in the resected specimen in as many as 50 % of patients initially thought to only have HGD. However, with improvements in endoscopic and imaging technology, endomucosal resection (EMR) and/or radiofrequency ablation is now preferred over resection if the lesion can be completely removed with negative margins [8]. Multi-focal HGD within a long segment of Barrett's esophagus and HGD not amenable to complete endomucosal resection or ablation can be considered for esophagectomy given the increased risk for occult invasive carcinoma within the areas of dysplasia. Esophagectomy may also be considered for palliation of unresectable patients who are unable to tolerate oral/enteral intake or for those treated with definitive chemoradiation therapy that subsequently present with local recurrence. However, only a select few are able to tolerate a procedure of this magnitude given their debilitated state and higher risk of morbidity and mortality for what is commonly referred to as "salvage esophagectomy" [9]. Other less invasive therapies, such esophageal stenting and photodynamic therapy, are often better options for this patient population.

Though much less common, esophagectomy may be considered for the management of severe benign esophageal disease, such as end-stage achalasia, multiple failed prior anti-reflux procedures, strictures not amenable to dilation, and unrepairable esophageal perforations or those associated with underlying esophageal pathology (stricture, end-stage achalasia) [10]. The basic approach to esophagectomy remains the same with the exception of omitting the celiac and mediastinal lymph node dissection that is critical in patients undergoing resection for malignant disease.

Preoperative Evaluation

Preoperative work-up should include a physiologic assessment of the patient to determine their candidacy for resection, including cardiac risk stratification and selective pulmonary function testing (i.e., heavy smokers, known chronic pulmonary disease). All cases of suspected cancer should have tissue diagnosis obtained by biopsy with upper endoscopy, as well as a CT-PET scan and endoscopic ultrasonography for appropriate staging. Patients treated with neoadjuvant therapy are typically restaged with a CT or PET-CT approximately 4 weeks after completion of therapy to assess treatment effect and to rule out distant metastatic disease that would preclude resection. Nutritional status should be assessed by history and laboratory data (albumin, prealbumin) prior to treatment. If adequate caloric intake cannot be maintained, a feeding jejunostomy tube should be considered preoperatively (or prior to neoadjuvant therapy) and surgery delayed until the patient has been nutritionally optimized. Upper endoscopy is recommended immediately prior to or at the time of operation to note the exact location of pathology. The proximal and distal extent of tumor, extent of Barrett's esophagus, and presence of other pathology should be noted. Significant extension of tumor beyond the cardia of the stomach may require a gastrectomy for complete resection and colon interposition for reconstruction. Bronchoscopy is recommended for mid-esophageal squamous cell cancers, which are notorious for invasion into the airway (and therefore unresectable). Diagnostic laparoscopy or thoracoscopy should be considered in cases where there is a question of resectability. Patients with evidence of unresectable malignant disease or those who are unable to tolerate surgical resection should be referred for definitive chemoradiation therapy.

Operative Approach

A variety of esophagectomy surgical techniques have been described over the last century, all of which remain in use today. Each technique uses a different combination of approaches to the esophagus in order to accomplish the main steps of esophagectomy: esophageal and gastric mobilization, lymphadenectomy (in the case of malignant disease), resection of the esophagus and proximal stomach, reestablishment of gastrointestinal continuity (reconstruction), and adjuvant procedures (i.e. pyloric emptying procedure, feeding tube placement). The details of the most common techniques (i.e. Ivor Lewis, McKeown, Transhiatal, Sweet, and Minimally Invasive Esophagectomy) are reviewed later in this chapter, along with the advantages and disadvantages of each. The operation can be separated into stages based on the approach (neck, chest, or abdomen). The basic steps performed in each stage are similar, regardless of the technique used.

Abdomen

The abdominal portion is required for any esophagectomy, regardless of technique, and the basic steps are similar. These steps can be accomplished via an upper midline laparotomy, paramedian laparotomy (as part of a thoracoabdominal incision), or by laparoscopy. First, the abdomen is explored to rule out metastatic disease with careful attention paid to the liver, omentum, and peritoneum. Diagnostic laparoscopy may be performed first to avoid an unnecessary laparotomy should distant metastatic disease be encountered. The left lobe of the liver is retracted to expose the esophageal hiatus. The gastrohepatic ligament is opened to expose the right crus (Fig. 16.1), taking care to preserve a replaced left hepatic artery if present; an accessory left hepatic artery may be divided. The phrenoesophageal ligament is opened and the esophagus is mobilized circumferentially from the hiatus. The intrathoracic esophagus is mobilized, sweeping all periesophageal tissue toward the esophagus (Fig. 16.2). Borders of this dissection include the

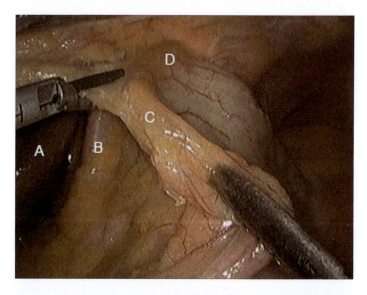

FIGURE 16.1 Division of the gastrohepatic ligament (*A* caudate lobe, *B* right crus, *C* divided gastrohepatic ligament, *D* esophageal hiatus)

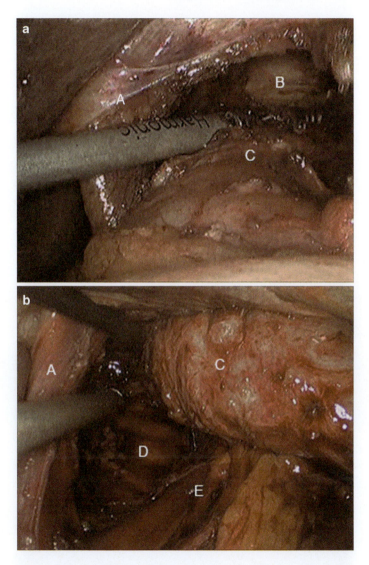

FIGURE 16.2 Esophageal mobilization from the abdomen. The *upper picture* demonstrates dissection along the pericardial plane anteriorly (*A* right crus, *B* pericardium, *C* distal esophagus) and the *lower picture* demonstrates dissection along the aortic plane posteriorly (*D* aortic plane, *E* left crus)

pericardium anteriorly, the aorta posteriorly, and the right and left pleura laterally. The short gastric vessels are then divided to mobilize the greater curve of the stomach. Care must be taken to identify and preserve the right gastroepiploic arcade, which will be the sole blood supply of the gastric conduit (Fig. 16.3). The gastrocolic attachments are divided from left to right beyond the pylorus, maintaining a distance of at least 1–2 cm from the right gastroepiploic vascular arcade. The stomach is retracted anteriorly and the posterior gastric attachments are divided, avoiding injury to the pancreas and splenic artery. The left gastric pedicle is then divided at its origin, making sure to mobilize all fatty and lymphatic tissue toward the specimen before division (Fig. 16.4). The right gastric artery may be preserved. Lymphatic tissue is also dissected off the superior aspect of the splenic artery and swept toward the specimen to obtain an adequate celiac lymphadenectomy. After the stomach has been completely mobilized, the pylorus should easily reach the right crus. If this is not the case, a Kocher maneuver is performed to gain additional mobilization/length. If desired, a

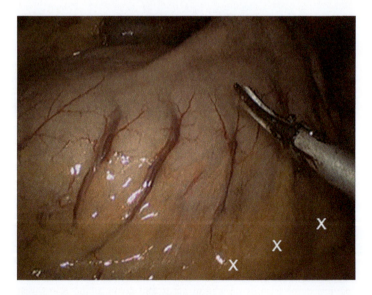

FIGURE 16.3 Right gastroepiploic arcade

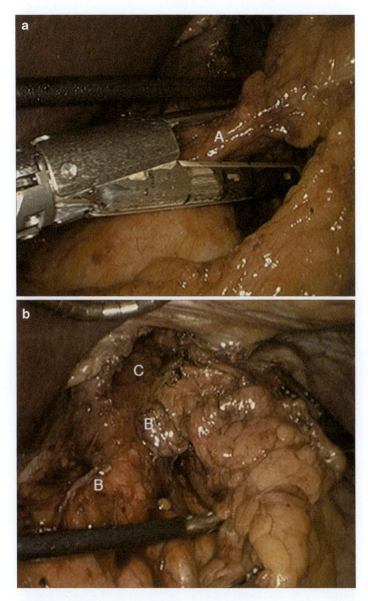

FIGURE 16.4 Division of the left gastric pedicle (*A* left gastric pedicle, *B* divided left gastric pedicle, *C* esophageal hiatus)

gastric-emptying procedure is then performed (i.e., pyloromy-otomy or pyloroplasty). Next, the gastric conduit is fashioned. The staple line is typically started at the third branch of the right gastric artery (Fig. 16.5). A linear stapler with a vascular load is placed across the lesser omentum, directed toward the lesser curve of the stomach, and deployed. The gastric tube is then created by orienting the stapler parallel to the greater curve and marching proximally with serially firings of the stapler, ending to the left of the esophagus (Fig. 16.6). Width of the conduit is varies by surgeon preference. A feeding jejunostomy tube is then placed, if desired (Fig. 16.7). Drains are typically not needed after completing the abdominal stage. If a cervical anastomosis is to be performed, the abdomen is left open and the neck dissection is begun. If an intrathoracic anastomosis is chosen, the conduit it secured to the specimen for later retrieval in the chest and the abdomen is closed.

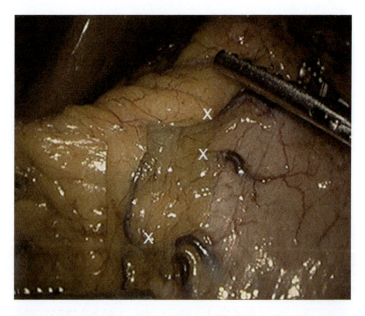

FIGURE 16.5 Branches of the right gastric artery along the lesser curve of the stomach

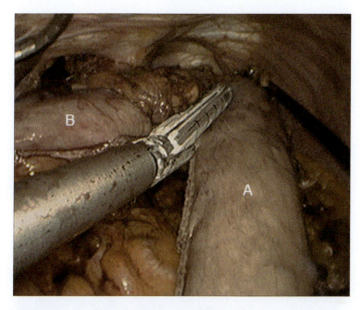

FIGURE 16.6 Creation of the gastric conduit (*A* gastric conduit, *B* specimen including proximal stomach and distal esophagus)

Chest

A transthoracic approach is used for the Ivor Lewis, McKeown, and Minimally Invasive Esophagectomy (MIE) techniques. The basic principles for safe dissection are the same whether performed via thoracotomy, thoracoscopy or robotically. Esophageal mobilization and creation of an intrathoracic anastomosis is typically performed through the right chest. After the right lung has been isolated, the inferior pulmonary ligament is divided and the lung is retracted away. Esophageal mobilization is begun by opening the mediastinal pleura at the junction of the pleura and the lung, anterior to the esophagus, from the diaphragm proximally to the azygous vein. Periesophageal tissue is then swept off the avascular plane along the pericardium toward the esophagus (Fig. 16.8). Dissection is carried superiorly from the

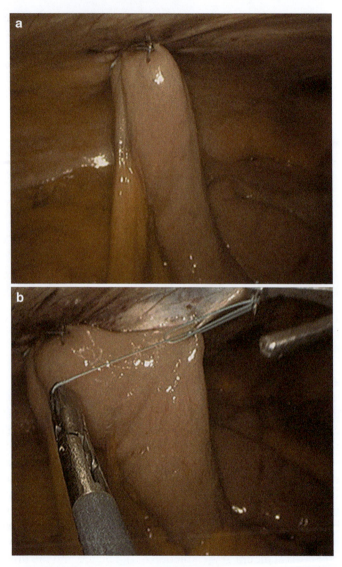

FIGURE 16.7 Laparoscopic jejunostomy tube placement. The *upper picture* demonstrates a loop of jejunum approximately 40 cm distal to the ligament of Treitz tacked up to the abdominal wall. A jejunostomy feeding tube is passed into the distal limb. The *lower picture* demonstrates completion of the jejunostomy tube with an anti-torsion stitch placed 3 cm from the tube entry site

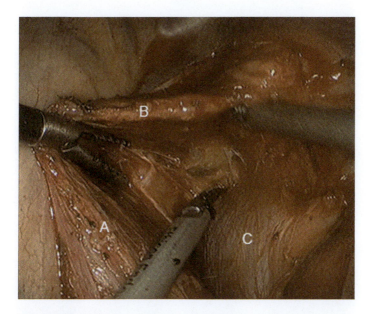

FIGURE 16.8 Mobilization of the intrathoracic esophagus along the pericardial plane (*A* esophagus, *B* periesophageal fat and lymph nodes, *C* pericardium)

inferior pulmonary vein, keeping dissection on the posterior aspect of the pericardium, until the bronchus intermedius is encountered. The airway is then traced back to the right main stem bronchus and subcarinal lymph node packet, which is harvested en bloc. The left main stem bronchus should then come into view. Care must be taken to avoid excess use of energy in this area to minimize the risk of thermal injury to the airway; therefore bronchial arterial branches should be clipped and divided rather than cauterized. The vagus nerve is encountered as dissection is carried proximally, which is divided close the esophagus to avoid traction injury to the right recurrent laryngeal nerve (RLN). The azygous vein is divided as it crosses over the esophagus to empty into the superior vena cava (Fig. 16.9) to facilitate mobilization of the esophagus up to the thoracic inlet

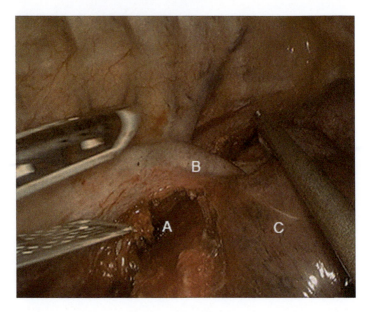

FIGURE 16.9 Division of the azygous vein as it arches over the esophagus (*A* esophagus, *B* azygous vein, *C* lung)

(Fig. 16.10). The mediastinal pleura overlying the posterior aspect of the esophagus is then opened from diaphragm to thoracic inlet. Posterior mobilization is carried out until the anterior/medial plane of dissection is met. Lymphatic and aortoesophageal branches along the posterior aspect of the esophagus should be clipped and divided. The posterior dissection should stay close to the esophagus to avoid injury to the main thoracic duct that lies within the fat posteriorly. Once the esophagus has been circumferentially mobilized, the conduit is retrieved from the abdomen and brought up into the chest. The esophagus is then transected proximal to the tumor to achieve appropriate margins. Intraoperative endoscopy may be performed to confirm the appropriate point of transection. The specimen is then removed and margins are checked by frozen section (Fig. 16.11). The esophagogastric intrathoracic anastomosis is then performed

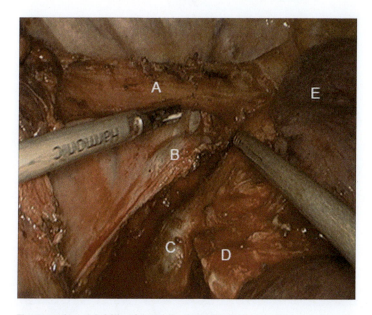

FIGURE 16.10 Mobilization of the intrathoracic esophagus up to the thoracic inlet (*A* esophagus, *B* divided azygous vein, *C* left main stem bronchus, *D* right main stem bronchus, *E* lung)

(discussed below). Drains and/or chest tubes are placed. If a cervical anastomosis is planned, the esophagus is not transected and only mobilization of the esophagus is carried out. The patient is then repositioned to perform the abdominal and cervical stages of the procedure.

Neck

A cervical approach is used for the Transhiatal, Sweet, and McKeown techniques. The MIE may also be performed with a cervical anastomosis. The left neck is preferred because of the more reliable, vertical course of the left RLN and because the esophagus is slightly deviated to the left in the neck. Injury to the RLN occurs primarily by excessive traction or

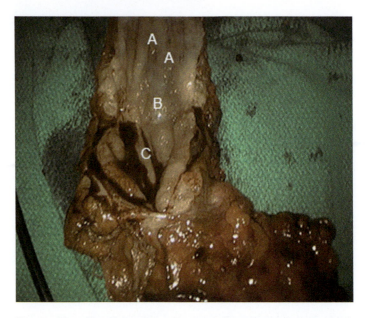

FIGURE 16.11 Esophagogastrectomy specimen opened on the back table to check gross margins prior to being sent for frozen section (*A* esophageal mucosa, *B* tumor, *C* gastric mucosa)

thermal injury from excessive electrocautery use. A 5–6 cm incision is made along the medial border of sternocleidomastoid muscle (SCM). The platysma is first divided and flaps are raised, followed by mobilization of the SCM laterally. Strap muscles are retracted medially. The anterior belly of the omohyoid muscle is typically divided. Dissection is continued medial to the internal jugular and carotid artery, retracting the vessels laterally with the SCM. The middle thyroid vein and inferior thyroid artery may be divided if needed for exposure. The thyroid and trachea are retracted medially and dissection is continued posteriorly down to the spine. The posterior aspect of the cervical esophagus is mobilized from the prevertebral fascia with blunt finger dissection until the esophagus can be hooked with the dissecting finger and retracted laterally into the wound (Fig. 16.12). The anterior aspect of the esophagus is carefully dissected away from the trachea, keeping dissection directly on the esophagus to

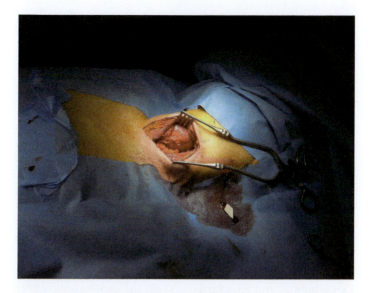

FIGURE 16.12 Left neck incision demonstrating exposure of the proximal esophagus

avoid injury to the RLN in the tracheoesophageal groove. Circumferential mobilization of the esophagus is carried distally into the thoracic inlet until the distal plane of dissection performed from the chest or abdomen is met. The esophagus can then be transected and the specimen removed through the abdominal or neck wound. Once the conduit has been passed up from below, the anastomosis can then be created (discussed below). The neck is closed in layers and a closed suction drain is placed next to the anastomosis.

Esophagogastric Anastomosis

Numerous techniques have been described for creation of the esophagogastric anastomosis, including hand-sewn, stapled, and combined techniques. If the proximal extent of disease is above 25 cm, a cervical anastomosis is recommended to assure adequate margins. Either a cervical or intrathoracic anastomosis can be performed for disease distal to 25 cm. The gastric conduit must pull up easily into the neck or chest to reach the transected esophagus without tension. However, pulling up excessive conduit can result in a redundant conduit that empties poorly.

Hand-sewn Anastomosis

A hand-sewn technique may be used for either a cervical or intrathoracic anastomosis. Most favor a two-layered anastomosis when the hand-sewn technique is used. The tip of the gastric conduit is opened anteriorly approximately 2 cm from the stapled edge. Full-thickness corner stitches are placed at 3 and 9 o'clock to approximate the transected esophagus and gastrotomy. The anastomosis is then started with interrupted 3–0 or 4–0 absorbable suture, taking seromuscular bites on the stomach side and muscularis propria (longitudinal and circular layers) on the esophageal side to create the outer layer back row. The inner layer is then constructed by placing interrupted simple sutures around the entire circumference with full-thickness bites on the stomach side and only mucosa on the esophageal side. The anterior, outer layer is then performed to complete the anastomosis. The anastomosis may also be done with a continuous, running technique.

Linear Stapled Anastomosis

A side-to-side linear-stapled technique may also be used to create either a cervical or intrathoracic anastomosis. The conduit must have 4–5 cm of overlap with the proximal esophagus. A gastrotomy is made on the anterior aspect of the conduit, approximately 5 cm from the tip. The esophagus is transected with an oblique angle (anterior aspect left longer than the posterior). The esophagus is overlapped with the gastric conduit (esophagus anterior to the conduit). Stay sutures are placed at the anterior corner of the esophagus and another from the posterior corner of the esophagus to the superior corner of the gastrotomy. A 3 cm linear stapler is positioned with one jaw in the esophagus and the other in the conduit with the tip of the stapler directed cephalad, then fired. The remaining open portion is closed with two running full-thickness sutures followed by an outer interrupted, circumferential seromuscular layer.

EEA/End-to-Side Stapled Anastomosis

An end-to-side stapled technique may be used for creation of an intrathoracic anastomosis and is the authors' favored technique [11]. The esophagus is divided at the desired level, typically superior to the divided azygous vein, with a linear stapler (Fig. 16.13). We prefer to use a 25-mm Orvil anvil (OrVil, Autosuture, Norwalk, CT, USA), which is a device that mounts the anvil on a 90-cm long polyvinyl chloride

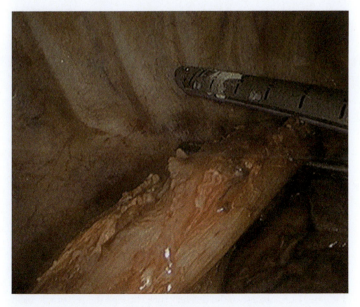

FIGURE 16.13 Division of the proximal esophagus above the azygous vein to complete the esophageal resection

delivery tube. The delivery tube is passed transorally, similar to a nasogastric tube, and advanced into the remaining proximal esophagus. A small opening is made in the center of the staple line of the divided esophageal stump and the delivery tube is pulled distally until the anvil shaft protrudes through the esophagotomy and the anvil head is seated in the distal stump (Fig. 16.14). The delivery tube is detached by cutting the securing stich and the tube is removed. The gastric conduit is then pulled up further into the chest to assure that it will reach the proximal esophagus. The tip of the conduit is opened parallel to the staple line enough to allow the head of a 25-mm EEA stapler (EEA XL 25-mm with 4.8-mm staples, autosuture, Norwalk, CT, USA) to be inserted (Fig. 16.15). Once the stapler head has been inserted into the gastrotomy, the conduit is pulled onto the stapler for a few centimeters. It

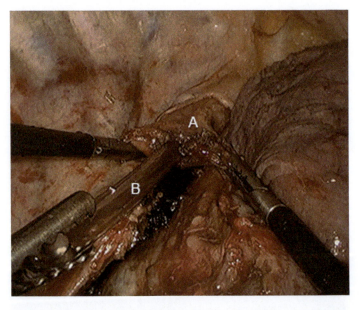

FIGURE 16.14 Passage of the delivery tube through the proximal esophageal stump for anvil placement using the OrVil device (*A* esophageal stump, *B* delivery tubing)

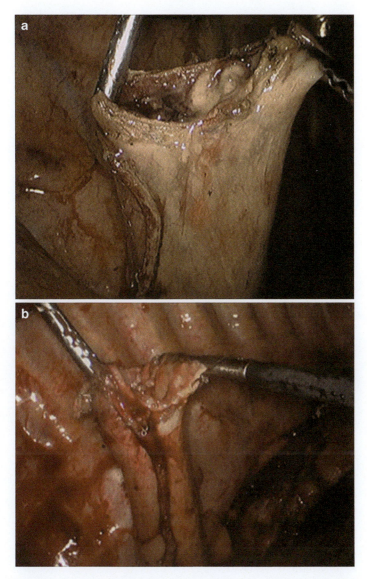

FIGURE 16.15 The gastric conduit is pulled up into the chest and opened along the staple line at the tip (**a**) the conduit is oriented with the staple line to the patient's right (facing the surgeon) (**b**) the EEA stapler head is then inserted into the conduit lumen (**c**) and the conduit is pulled up onto the stapler neck (**d**)

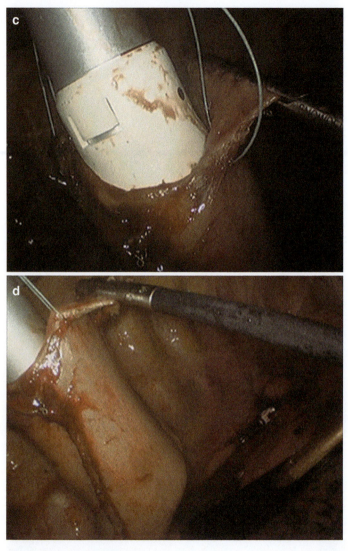

FIGURE 16.15 (continued)

is important to avoid twisting of the conduit once the stapler head is inserted, keeping the staple line to the patient's right (Fig. 16.15). The stapler pin is then brought out through the wall of the conduit opposite the staple line and docked with the anvil (Fig. 16.16). The stapler is fired after making sure surrounding tissue has been cleared. Once the stapler has been removed, two complete anastomotic rings (one from the esophagus side and the other from the gastric side) should be removed from the stapler. This creates an end (esophagus) to side (conduit) anastomosis, which avoids using the gastric conduit tip (which is usually slightly ischemic). The excess conduit is then resected with a linear stapler, making sure to avoid crossing of the staple lines (Fig. 16.17). The gastric conduit should appear well perfused and appropriately oriented with the staple line facing the surgeon (Fig. 16.18). Alternatively, the esophagus can be

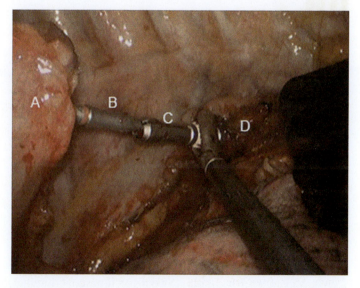

FIGURE 16.16 The pin of the EEA stapler is brought out the side of the gastric conduit opposite the staple line and docked with the anvil that has been seated in the proximal esophageal stump (*A* gastric conduit, *B* EEA stapler pin, *C* anvil, *D* proximal esophageal stump)

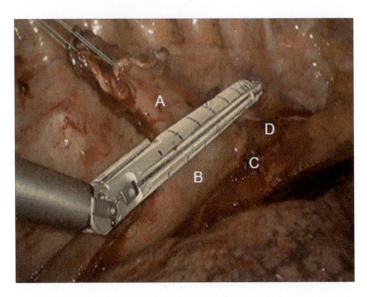

FIGURE 16.17 Once the end-to-side esophagogastric anastomosis is completed, the excess conduit/conduit tip is resected, making sure not to cross the staple lines (*A* excess conduit/conduit tip, *B* gastric conduit, *C* esophagogastric anastomosis, *D* proximal esophagus)

transected with scissors and a 25-mm or 28-mm EEA stapler anvil is placed into the esophagus and secured with two purse string sutures. All layers of the esophagus, including the mucosa, should be incorporated into the purse string. Once the anvil is secured, the end-to-side esophagogastric anastomosis is completed, as described above.

Operative Techniques

Throughout the last century, a number of esophagectomy techniques have been popularized, including Transhiatal, Ivor Lewis, McKeown (or 3-hole), Sweet (or thoracoabdominal) and Minimally Invasive Esophagectomy (MIE) techniques. Significant controversy persists regarding which open approach is best. The MIE has been developed over the last two decades, but its definition remains vague (i.e. hybrid,

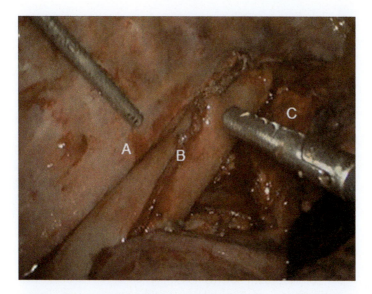

FIGURE 16.18 Complete end-to-side, intrathoracic esophagogastric anastomosis (*A* spine, *B* gastric conduit, *C* airway)

hand-assisted, laparoscopic, thoracoscopic, and robotic techniques), making comparison with open approaches difficult. Factors to consider when deciding between these operative strategies include surgeon experience, tumor location, pulmonary reserve, history of previous operations, indication (malignant or benign pathology), and availability of conduit for reconstruction. The basic principles and steps of each approach were reviewed previously. The steps specific to each technique and the strengths/ weaknesses of each are discussed in the following section.

Ivor Lewis Esophagectomy (ILE)

The ILE consists of an upper midline laparotomy followed by repositioning and right thoracotomy for resection and reconstruction with an intrathoracic anastomosis. With the patient supine, the abdominal stage is performed first. After ruling out metastatic disease, the stomach is mobilized, the left gastric is pedicle divided and celiac lymphadenectomy are performed, the gastric conduit is created, and adjunct procedures (i.e. pyloroplasty and J-tube) completed. The tip of the conduit is attached to the specimen for later retrieval in the chest. The abdomen is closed and the patient is repositioned in the left lateral decubitus position. Single-lung ventilation is initiated (a double-lumen endotracheal tube or bronchial blocker is required to isolate the right lung). Following right thoracotomy, the intrathoracic esophagus is mobilized and mediastinal lymphadenectomy is performed. The conduit is then pulled up into the chest, the esophagus is transected proximal to the disease, and the specimen is removed. The intrathoracic esophagogastric anastomosis is then performed. After the chest has been washed out, drains/chest tubes are placed and the chest is closed.

ILE is an ideal operative strategy for mid-esophageal and distal esophageal tumors, as this approach allows excellent visualization for complete mobilization of the esophagus and lymphadenectomy. The number of lymph nodes harvested tends to be greater with a thoracic approach and the risk of vocal cord paralysis is lower by avoiding the neck dissection needed for a cervical anastomosis [5, 12]. Anastomotic leaks are less common, presumably due to less tension on the intrathoracic anastomosis in comparison to a cervical anastomosis where the conduit must be pulled up for a greater distance [12, 13]. Historically, intrathoracic anastomotic leaks tended to result in greater morbidity due to associated mediastinal sepsis or empyema. However, appropriately placed drains and percutaneous drainage techniques have resulted in less morbidity from intrathoracic leaks in the current era. Pulmonary complications and more postoperative pain are the primary negatives of the ILE, attributed mainly to the thoracotomy.

Transhiatal Esophagectomy (THE)

THE consists of an upper midline laparotomy combined with a left neck incision for creation of a cervical anastomosis. The patient is placed in the supine position and both the neck and abdomen are prepped into the field. Only a single-lumen endotracheal tube is needed. The abdominal stage is carried out in similar fashion to the ILE, however much of the intra-thoracic esophageal mobilization is performed by blunt dissection. As much of the esophageal mobilization as possible is performed under direct vision from the abdomen and neck to divide aortoesophageal branches and other attachments. The remaining mobilization is performed blindly with the surgeon's left hand inserted through the neck incision and the right hand through the abdominal incision. Blunt dissection is performed to free up any remaining attachments until the dissection planes from above and below are met. Bleeding is not uncommon during the blunt dissection, as aortoesopha-geal branches are blindly avulsed. However, most bleeding is stopped by packing the mediastinum. Once the esophagus is completely mobilized, it is divided in the neck proximally and the specimen is removed through the abdominal wound. The conduit is then brought up into the neck to create the cervical anastomosis. One technique used to bring the conduit up into the neck is to pass a Penrose drain or chest tube from the neck to the abdomen. The tip of the conduit is attached to the tube or drain and the conduit is then gently pushed/pulled up through the mediastinum and delivered into the neck. The cervical esophagogastric anastomosis is then performed.

THE is a useful technique for benign disease that does not require a lymphadenectomy, but may also be used for malignant lesions located in the middle and lower esopha-gus. However, THE may be contraindicated for bulky tumors in the middle esophagus that may be adherent to mediastinal structures. Avoiding a thoracotomy has resulted in fewer pulmonary complications and less postoperative pain, which makes the THE an ideal approach for those with significant pulmonary disease [12, 13]. Operative time tends to be shorter, as there is no need to reposition the patient during the course of the procedure. Cervical anastomotic leaks tend to be associated with less morbidity, as simple opening of the wound is all that is needed in most cases and contamination of the mediastinum or pleural space is uncommon. Downsides of THE include harvesting of fewer lymph nodes, greater blood loss, and higher incidence of injury to intrathoracic structures due to the blunt mediastinal dissection [6, 12, 13]. Although cervical anastomotic leaks tend to be easier to manage in the peri-operative period and are associated with less morbidity, they occur more frequently and also develop strictures at a higher rate. The higher leak and stricture rate of cervical anastomoses are presumably from increased tension placed on the anastomosis. The neck dissection also increases the risk of recurrent laryngeal nerve injury, which is commonly associated with postoperative aspiration.

McKeown (Three-Hole) Esophagectomy

Three incisions are required for the McKeown technique: a right thoracotomy, an upper midline laparotomy, and a left neck incision. The right chest is entered first to carry out mobilization of the intrathoracic esophagus and mediastinal lymphadenectomy. Once the esophagus has been mobilized, the chest is closed without dividing the esophagus. The patient is then placed in the supine position and the remainder of the procedure is carried out in similar fashion to the THE. However, blunt mediastinal dissection is not required, as the intrathoracic esophagus has already been completely mobilized.

The McKeown esophagectomy has both the advantages and disadvantages of the ILE and THE. An additional incision increases the chance of wound complications and increased postoperative pain. A unique advantage to this technique is that pathology at any level can be addressed.

Sweet or Left Thoracoabdominal Esophagectomy

The Sweet technique utilizes a left thoracoabdominal incision and neck incision for creation of a cervical anastomosis, as the aortic arch prevents creation of a high intrathoracic anastomosis. The patient is positioned in a modified right lateral decubitus position with the abdomen and hips tilted slightly posteriorly. Left lung is isolation is required. The incision extends from just below the scapular tip, along the 6th or 7th intercostal space, across the costal margin, and then obliquely onto the upper abdomen in a paramedian fashion. The abdominal portion of the incision is made first and once resectability is confirmed, the thoracotomy is made and the incisions are connected by sharply dividing the costal margin. The diaphragm is incised circumferentially for 8–10 cm, leaving a 2 cm cuff for closure. This excellent exposure allows for completion of both the abdominal and chest stages through a single incision. After resection, the conduit is passed beneath the aortic arch and the cervical stage with a cervical anastomosis is completed. The diaphragm is closed and the costal margin is reapproximated with figure-of-eight sutures. The thoracoabdominal incision is then closed in layers after drains are placed.

The Sweet esophagectomy is ideal for locally advanced distal esophageal tumors, such as tumors invading the diaphragmatic hiatus, as this wide exposure provides optimal access to the hiatus and gastroesophageal junction (Fig. 16.19). The main disadvantages of this technique include increased postoperative pain owing to the large incision, as well as risk of costal arch dehiscence and diaphragm dysfunction.

Minimally Invasive Esophagectomy (MIE)

The MIE is technically challenging and requires significant minimally invasive surgical expertise. The learning curve is steep with an estimated 35–40 MIE's needed for a surgeon to become proficient from a technical and patient-care standpoint [14]. Although open esophagectomy techniques continue to be favored by the majority of surgeons today, the number of centers performing MIE continues to increase [6]. A totally minimally invasive esophagectomy is performed with only laparoscopy and thoracoscopy, avoiding rib spreading, rib resection, or hand-assistance and is the authors' favored technique when technically feasible. Hybrid procedures are those in which either the abdominal phase or the thoracic phase is performed open. Alternatively, a

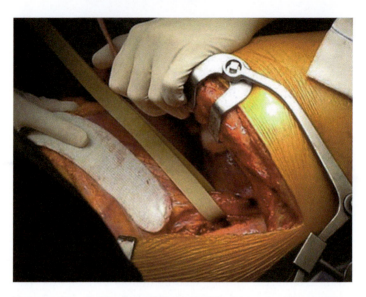

FIGURE 16.19 A left thoracoabdominal incision provides excellent exposure to the distal esophagus and hiatus

hand-assisted port may be added to facilitate the operation. The steps of the procedure are identical to that of the ILE if the anastomosis is to be placed in the chest. If a cervical anastomosis is needed, a neck incision is added and the steps are carried out in similar fashion to the McKeown or transhiatal esophagectomy techniques. Port size and location is variable by surgeon. Five to six ports are typically used for the abdominal stage and 4–5 ports are used for the chest stage (Fig. 16.20). A diaphragm retraction stitch placed in the tendinous portion of the diaphragm can be used to improve visualization of the distal esophagus during the thoracoscopic approach (Fig. 16.21). The specimen is removed through the neck wound for a McKeown or transhiatal MIE, while one of the chest port sites is extended to 4-cm and the specimen is removed without rib spreading for an Ivor Lewis MIE. Proper port placement is critical, making sure ports are spaced sufficiently enough apart to avoid

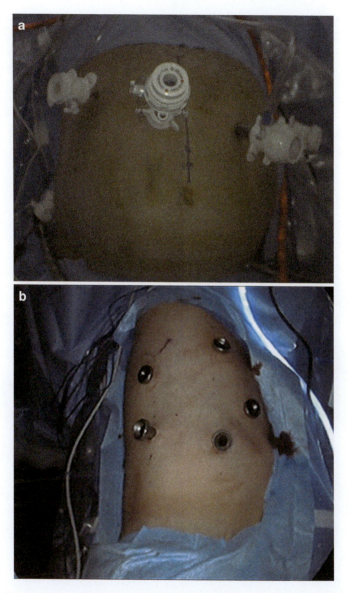

FIGURE 16.20 Port placement for laparoscopic-thoracoscopic Ivor Lewis MIE. The *upper picture* demonstrates port placement for the laparoscopic approach to the abdomen. The *lower picture* demonstrates port placement in the right chest for the thoracoscopic approach

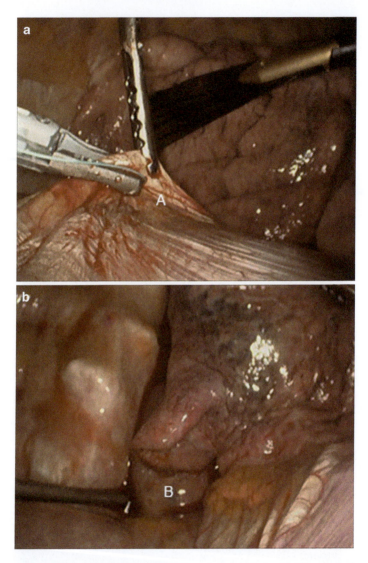

FIGURE 16.21 Diaphragm stitch placed to improve visualization of the distal esophagus (*A* tendinous portion of diaphragm, *B* distal esophagus)

crossing of instruments and poor angles. The majority of images provided in this chapter were obtained from laparo-scopic-thoracoscopic MIE's, demonstrating the excellent visualization provided during these operations. A high-defi-nition camera with an angled 30- or 45° scope typically pro-vides the best views.

Advantages and disadvantages are similar to the corre-sponding open technique used for MIE. Additional advantages of the minimally-invasive approach include less postoperative pain, fewer pulmonary complications, less intraoperative blood loss, and shorter lengths of stay [5, 6, 15]. Although there is no absolute contraindication to MIE, relative contraindications include a history of multiple prior thoracic or abdominal sur-geries, bulky T3 or T4 tumors, preoperative radiation therapy, and morbid obesity. Resectable T4 tumors invading surround-ing structures are likely best approached in an open fashion. It is recommended that surgeons earlier on in their learning curve select early stage esophageal tumors, such as Barrett's esophagus with HGD, T1 (invading the lamina propria or sub-mucosa), or T2 (invading muscularis propria) lesions without previous neoadjuvant therapy.

References

1. Ochsner A, Debakey M. Surgical aspects of carcinoma of the esophagus: review of the literature and report of four cases. J Thorac Cardiovasc Surg. 1941;10:401–45.
2. Earlam R, Cunha-Melo JR. Oesophageal squamous cell carci-noma: I. A critical review of surgery. Br J Surg. 1980;67(6): 381–90.
3. Birkmeyer JD, Siewers AE, Finlayson EV, et al. Hospital volume and surgical mortality in the United States. N Engl J Med. 2002;346:1128–37.
4. Wright CD, Kucharczuk JC, O'Brien SM, et al. Predictors of major morbidity and mortality after esophagectomy for esopha-geal cancer: a society of thoracic surgeons general thoracic sur-gery database risk adjustment model. J Thorac Cardiovasc Surg. 2009;137:587–95.

5. Luketich JD, Pennathur A, Awais O, et al. Outcomes after minimally invasive esophagectomy: review of over 1000 patients. Ann Surg. 2012;256:95–103.
6. Schuchert MJ, Luketich JD, Landreneau RJ. Management of esophageal cancer. Curr Probl Surg. 2010;47(11):845–946.
7. Kassis ES, Kosinski AS, Ross P, et al. Predictors of anastomotic leak after esophagectomy: an analysis of the society of thoracic surgeons general thoracic database. Ann Thor Surg. 2013; 96(6):1919–26.
8. NCCN Clinical Practice Guidelines in Oncology. Esophageal and esophagogastric junction cancers (version 1.2014). http://www.nccn.org/professionals/physician_gls/pdf/esophageal.pdf. Accessed 27 July 2014.
9. Swisher SG, Wynn P, Putnam JB, et al. J Thorac Cardiovasc Surg. 2002;123:175–83.
10. Orringer MB, Marshall B, Iannettoni MD. Transhiatal esophagectomy for treatment of benign and malignant esophageal disease. World J Surg. 2001;25(2):196–203.
11. Campos GM, Jablons D, Brown LM, Ramirez RM, Rabl C, Theodore P. A safe and reproducible anastomotic technique for minimally invasive Ivor Lewis oesophagectomy: the circular-stapled anastomosis with the trans-oral anvil. Eur J Cardiothorac Surg. 2010;37(6):1421–6.
12. Boshier PR, Anderson O, Hanna GB. Transthoracic versus transhiatal esophagectomy for the treatment of esophagogastric cancer: a meta-analysis. Ann Surg. 2011;254(6):894–906.
13. Hulscher JB, Tijssen JG, Obertop H, et al. Transthoracic versus transhiatal resection for carcinoma of the esophagus: a meta-analysis. Ann Thorac Surg. 2001;72(1):306–13.
14. Tapias LF, Morse CR. Minimally invasive Ivor Lewis esophagectomy: description of a learning curve. J Am Coll Surg. 2014; 218(6):1130–40.
15. Biere SS, van Berge Henegouwen MI, Mass KW, et al. Minimally invasive versus open oesophagectomy for patietns with oesophageal cancer: a multicentre, open-label, randomised controlled trial. Lancet. 2012;379:1887–92.

Chapter 17
Gastric and Duodenal Surgery

Patrick J. Shabino, Jad Khoraki, and Guilherme M. Campos

Abstract While gastric and duodenal surgeries for peptic ulcer disease (PUD) were, until the late 1980s, among the most common general surgical procedures; now surgery is reserved for tumors, gastroparesis and infrequent complications of PUD such as perforation and obstruction. This dramatic change in the indications for gastric and duodenal surgery has occurred because of the discovery of Helicobacter Pylori as the main causative agent of PUD and the introduction of effective drug therapies to eliminate the bacteria and reduce gastric acid secretion. In this chapter we will detail the

P.J. Shabino, MD
Department of Surgery, University of Wisconsin School of Medicine and Public Health, University of Wisconsin, Madison, WI, USA

J. Khoraki, MD
Department of Surgery, University of Wisconsin School of Medicine and Public Health, Madison, WI, USA
Department of Surgery, University of Wisconsin Hospital and Clinics, Madison, WI, USA

G.M. Campos, MD, FACS (✉)
Division of Bariatric and Gastrointestinal Surgery, Department of Surgery, Virginia Commonwealth University, 1200 East Broad Street, PO Box 980519 Richmond, Virginia 23298, USA
e-mail: guilherme.campos@vcuhealth.org

H. Chen (ed.), *Illustrative Handbook of General Surgery*,
DOI 10.1007/978-3-319-24557-7_17,
© Springer International Publishing Switzerland 2016

indications and technical aspects of the most common gastric and duodenal operations for complications of PUD and other benign and malignant gastric diseases. Duodenal surgery for other indications is discussed elsewhere in this text.

Keywords Peptic Ulcer Disease • Gastric ulcer • Duodenal perforation • Gastrointestinal bleeding • Gastric surgery • Duodenal surgery

Pyloroplasty

Indications

Current indications for a pyloroplasty include diabetic, idiopathic and post-surgical gastroparesis, pyloric stenosis from PUD and as a concurrent procedure with esophagectomy with gastric pull-up or truncal vagotomy. Gastroparesis is a challenging condition to treat and is frequently seen in patients with type I and type II diabetes; however the etiology of many patients' gastroparesis remains unknown (idiopathic gastroparesis). Post-surgical gastroparesis is seen following truncal vagotomy for ulcer disease or following inadvertent vagotomy during procedures at the gastro-esophageal junction such as laparoscopic hiatal hernia repair or anti-reflux procedures. In the past, peptic ulcer disease causing scarring of the pylorus and subsequent chronic gastric outlet obstruction was a common cause of delayed gastric emptying and an indication for pyloroplasty. However, the introduction of effective drug therapy to eradicate H. pylori as well as antihistamine agents and proton pump inhibitors has made this indication quite rare.

Drug therapy for diabetic, idiopathic or post-surgical gastroparesis is the first line of treatment, but often fails in alleviating patient's symptoms that may require frequent hospital admissions for re-hydration and intravenous medications. Other treatment options for gastroparesis include insertion of feeding tubes (gastrostomy or jejunostomy), implantable gastric electrical stimulation, endoscopic intrapyloric injection of botulinum toxin, or partial gastrectomy, but results vary significantly, and none are without the possibility for complications [1]. Pyloroplasty has also been used with some success in patients with diabetic or idiopathic gastroparesis [2].

Pyloroplasty involves creation of a full thickness division of the pylorus and subsequent closure to open the pylorus and should be distinguished from pyloromyotomy. Pyloromyotomy is usually reserved for the treatment of pyloric stenosis in pediatric patients where only a partial thickness incision through serosa and muscular fibers is made while not opening the underlying mucosa.

There are three main techniques used to attempt to improve pyloric emptying: Heineke-Mikulicz and Finney pyloroplasties and Jaboulay gastroduodenostomy. In addition to treating poor gastric emptying, the Heineke-Mikulicz pyloroplasty is the preferred approach to duodenal bleeding from the gastro-duodenal artery as provides access to the bleeding vessel while allowing subsequent closure without narrowing of the pylorus and proximal duodenum. The Finney pyloroplasty or Jaboulay gastroduodenostomy are preferred when scarring of the pylorus (usually due to peptic ulcer disease) extends into the duodenal bulb and a more extensive surgical repair is required.

All pyloroplasties may be performed with an open approach through an upper midline incision or via laparoscopy, depending on the indication and available expertise. All of these interventions have the possibility for complications such as leak, bile reflux, diarrhea and dumping symptoms.

Heineke-Mikulicz Pyloroplasty

A Heineke-Mikulicz pyloroplasty is the most common type of pyloroplasty performed. The anterior wall of the stomach and junction with the duodenum are identified. A Kocher maneuver may be performed, to allow a tension free anastomosis, by incising the peritoneum lateral to the duodenum and dissecting in the avascular plane posterior to the duodenal sweep.

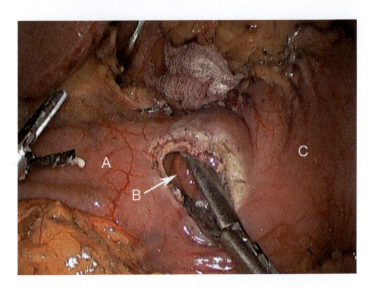

FIGURE 17.1 Laparoscopic pyloroplasty with longitudinal incision across pylorus (*A* duodenum, *B* pylorotomy, *C* stomach)

Two stay sutures may be placed superiorly and inferiorly to the longitudinal axis of the pylorus. An incision is made starting approximately 2 cm proximal to the pylorus and proceeding longitudinally through the pylorus to a point 1 or 2 cm distal on the duodenum. The bowel lumen is opened and examined; hemostasis is obtained (Fig. 17.1). In order to avoid narrowing the bowel lumen, the longitudinal incision is closed in a transverse fashion (Fig. 17.2). This is accomplished with a one or two layer closure. The inner layer is completed with a running or interrupted full-thickness stitch using absorbable monofilament suture, while the outer layer is completed using interrupted sero-muscular stitches (Fig. 17.3).

As with other laparoscopic foregut procedures, patient positioning is critical. Low lithotomy position allows the surgeon to position themselves with better access to the area of interest. The laparoscope monitor should be positioned at the head of the surgical table. The technique is similar to that described in the open case however may benefit from

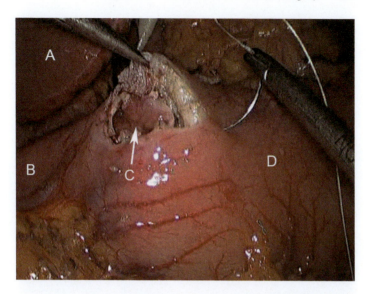

FIGURE 17.2 Closure of enterotomy proceeds transversely; retraction with atraumatic grasper replaces preplaced stay sutures (*A* liver, *B* duodenum, *C* pylorotomy, *D* stomach)

placement of a liver retractor to assist in visualization. An endostitch or similar endoscopic suturing device maybe used to assist in intracorporeal suturing of the enterotomy.

Regardless of the approach used, care should be taken to avoid narrowing the gastric outlet with the closure of the enterotomy. If the cause of gastric outlet obstruction is unclear luminal biopsy should be taken at the time of the procedure.

Finney Pyloroplasty

A Finney Pyloroplasty is better suited to more extensive pyloric narrowing and is conceptually similar to a side-to-side bowel anastomosis. This technique can be used either with an open or laparoscopic approach. Mobilization of the duodenum by a Kocher maneuver is essential to allow approximation of

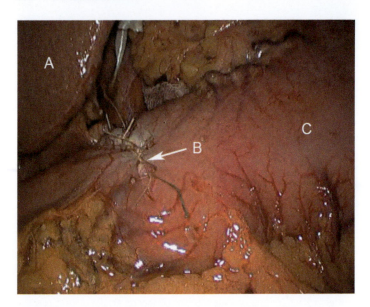

FIGURE 17.3   Completed pyloroplasty (*A* liver, *B* closed enterostomy, *C* stomach)

the suture line without undo tension. An incision is made along the anterior wall of the stomach starting 5 cm proximal to the pylorus and extending longitudinally 5 cm distal on the duodenum. A stay suture is placed at the pylorus superior to the incision; this will form the apex of the anastomosis. Another stitch then joins the distal end of the incision in the duodenum to the proximal end in the stomach thus approximating a cut edge of duodenum to a cut edge of stomach both posteriorly and anteriorly. These edges can then be anastomosed in one or two layers. Again care should be taken with two layer closure not to narrow the new lumen created.

Jaboulay Gastroduodenostomy

A Jaboulay gastroduodenostomy bypasses the area of pyloric narrowing and is best suited to cases where there is active inflammation at the pylorus or the proximal duodenum or an extensive segment of narrowing. Mobilization of the duodenum by a Kocher maneuver is also essential to allow approximation of the suture line without undo tension. Following mobilization of the duodenum the pylorus is left intact and the most proximal area of healthy appearing duodenum is approximated to the distal antrum with a back wall of sero-muscular interrupted silk sutures which will form the second layer of the posterior aspect of the anastomosis. The approximated gastric and duodenal walls are then incised and a full thickness anastomosis is performed using absorbable monofilament suture. The second layer of the anterior aspect of the anastomosis is then completed with interrupted silk Lembert stitches.

Graham Patch

Indications

Perforated peptic duodenal ulcers remain a common cause of pneumoperitoneum, necessitating emergent surgical treatment. Given the emergent nature of the patient's presentation, as well as improvements in medical management of peptic duodenal ulcer disease, a Graham patch repair without any other surgical intervention to reduce gastric acid production is usually preferred to treat perforated duodenal ulcers. For patients with a perforated gastric ulcer, a partial gastrectomy is the optimal treatment, however if the patients clinical status will not allow a formal resection, a wedge resection may be performed. Given the risk that a gastric perforation represents a gastric cancer, simple closure is only an option when the patient's condition is so poor that the surgeon judges it unsafe to proceed with either of the first two options.

A laparoscopic approach is safe when patient condition is stable and may decrease peri-operative morbidity [3]. Data from the National Surgical Quality Improvement Program demonstrated reduction in duration of inpatient stay with the

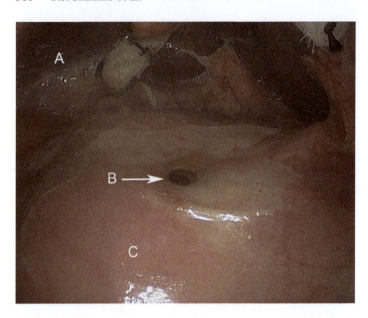

FIGURE 17.4 Duodenal ulcer with perforation (*A* liver, *B* duodenal perforation, *C* duodenum)

laparoscopic approach; however that finding is tempered by the fact that patients offered the open approach may have worse general medical condition at baseline [4].

Surgical Technique – Graham Patch

The traditional approach to the procedure is through an open upper midline incision although this may now be approached with laparoscopy. The wall of the stomach and duodenum are inspected for evidence of perforation. Once the defect is visualized on the duodenum (Fig. 17.4), a healthy portion of omentum is identified and mobilized so it can reach the defect without tension. Interrupted full thickness stay sutures of silk, vicril or PDS are placed bridging the defect, taking care not to incorporate the posterior bowel wall (Fig. 17.5). These sutures are only approximated after the mobilized

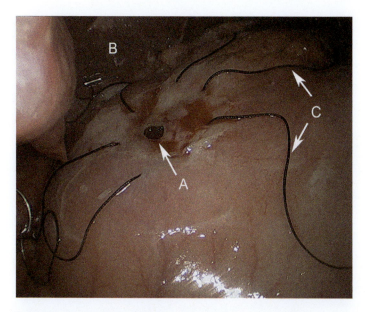

FIGURE 17.5 Stay sutures placed across ulcer defect with wide full thickness bites (*A* duodenal ulcer, *B* liver, *C* stay sutures)

portion of omentum is brought on top of the perforation and then secured within the loop of the sutures as they are tied. The basic concept of the Graham Patch is to 'patch' the perforation with the omentum and not to close the defect by approximating it with the sutures. Attempts to close the perforation primarily may lead to duodenal stenosis or tearing of the inflamed tissues. Care is taken to avoid securing the omentum too tightly and compromising blood flow to the omental patch (Fig. 17.6). The abdominal cavity is then irrigated and suctioned clean.

As is seen in other cases of foregut surgery, positioning of the operator to reach the superior portion of the abdomen is essential. The patient positioning should be performed as described in the preceding section. Standard laparoscopic sutures with a SH needle and 2 or 3-0 sutures should be used; the endostitch or similar laparoscopic suturing device should be avoided as their needles are bulkier and may disrupted the inflamed tissues.

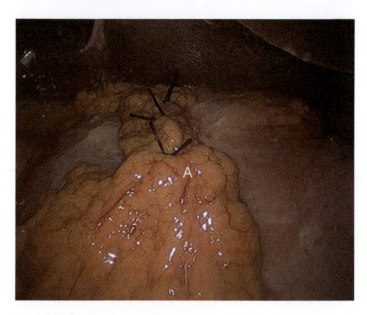

FIGURE 17.6 Completed graham patch (*A* tongue of omentum)

Vagotomy and Antrectomy

Indications

Typically reserved for recalcitrant peptic ulcer disease, the use of vagotomy and antrectomy is rare nowadays as medical therapy has improved. While vagotomy with antrectomy is quite effective in cases of persistent peptic ulcer disease with an estimated rate of recurrence of 0–2 %, it has potential for substantial morbidity. Surgery is reserved for those patients with recalcitrant disease or contraindication to medical therapy [5, 6]. When considering patients for surgical treatment of peptic ulcer disease, other causes of ulceration including neoplasm, Crohn's disease and gastrinoma, should be excluded.

Vagotomy interrupts neural stimulation of acid secretion from parietal cells as promoted by acetylcholine release at the cell membrane. Three types of vagotomy were commonly used; truncal, selective or highly selective vagotomy. The pylorus is denervated with a truncal vagotomy, necessitating a gastric emptying procedure such as a pyloroplasty. Selective or highly selective vagotomies are almost never used in current surgical practice.

Antrectomy focuses on removing the site of gastrin production from antral G cells which subsequently stimulates acid secretion. The sites of mucosal injury and ulceration may also be resected with antrectomy, further promoting cure.

Surgical Technique – Vagotomy

Truncal Vagotomy

Truncal Vagotomy focuses on identifying and dividing the left and right vagus above the level of the crura. This procedure has moved to the forefront of surgical management of peptic ulcer disease as the incidence of elective surgery for this problem fades and with it surgeon experience with selective vagotomy. Of note, this procedure warrants a concurrent gastric emptying procedure as the pylorus is denervated along with the acid secreting parietal cells.

Via an upper midline laparotomy incision or laparoscopic surgery, the gastrohepatic ligament in incised and the esophageal hiatus is identified. Phrenoesophageal attachments are divided and the esophagus is encircled. Gentle spreading along the anterior esophagus will reveal the left vagus nerve. The right vagus is identified tracking posteriorly alongside the esophageal wall. Each nerve should be isolated, clipped proximally and distally and a 1 cm segment resected between the clips and sent to pathology for review. The nerves must be transected above the level of the hiatus so as to ensure the criminal nerve of grassi does not remain intact and cause recurrence.

Surgical Technique – Antrectomy

Antrectomy targets the site of gastrin production. At the completion of the procedure, the resected specimen should represent about 35 % of the total stomach. After visualizing the upper abdomen through an upper midline incision or via laparoscopy and retracting the liver, the gastrohepatic ligament is incised and the left gastric artery is ligated. The gastrocolic ligament is carefully dissected proximal to the main gastroepiploic arcade. Branching vessels to the greater curvature of the stomach are ligated. The dissection along the greater curve continues proximally to a point across the organo-axis from the incisura and distally to the pylorus. The stomach can then be transected proximally from the end of the proximal dissection along the greater curvature to the midpoint of the lesser curve. The antrum extends more proximally along lesser curve necessitating the more proximal resection on this aspect of the stomach. The antrum is then lifted anteriorly and dissected away from the pancreas posteriorly. The antrectomy is completed with transection of the duodenum just distal to the pylorus. A distal margin should be sent to confirm the presence of Brunner's glands to avoid retained antrum. Kocherization of the duodenum may be a reasonable step prior to duodenal transection depending on the plan for reconstruction of continuity. Gastrointestinal continuity is restored either with a gastro-duodenostomy (Billroth I anastomosis) or a gastrojejunostomy (Billroth II or Roux-en-Y anastomosis).

Gastric Wedge Resection, Partial, Sub-total and Total Gastrectomy

Indications, Extent of Gastric Resection, Lymphadenectomy, and Reconstructions

Gastric neoplasms represent the most common indication for gastric resection. Masses in the stomach typically fall into one of three groups: gastric adenocarcinoma, gastrointestinal stromal tumor (GIST) and lymphoma. While lymphoma is typically treated non-operatively, both GIST and adenocarcinoma are indications for gastric resection. The majority of patients with gastric masses will present with epigastric fullness, dyspepsia, pain or bleeding. The evaluation of a gastric mass can include cross-sectional imaging with computed tomography, endoscopy with cold forceps biopsy, and/or endoscopic ultrasound with fine needle aspiration (FNA) biopsy [7].

The extent of gastric resection and type of lymphadenectomy should be chosen based on individual patient and tumor characteristics. Wedge resection is reserved for selected GIST that can be completely excised without a formal resection, partial gastrectomy can be used for GIST or rare complications from PUD and subtotal or total gastrectomies are the preferred options for patients with gastric adenocarcinoma.

GISTs are rare tumors that are typically located in the stomach. These tumors arise from the cells of Cajal which are part of the autonomic nervous system of the stomach. These tumors express Kit protein, a tyrosine kinase receptor, and many express CD34. Diagnosis is confirmed with FNA. Surgery is indicated with goal of a grossly negative margin, and non-anatomical wedge resections are usually employed [8]. Care is taken to not to spill tumor contents during resection out of concern for seeding the peritoneal cavity. GISTs usually do not spread via the lymph system, therefore lymphadenectomy is not indicated. Imatinib mesylate is commonly used as neoadjuvant therapy from 3 to 6 months to decrease tumor size and/or allow for wedge or complete resections. Imatinib is also used as adjuvant therapy after surgery in many cases.

The incidence of gastric adenocarcinoma has declined in the past century. Epidemiologic studies have linked this disease to a diet high in nitrates, lower socioeconomic status, Helicobacter pylori, chronic atrophic gastritis and Asian heritage. Gastric adenocarcinoma diagnosis is confirmed with endoscopic biopsy, and patients should be evaluated for precise location and extent of the tumor and metastatic disease with computed tomography of the chest and abdomen. If no evidence of metastatic disease is found, endoscopic ultrasonography should be performed to assess depth of invasion and to evaluate regional lymph node basins. Should involvement of the aorta, vena cava or celiac axis be identified the tumor is considered unresectable [7].

The extent of gastric resection is chosen based on tumor location. A sub-total gastrectomy is usually chosen for patients with tumors below the incisura angularis and at least 6 cm from the GE junction. A total gastrectomy is typically needed for patients with tumor above the incisura angularis, in the gastric body or fundus or less than 6 cm from the GE junction.

Gastric adenocarcinoma readily metastasizes via the lymph system and lymphadenectomy is recommended during surgical resection with curative intent. The extent of lymphadenectomy has been controversial for many years, and early data from studies performed in western countries (the Dutch D1D2 gastric cancer trial [9] and the MRC Trial [10]) showed that a more limited lymphadenectomy (D1) was associated with improved peri-operative outcomes and similar oncologic outcomes. However since that time, other studies and also a 15 year follow up of the Dutch D1D2 Trial have demonstrated a benefit to accurate staging and also to survival with a D2 lymph node dissection [11–14]. A D2 lymph nodal dissection involves omentectomy with clearance of the peri-gastric, hepatic artery, porta-hepatis, splenic, right gastroepiploic, sub-pyloric and base of left gastric artery/celiac lymph nodes. The addition of splenic hilum nodes (level 10), splenectomy and/or distal pancreatectomy, or a peri-aortic lymph nodal dissection (D3 lymph node dissection) has been shown to increase peri-operative morbidity without improving survival [15]. As such, most centers specialized in gastric cancer treatment do advocate for a complete D2 lymphadenectomy (without level 10, splenectomy and/or distal pancreatectomy) when performing gastrectomy for cancer with curative intent.

After a formal resection of any extent (antrectomy, partial, sub-total or total gastrectomies), a reconstruction of enteric continuity may be accomplished by a gastroduodenostomy (Bilroth I), a gastrojejunostomy (Bilroth II or Roux-en-Y) or a esophagojejunostomy. With any form of pyloric resection and subsequent reconstruction, dumping syndrome may result and patients may experience postprandial diaphoresis, dizziness, flushing and palpitations. Another important technical aspect of any gastrectomy, is to ascertain that the distal transection site is actually made after the pylorus in the pliable duodenum. If the distal transection is erroneously done before the pylorus, it will leave a small portion of gastric antrum; condition referred to as "retained antrum". This becomes important when a BII or Roux-en-Y reconstruction is chosen as the G cells at the blind "retained" antral margin will not be exposed to any acid from the proximal stomach, thus leading to unopposed secretion of gastrin, that in turn may stimulate any remnant of parietal cell mass to secrete excess acid; leading to gastrojejunal ulcerations at the new reconstruction site. Paying close attention to surgical landmarks and sending a distal resection margin for frozen section to identify duodenal Brunner's glands helps to avoid this complication.

In the setting of benign disease or disease allowing for only an antrectomy, a Bilroth I (BI) gastroduodenostomy reconstruction is preferred. This technique is almost never used nowadays, such are the paucity of cases in which it can be employed. Mobilization of the duodenum by a Kocher maneuver usually allows a BI gastroduodenostomy without undue tension. If unable to create a Bilroth I gastroduodenal anastomosis without tension, a Bilroth II or Roux-en-Y gastrojejunostomy must be used.

When a BII reconstruction is chosen, the first loop of jejunum after the ligament of Treitz that will comfortably reach the gastric remnant without tension is identified and mobilized. One can chose a retrocolic or antecolic fashion and create the anastomosis on the anterior or posterior surface of the gastric remnant. A retrocolic approach produces the shortest distance to the gastric remnant and a posterior anastomosis may facilitate drainage. An antecolic limb may have a smaller risk of post-operative obstruction and may be preferred in gastric cancer cases in which local recurrence is possible. The gastrojejunostomy should be iso-peristaltic. The anastomosis may be performed with hand sewn, linear or circular-stapled techniques. A nasogastric tube may be placed and positioned through the gastrojejunostomy.

With a BII reconstruction bile always will flow through the gastric remnant and produces gastritis and in many patients epigastric pain. A Braun enteroenterostomy following Bilroth II may decrease the incidence of bile reflux [16]. Bile reflux is avoided with a properly done and functional Roux-en-Y reconstruction. If severe bile reflux symptoms develop following a Bilroth II, conversion to Roux-en-Y need be considered.

Obstruction following antrectomy with Bilroth II or Roux-en-Y reconstruction poses particular dangers. Obstruction of the afferent loop may occur due to a multitude of causes and lead to duodenal distension. Most concerning in the immediate post-operative period, afferent loop obstruction may progress to duodenal stump leak. The finding of acute afferent loop distension is a surgical emergency. Operative correction of the inciting defect (redundant afferent limb, internal hernia, adhesions, volvulus) must be undertaken promptly.

Gastric Wedge Resection

In the setting of benign disease or GISTs an anatomic resection may not be necessary. Survival following GIST resection requires microscopically negative margins but a lymphadenectomy is usually not necessary [8]. As such as gastric wedge resection is an appropriate option when the disease is remote from the pylorus and gastroesophageal junction. Lesions located on the greater or lesser curve can be removed with relative ease laparoscopically with intraoperative endoscopy to assist in identifying the lesions. Anterior lesions may be elevated with stay sutures and similarly wedged with a linear stapler. Posterior lesions require dissection of the greater curve from its attachments and elevation to allow the lesion to be isolated and removed with a linear stapler.

Subtotal Gastrectomy

The procedure begins with inspection of the peritoneal cavity and peritoneal washings which are sent for pathologic review. If evidence of metastasis is identified the case is halted. If no evidence of metastatic disease is identified, the procedure continues with omentectomy (Fig. 17.7). An endoscopic energy and vessel sealing device may aid in this dissection.

The surgeon should divide the left gastric, right gastric and right gastroepiploic vessels at their base and excise the surrounding lymph node basins. The base of the right gastroepiploic vessels is exposed by elevating the right gastroepiploic arcade and the greater curvature of the stomach (Fig. 17.8). The right gastroepipolic is divided at its base and the lymph nodes in this region are taken with the gastric specimen (Fig. 17.9). To reach the left gastric artery vessels, the gastrohepatic ligament is incised in the lesser curve of the stomach (Fig. 17.10). The left gastric artery and vein are divided at

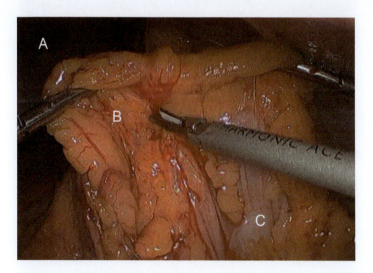

FIGURE 17.7 Omentectomy (*A* liver, *B* omentum, *C* transverse colon)

316   P.J. Shabino et al.

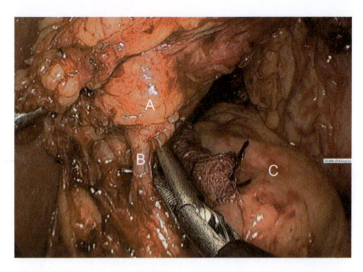

FIGURE 17.8 Right gastroepiploic nodal basin (*A*) and artery (*B*) isolated for division (*C* pancreas)

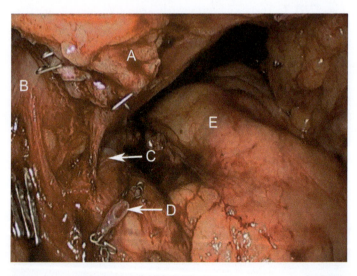

FIGURE 17.9 Dissection of the Right Gastro-epiploic nodal basin and artery – final aspect (*A* node tissue, *B* duodenum, *C* gastroduodenal artery, *D* transected stump of right gastroepiploic artery, *E* pancreas)

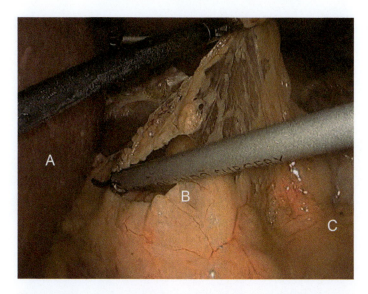

FIGURE 17.10 Gastrohepatic ligament incised (*A* liver, *B* gastrohepatic ligament, *C* stomach)

their base with a linear stapler and lymph nodes in this region are taken with the gastric specimen. All lymphatic tissue is carefully dissected free from the anterior surface of the celiac axis. This dissection is carried over the common hepatic artery to the right of the porta hepatis and above the splenic artery, close but not into the splenic hilum.

After the duodenum has been mobilized and dissected away from the pancreas and GDA, lymphatic tissue is resected from the sub-pyloric region, and anterior and superior to the pancreas. The duodenum is divided with a GIA stapler (Fig. 17.11). Then most of the stomach is removed by transecting at a proximal level to leave only the gastric fundus (Fig. 17.12), which sole blood supply will come from the short gastric vessels. Gastrointestinal continuity is restored with a gastrojejunostomy (Classic Billroth II or Roux-en-Y anastomosis). A Roux-en-Y reconstruction is preferred: after completion of the gastric resection, an appropriate segment of jejunum is identified and transected with a linear stapler about 30 cm from the ligament of Treitz (Fig. 17.13). The

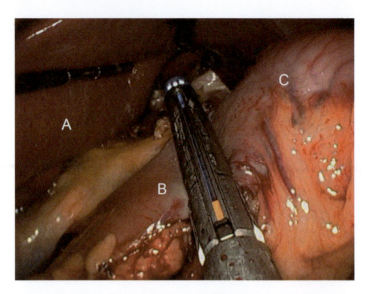

FIGURE 17.11 Duodenum is divided (*A* liver, *B* duodenum, *C* stomach)

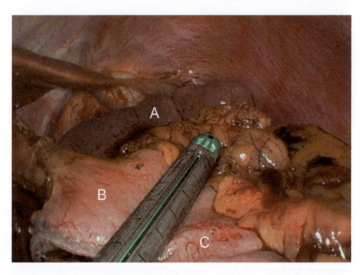

FIGURE 17.12 Stomach transection (*A* spleen, *B* gastric pouch, *C* resected stomach)

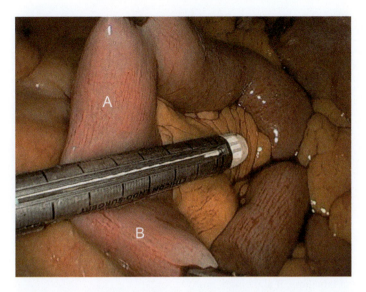

FIGURE 17.13 Division of jejunum creating biliopancreatic and alimentary limbs (*A* biliopancreatic limb, *B* alimentary limb)

mesentery is then divided to allow the alimentary jejunal limb (the distal limb) to reach comfortably the upper abdomen and the gastric remnant. The proximal limb (bilio-pancreatic limb) is then reconnected to the alimentary limb 60–70 cm distal to the proximal end of the alimentary limb. The jejunojejunostomy connecting the alimentary to the biliopancreatic limb may be created immediately after transecting the jejunum. We favor a side-to-side linear stapled jejunojejunostomy (Fig. 17.14). The resulting mesenteric defect is then closed with a running locking stitch (Fig. 17.15). Debate exists whether an antecolic or retrocolic alimentary limb is superior. An antecolic approach is shown. The alimentary limb is laid adjacent to the gastric remnant after it has been brought over the transverse colon. The anastomosis may be completed in hand sewn, linear or circular-stapled fashion. In the circular stapled technique a 25 mm anvil is passed trans-orally and the stapler is passed trans-abdominally and into the cut end of alimentary limb (Fig. 17.16). The stapler and anvil are mated

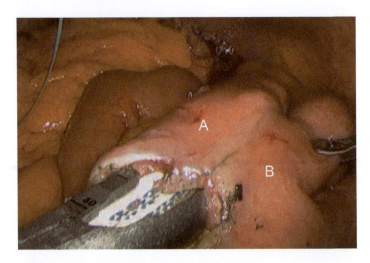

FIGURE 17.14 Side-to-side stapled Jejunojejunostomy (*A* biliopancreatic limb, *B* alimentary limb)

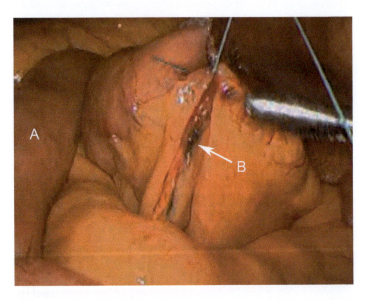

FIGURE 17.15 Jejunojejunostomy mesenteric defect is closed (*A* jejunum, *B* mesenteric defect)

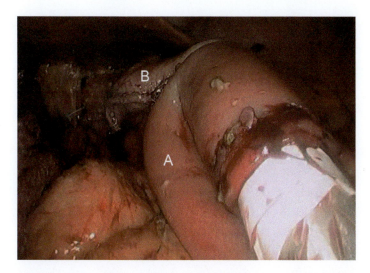

FIGURE 17.16 Creation of a gastrojejunostomy following subtotal gastrectomy (*A* alimentary limb, *B* gastric pouch)

through the wall of jejunum and the anastomosis is created. The remaining jejunal stump is then resected with a linear stapler to complete the anastomosis (Fig. 17.17). Stay sutures are placed on either side of the anastomosis to relieve tension. The anastomosis is tested by submerging it under instilled irrigation and insufflating air via the nasogastric tube, taking care to obstruct the alimentary limb to prevent air from insufflating a large portion of small bowel. After appropriate insufflation of the anastomosis, air bubbles will be observed if there is an anastomotic leak.

Total Gastrectomy

Laparoscopic resection seem to have comparable oncologic outcomes to open surgery with fewer post-operative complications and is preferable in selected cases when expertise is available [17, 18]. The procedure begins with omentectomy and the attachments of the omentum to the

322   P.J. Shabino et al.

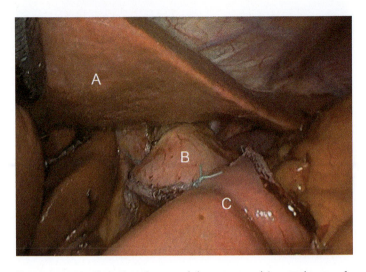

FIGURE 17.17 Completed gastrojejunostomy (*A* gastric pouch, *B* alimentary limb)

underlying transverse colon from the splenic flexure to the hepatic flexture are divided (Fig. 17.18). The gastrohepatic ligament is divided the phrenoesophageal ligament and peritoneal coverage of the right and left crus are incised (Fig. 17.19 and 17.20) .

The distal esophagus is exposed with dissection in the avascular plan between the esophagus and right crus. The gastrosplenic ligament, short gastric vessels and posterior attachments of the stomach to the pancreas are divided up to the left crus (Fig. 17.21). A retro-esophageal window is created through which a penrose drain is passed to allow retraction and dissection of the distal esophagus (Fig. 17.22). Attachments around the gastroesophageal junction and distal esophagus are completely divided.

The dissection continues by exposing the main gastric vessels to their base along with their surrounding lymph tissue. The posterior stomach is separated from the pancreas. The stomach is elevated and the dissection continues at the base of the left gastric vessels. The peritoneal coverage of the

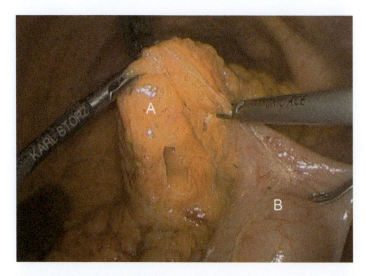

FIGURE 17.18 Omentum dissected away from transverse colon (*A* omentum, *B* colon)

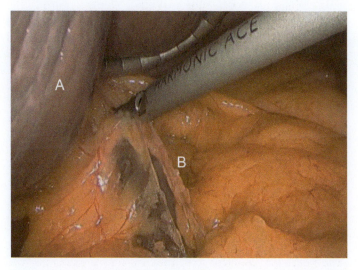

FIGURE 17.19 Gastrohepatic ligament incised (*A* liver, *B* gastrohepatic ligament)

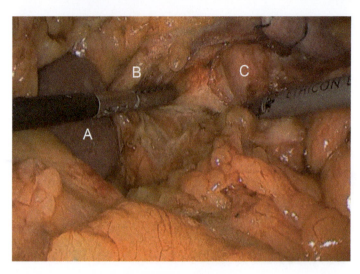

FIGURE 17.20 Right crus dissection. Begin to mobilize esophagus (*A* caudate lobe of liver, *B* right crus, *C* esophagus)

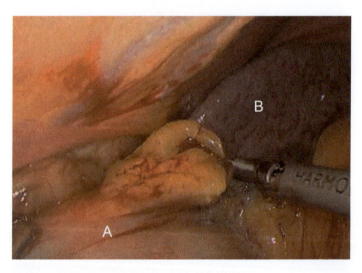

FIGURE 17.21 Gastrosplenic divided to *left* crus (*A* stomach, *B* spleen)

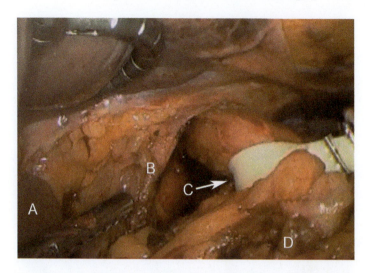

FIGURE 17.22 Esophagus following posterior tunnel. 360° control obtained and caudad retraction applied to penrose (*A* caudate lobe of liver, *B* right crus, *C* penrose drain around GE junction, *D* stomach)

pancreas is opened and dissected from left to right. This is carried over the hepatic artery to the porta hepatis as described previously. Lymphoid tissue is dissected from the celiac axis superiorly. The left gastric vessels are divided at their base with a vascular stapler load (Fig. 17.23).

The posterior aspect of the duodenum is mobilized and the right gastroepiploic is dissected to its base and divided (Fig. 17.24). The duodenum is divided with a linear stapler (Fig. 17.25). Ideally a 6 cm margin from tumor to esophageal transection should be obtained. Prior to transection, stay sutures can be placed on the distal esophagus at the 3 o'clock and 9 o'clock positions to allow retraction into the abdominal cavity. The distal esophagus is then transected (Fig. 17.26). The specimen is removed from the peritoneal cavity. With the laparoscopic approach, the left lower quadrant incision is enlarged and a wound protector place to allow the specimen

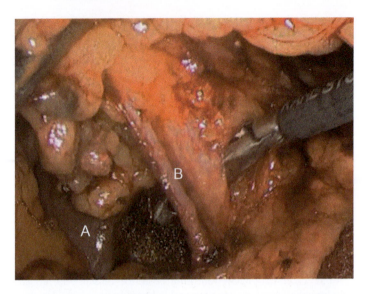

FIGURE 17.23 Left gastric artery identified and transected with vascular stapler load (*A* caudate lobe of liver, *B* left gastric artery)

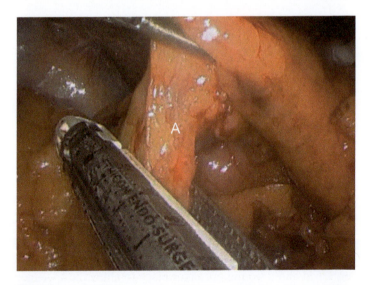

FIGURE 17.24 Nodal tissue mobilized anteriorly with specimen. Dissection carried to base of *right* gastroepiploic vessels (*A* right gastroepiploic vessels)

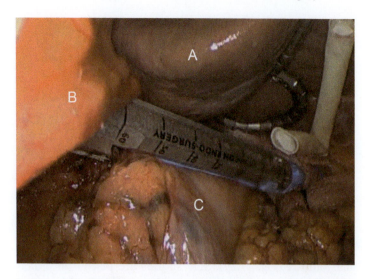

FIGURE 17.25 Division of the duodenum with endoscopic linear stapler (*A* liver, *B* falciform ligament, *C* antrum)

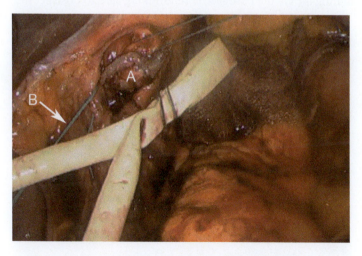

FIGURE 17.26 Division of the esophagus; note preplaced stay sutures at 3 and 9 o'clock position to maintain intra-abdominal esophagus length (*A* transected proximal esophagus, *B* stay suture)

to be removed. Proximal and distal margins are sent to pathology for frozen section evaluation of margins. The

The case is completed with Roux-en-Y reconstruction. The jejunojejunostomy and closure of the mesenteric defect are done using similar techniques than the one used for a subtotal gastrectomy described above. The esophagojejunostomy may be done using handsewn, circular or linear stapled techniques. The alimentary jejunal limb is laid adjacent to the stapled end of esophagus after the jejunum has been brought over the colon. In the circular stapled technique the anvil is passed trans-orally and the stapler is passed trans-abdominally and into the cut end of alimentary limb (Fig. 17.27). The stapler and anvil are mated through the wall of jejunum and the anastomosis is created (Fig. 17.28). The remaining jejunal stump is then resected with a linear stapler to complete the anastomosis (Fig. 17.29). Stay sutures are placed on either side of the anastomosis to relieve tension. The anastomosis is tested by submerging it under instilled irrigation and insufflating air via the nasogastric tube, taking care to obstruct the

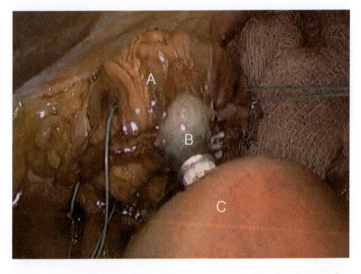

FIGURE 17.27 Esophagojejunostomy created with circular stapler after passing anvil via transoral route (*A* esophagus, *B* mated stapler, *C* jejunum)

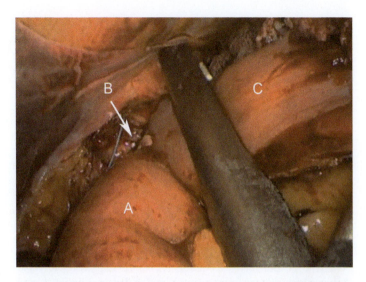

FIGURE 17.28 Completion of the esophagojejunostomy with transection of the jejunal stump (*A* alimentary limb, *B* esophagojejunostomy, *C* jejunal stump)

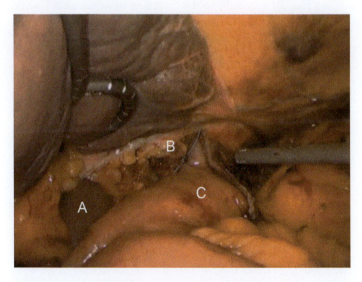

FIGURE 17.29 Completed esophagojejunostomy – Final aspect (*A* caudate lobe of liver, *B* esophagus, *C* jejunum)

alimentary limb to prevent air from insufflating a large portion of small bowel. After appropriate insufflation of the anastomosis, air bubbles will be observed if there is an anastomotic leak. A nasogastric tube should be carefully placed through the completed anastomosis.

References

1. Tack J, Vanormelingen C. Management of Gastroparesis: Beyond Basics. Curr Treat Options Gastroenterol. 2014;12(4):468–477.
2. Toro J, Lytle N, Patel A, et al. Efficacy of laparoscopic pyloroplasty for the treatment of gastroparesis. J Am Coll Surg. 2014;218:652–60.
3. Lau H. Laparoscopic repair of perforated peptic ulcer. Surg Endosc. 2004;18:1013–21.
4. Byrge N, Barton R, Enniss T, Nirula R. Laparoscopic versus open repair of perforated gastroduodenal ulcer: a national surgical quality improvement program analysis. Am J Surg. 2013;206:957–62.
5. Lagoo J, Pappas T, Perez A. A relic or still relevant: the narrowing role for vagotomy in the treatment of peptic ulcer disease. Am J Surg. 2014;207:120–6.
6. Schroder V, Pappas T, Vaslef S, et al. Vagotomy/drainage is superior to local oversew in patients who require emergency surgery for bleeding peptic ulcers. Ann Surg. 2014;259:1111–8.
7. Lightdale C. Endoscopic ultrasonography in the diagnosis, staging and follow-up of esophageal and gastric cancer. Endoscopy. 1992;1:297–303.
8. DeMatteo R, Lewis J, Leung D, et al. Two hundred gastrointestinal stromal tumors – recurrence patterns and prognostic factors for survival. Ann Surg. 2000;231(1):51–8.
9. Bonenkamp J, Hermans J, Sasako M, et al. Extended lympho-node dissection for gastric cancer. Dutch gastric cancer group. N Engl J Med. 1999;340:908–14.
10. Cuschieri A, Weeden S, Fielding J, et al. Patient survival after D1 and D2 resections for gastric cancer: long-term results of the MRC randomized surgical trial. Surgical Co-operative Group. Br J Cancer. 1999;79:1522–30.
11. Smith D, Schwarz RR, Schwarz RE. Impact of total lymph node count on staging and survival after gastrectomy for gastric can-

cer: data from a large US-population database. J Clin Oncol. 2005;11:439–49.

12. Schwarz R, Smith D. Clinical Impact of lymphadenectomy extent in resectable gastric cancer of advanced stage. Ann Surg Oncol. 2007;14:317–28.

13. Wu C, Hsiung C, Lo S, et al. Nodal dissection for patients with gastric cancer: a randomized controlled trial. Lancet Oncol. 2006;7:309–15.

14. Songun I, Putter H, Kranenbarg E, et al. Surgical treatment of gastric cancer: 15-year follow-up results of the randomized nationwide Dutch D1D2 trial. Lancet Oncol. 2010;11:439–49.

15. Sasako M, Sano T, Yamamoto S, et al. D2 lymphadenectomy alone or with para-aortic nodal dissection for gastric cancer. N Engl J Med. 2008;359(5):453–62.

16. Vogel S, Drane W, Woodward E. Clinical and radionuclide evaluation of bile diversion by Braun enteroenterostomy: prevention and treatment of alkaline reflux gastritis. An alternative to Roux-en-Y diversion. Ann Surg. 1994;219(5):458–65.

17. Lee J, Yom C, Han H. Comparison of long-term outcomes of laparoscopy-assisted and open distal gastrectomy for early gastric cancer. Surg Endosc. 2009;23(8):1759–63.

18. Zhao Y, Yu P, Hao Y, et al. Comparison of outcomes for laparoscopically assisted and open radical distal gastrectomy with lymphadenectomy for advanced gastric cancer. Surg Endosc. 2011;25(9):2960–6.

Part IV
Small Bowel and Appendix Surgery

Luke M. Funk

Chapter 18
Meckel's Diverticulum

Jocelyn F. Burke and Charles M. Leys

Abstract Located on the anti-mesenteric border of the distal ileum, Meckel's diverticulum is the most commonly encountered congenital anomaly of the GI tract. Patients with a Meckel's diverticulum may develop symptoms related to diverticulitis, bowel obstruction or GI bleeding. An inflamed diverticulum will present with localized peritonitis and can be identified with ultrasound or CT scan imaging. To investigate whether GI bleeding is due to a Meckel's diverticulum, patients are typically evaluated with a nuclear medicine technetium 99 m pertechnetate scan, known as a Meckel's scan. Presence of a symptomatic diverticulum is most often confirmed by diagnostic laparoscopy, and treatment involves either diverticulectomy or segmental small bowel resection.

Keywords Distal Ileum • Congenital Anomaly • Diverticulitis • Bowel Obstruction • GI Bleeding • Pertechnetate Scan • Meckel's Scan • Diverticulectomy • Small Bowel Resection

J.F. Burke, MD • C.M. Leys, MD, MSCI (✉)
Department of Surgery, University of Wisconsin
Hospital and Clinics, Madison, WI, USA
e-mail: Leys@surgery.wisc.edu

H. Chen (ed.), *Illustrative Handbook of General Surgery*,
DOI 10.1007/978-3-319-24557-7_18,
© Springer International Publishing Switzerland 2016

Indications

Meckel's diverticulum is the most frequently encountered congenital anomaly of the gastrointestinal (GI) tract, occurring in approximately 2 % of the population. It results from failure of the embryonic omphalomesenteric (or vitelline) duct to involute, leading to the presence of a true diverticulum. It is located on the anti-mesenteric border on the distal ileum approximately 60 cm proximal to the ileocecal valve [1]. Approximately 25 % of the diverticula have a persistent fibrous attachment to the umbilicus.

Meckel's diverticulum can present in a variety of ways, but the three most common manifestations are lower intestinal bleeding, intestinal obstruction, and diverticular inflammation. Bleeding is due to associated heterotopic tissue, most commonly gastric mucosa, which produces acid and leads to peptic ulceration of the adjacent small bowel mucosa. This classically results in a painless rectal bleeding with bright red or maroon colored stools. Obstruction can present as intussusception with a diverticulum as the lead point or as volvulus around a remnant fibrotic band adherent to the umbilicus. Finally, inflammation and possible perforation of the diverticulum presents with focal peritoneal signs and symptoms similar to appendicitis. Therefore, in a patient diagnosed with appendicitis but found to have a grossly normal appendix intra-operatively, a search for a possibly inflamed Meckel's diverticulum should be conducted. The mechanism for this inflammation can be luminal obstruction, as with appendicitis, or may be due to associated heterotopic gastric or pancreatic tissue.

Much debate exists regarding the appropriate treatment of a diverticula encountered incidentally during an operation for another indication. Some authors recommend routine resection due to concern for potential malignancy and the low morbidity associated with resection [2]. Others recommend a more selective approach, based on diverticulum and patient characteristics that increase the probability of developing symptoms. Specifically, the risk of developing symptoms is elevated in younger patients, males, and with diverticula that are >2 cm in length, narrow-based, or contain heterotopic tissue [3].

Preoperative Imaging and Preparation

The ability to conclusively diagnose a Meckel's diverticulum preoperatively is limited. The diagnosis is most often based on a high index of suspicion and confirmed intra-operatively. In patients with a bowel obstruction and no previous abdominal operation, the presence of a Meckel's diverticulum should be considered. In patients presenting with focal peritonitis, ultrasound (US) or computed tomography (CT) scan may identify a tubular, inflamed midline mass, suggesting the diagnosis of Meckel's diverticulitis (Fig. 18.1).

Patients with evidence of lower GI bleeding should undergo a thorough workup for other causes of bleeding, including a detailed history and physical and placement of a nasogastric tube to rule out upper GI source. To evaluate for a Meckel's diverticulum as a bleeding source, a nuclear medicine Technetium (Tc)-99 m pertechnetate scan is the preferred test (Fig. 18.2). The Tc-99 m is taken up by gastric mucosa, so this scan will only identify a diverticulum containing heterotopic gastric mucosa. Sensitivity for this test ranges from 60 % historically to over 90 % in a recent study [4]. Regardless, some diverticula will be missed with this test, so diagnostic laparoscopy is indicated in a highly suspicious case of painless rectal bleeding, even if the "Meckel's scan" is negative.

Pre-operative preparation for patients presenting with a symptomatic Meckel's diverticulum includes intra-venous fluid resuscitation and a 2nd-generation cephalosporin. In cases of diverticulitis, which can be perforated, broad-spectrum gram-negative and anaerobe coverage should be utilized. In the setting of obstruction, nasogastric tube decompression is helpful. If symptomatic from severe anemia, the patient may require packed red blood cell transfusion.

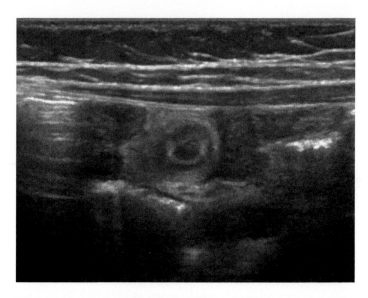

FIGURE 18.1 Ultrasound image of a thickened tubular structure with gut signature in the right mid-abdomen, distant from the cecum, representing an inflamed Meckel's diverticulum (Image credit: Kara Gill, MD)

Description of the Procedure

In many cases, the diagnosis is suspected but not known, so it is often advantageous to begin with a diagnostic laparoscopy to confirm the diagnosis [5–8]. Laparoscopic exploration for a suspected or confirmed Meckel's diverticulum is typically performed with standard umbilical access through either a periumbilical or midline umbilical incision. Since the diverticulum may be adherent to the underside of the umbilicus, the fascia and peritoneum should be entered with a careful open cutdown approach. As the umbilical stalk is explored in this manner, a remnant fibrous cord may be identified, allowing an adherent diverticulum to be pulled up and out of the wound.

If the diverticulum is not immediately identified, laparoscopy proceeds using either a single-site or standard three port set up. In the three port approach, the additional 5 mm ports

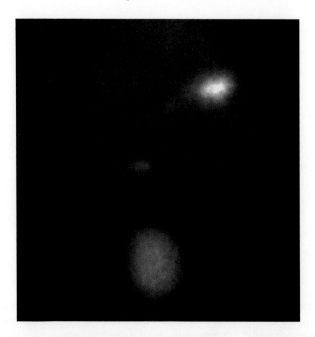

FIGURE 18.2 Technetium (Tc)-99 m pertechnetate nuclear medicine scan ("Meckel's scan"). The tracer is taken up by gastric mucosa, which is commonly present in Meckel's diverticula and causes peptic ulceration and bleeding. Radiotracer is readily seen in the stomach and bladder, with the Meckel's diverticulum revealed as a small focus of abnormal uptake in the right mid-abdomen after 30 min (Image credit: Kara Gill, MD)

are typically placed in the left lower quadrant and left suprapubic location, similar to the placement for a laparoscopic appendectomy. The patient is positioned in Trendelenburg and tilted left side down. This set up and position allows easy identification of the cecum and terminal ileum, which is then run proximally to look for the diverticulum. If the diverticulum is densely adherent to the abdominal wall at the umbilicus, the laparoscope can be moved to the left lower quadrant port site to visualize and divide this attachment.

After the diverticulum is identified, options for removal are simple diverticulectomy or segmental small bowel resection.

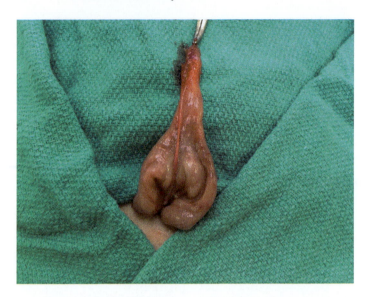

FIGURE 18.3 Meckel's diverticulum and segment of ileum has been delivered through a small umbilical midline incision. Note the small mesenteric vessel coursing up along the diverticulum

In most cases, a simple diverticulectomy can be performed using a GIA stapling device either intra- or extra-corporeally. The staple line should be oriented transversely to avoid narrowing the ileal lumen. In an infant or small child, the diverticulectomy is more easily accomplished by eviscerating the segment of ileum and amputating the diverticulum with a stapler extra-corporeally (Figs. 18.3, 18.4, and 18.5). In an older child or adult with more abdominal domain, an endo-GIA stapler may be utilized for an intra-corporeal diverticulectomy, similar to a laparoscopic appendectomy. The mesenteric vessel to the diverticulum must be controlled with either suture, staples, or any available energy device. In cases of GI bleeding, it is important to be aware that the bleeding ulcer is often located in the adjacent ileum, so a short segment bowel resection with primary anastomosis is generally recommended to avoid the pitfall of recurrent bleeding. Alternatively, a V-shaped cuff of adjacent ileum can be

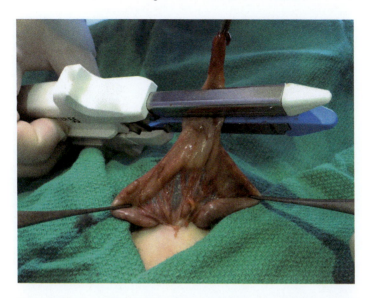

FIGURE 18.4 A standard GIA stapler is placed across the base of the diverticulum, transverse orientation relative to the ileum, with great care to avoid narrowing the small bowel lumen. The diverticular mesenteric vessel has been cauterized

excised with the diverticulum, and the remaining enterotomy closed transversely with sutures after inspecting the ileum for ulcers. The resected specimen should be opened prior to sending it to pathology to confirm that it contains the ulcer.

Postoperative Care

Most patients who have undergone Meckel's diverticulectomy can be treated using standard postoperative regimens. Those treated laparoscopically and without contamination, rupture, or obstruction can be managed with early diet advancement and without nasogastric tube. Early ambulation should be encouraged. A typical postoperative length of hospital stay is approximately 2–5 days [7]. Postoperative complications are uncommon, but include wound infection, bleeding,

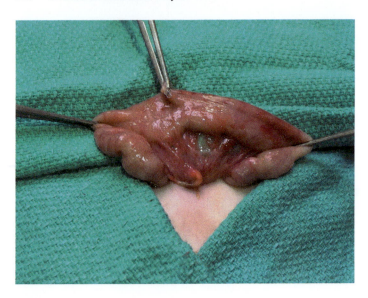

FIGURE 18.5 The transverse staple line remaining on the ileum after completing the diverticulectomy

and the small risk of bowel obstruction from post-operative adhesions. Anastomotic leak or stricture should be rare.

References

1. Pepper VK, Stanfill AB, Pearl RH. Diagnosis and management of pediatric appendicitis, intussusception, and Meckel diverticulum. Surg Clin North Am. 2012;92(3):505–26, vii.
2. Thirunavukarasu P, Sathaiah M, Sukumar S, et al. Meckel's diverticulum – a high-risk region for malignancy in the ileum. Insights from a population-based epidemiological study and implications in surgical management. Ann Surg. 2011;253(2):223–30.
3. Park JJ, Wolff BG, Tollefson MK, Walsh EE, Larson DR. Meckel diverticulum: the Mayo clinic experience with 1476 patients (1950–2002). Ann Surg. 2005;241(3):529–33.
4. Sinha CK, Pallewatte A, Easty M, et al. Meckel's scan in children: a review of 183 cases referred to two paediatric surgery specialist centres over 18 years. Pediatr Surg Int. 2013;29(5):511–7.

5. Tam YH, Chan KW, Wong YS, et al. Single-incision laparoscopic surgery in diagnosis and treatment for gastrointestinal bleeding of obscure origin in children. Surg Laparosc Endosc Percutan Tech. 2013;23(3):e106–8.
6. Huang CC, Lai MW, Hwang FM, et al. Diverse presentations in pediatric Meckel's diverticulum: a review of 100 cases. Pediatr Neonatol. 2014.
7. Ruscher KA, Fisher JN, Hughes CD, et al. National trends in the surgical management of Meckel's diverticulum. J Pediatr Surg. 2011;46(5):893–6.
8. Chan KW, Lee KH, Mou JW, Cheung ST, Tam YH. Laparoscopic management of complicated Meckel's diverticulum in children: a 10-year review. Surg Endosc. 2008;22(6):1509–12.

Chapter 19
Small Bowel Resection

Laura E. Fischer and Luke M. Funk

Abstract Small bowel resection is a common procedure which is performed for a wide variety of indications in all age groups. Multiple different techniques to accomplish a small bowel resection and anastomosis have developed over the last 200 years, including the open versus laparoscopic approach, single versus double layer, and hand-sewn versus stapled anastomosis. In general, the various surgical techniques are similar in outcome as long as common principles are followed: adequate exposure, gentle tissue handling, absence of tension, and adequate tissue oxygenation.

Keywords Small Intestine • Resection • Anastomosis • Laparoscopy • Stapled • Hand-sewn

L.E. Fischer, MD, MS
Department of Surgery, University of Wisconsin,
Madison, WI, USA

L.M. Funk, MD, MPH (✉)
Department of Surgery, University of Wisconsin School
of Medicine and Public Health, H4/728 Clinical Science Center,
600 Highland Avenue, Madison, WI 53792-7375, USA
e-mail: funk@surgery.wisc.edu

H. Chen (ed.), *Illustrative Handbook of General Surgery*,   345
DOI 10.1007/978-3-319-24557-7_19,
© Springer International Publishing Switzerland 2016

Indications

Small bowel resection is a common procedure in all surgical populations for a wide variety of indications including malignancy, obstruction, ischemia, traumatic injury, hemorrhage, fistula, stricture, and congenital anomalies. There are multiple ways to complete a small bowel resection, but the general concepts for a successful anastomosis such as adequate exposure, gentle tissue handling, absence of tension, and adequate tissue oxygenation remain the same [1].

Preoperative Preparation

Pre-operative imaging should be completed as needed to delineate the nature and location of the problem in question. Common imaging studies include abdominal X-rays (upright, supine, and occasionally left lateral decubitus) computed tomography of the abdomen and pelvis with intravenous and oral contrast, and upper gastrointestinal X-ray series. The patient should be made NPO 12 h prior to an elective procedure. If the patient is undergoing an emergent procedure, a nasogastric tube should be placed to empty the stomach prior to induction of general anesthesia. In general, a bowel preparation is not necessary for a small bowel resection and anastomosis, but this is within the purview of the operating surgeon. An epidural can be considered for post-operative pain control if an open procedure with a midline laparotomy is planned.

Positioning and Anesthesia

All patients should undergo induction of general anesthesia with endotracheal intubation. Rapid sequence induction is used for emergent procedures in which the patient has not been made NPO for 12 h to reduce the risk of aspiration of gastric contents. An assistant can provide cricoid pressure to further reduce the risk of gastroesophageal reflux into the oropharynx. The patient should be placed in the supine position. For an open procedure, the arms are secured on padded arm boards at a 90° angle to the body's axis. For laparoscopic procedures, one or both arms can be tucked to the patient's side to maximize the range of the surgeon's position. An orogastric or nasogastric tube is placed to decompress the stomach and proximal small bowel during the procedure, if not placed pre-operatively. Sequential compression devices should be placed on the lower legs bilaterally for deep vein thrombosis prophylaxis and subcutaneous heparin can be administered as long as there are no specific contraindications, such as current hemorrhage or recent cerebrovascular accident. A foley catheter should be placed for urinary drainage and monitoring of urine output if the procedure is emergent or is expected to last more than a couple of hours. The abdominal skin should be widely prepped after hair has been clipped short using an atraumatic electric clipper [2]. A single dose of antibiotics should be administered within 1 h of incision [3]. We typically use a second generation cephalosporin.

Description of the Procedure

Open Small Bowel Resection

The classic approach for a small bowel resection is via an open approach. An open procedure should also be performed when the patient is hemodynamically unstable or is medically unable to tolerate intra-abdominal insufflation. Massive bowel dilation and extensive adhesive disease are relative contraindications to laparoscopy. A vertical midline incision in preferred in patients over the age of 2 (for children less than 2, a transverse abdominal incision is often preferred due to the proportionally larger transverse length of a young child's abdomen). The incision is often started at the level of the umbilicus and can be extended superiorly or inferiorly depending on the location of the surgical problem. Once an incision of appropriate length is created, retractors such as a Bookwalter or Balfour can be placed to enhance exposure of the operative field. The small bowel can then be eviscerated from the abdominal cavity. Adhesiolysis can be performed using a Metzenbaum scissors and gentle retraction or using a dissecting forceps (e.g. Westphal dissector or a right angle clamp) and Bovie cautery to mobilize the entire length of small bowel. The diseased area of small bowel is then identified and resection margins determined. It is critical to run the entire length of small bowel from the ligament of Treitz to the ileocecal valve to ensure the unresected bowel appears normal and to determine the length of remaining bowel after the proposed resection. In general, attempts are made to preserve a minimum of 30 % or at least 100 cm of small bowel to prevent short bowel syndrome [4]. This is of particular importance if the ileocecal valve has been resected. In patients who may require multiple bowel resections over their lifetime, such as Crohn's disease, resection of bowel is minimized as much as possible.

Prior to performing the bowel resection, sterile towels are placed beneath and around the area to be resected to minimize contamination of the surgical field due to spillage of intraluminal contents. The bowel resection can be performed with a stapling device or sharply with a scalpel between two non-crushing bowel clamps. The mesentery is then divided using an energy device, such as the LigaSure™ (Covidien, Mansfield MA) or the Harmonic Ultrasonic© scalpel (Ethicon, Cincinnati OH). Alternatively, sections of mesentery can be clamped and sharply divided with a Metzenbaum scissors (Fig. 19.1). Silk or Vicryl ties can then be used to permanently ligate blood vessels. In cases where the patient is hemodynamically unstable, a gastrointestinal anastomosis (GIA) stapler with vascular loads can be used to remove the damaged portion of bowel within a few minutes. It is important to divide the mesentery more proximally when resecting a malignant tumor to obtain an appropriate number of lymph nodes to guide further oncologic management. If the patient is hemodynamically unstable, the stapled ends of

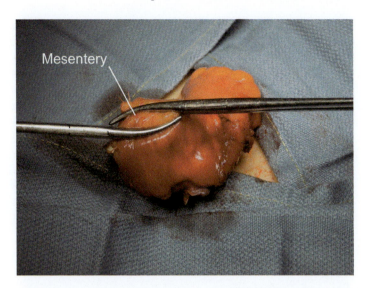

FIGURE 19.1 Metal clamps are placed across the distal mesentery in opposite directions with their tips pointing inwards. A Metzenbaum scissors is then used to divide the mesentery sharply. Silk or Vicryl ties are used to ligate the mesenteric vessels. This mesenteric division should occur more proximally when resecting small intestine to remove a malignancy

the small bowel can be left in discontinuity while the patient is taken to the ICU for resuscitation with a plan for a delayed anastomosis. With either immediate or delayed anastomosis after a traumatic injury, the leak rate for small bowel anastomoses was only 3 % in one series [5].

Hand-Sewn Technique

If the patient is hemodynamically stable, the bowel anastomosis can be performed using either a hand-sewn or stapled technique. A hand-sewn anastomosis may be performed in an end-to-end fashion in either one or two layers, as long as the bowel diameters are approximately equal. Alternatively, a side-to-side (functional end-to-end) or end-to-side hand-sewn anastomosis may be performed. There is no difference in leak rate between single and double layer anastomoses [6, 7]; this can be left to surgeon preference. A single layer anastomosis or the inner layer of a two layer anastomosis can be performed with either a running transmural technique or using interrupted sutures. We prefer to use monofilament absorbable suture, often 2-0 or 3-0 polydioxanone (PDS®) suture (Ethicon, Cincinnati OH). It is critical to take full thickness bites to prevent anastomotic breakdown or leakage as the submucosal layer of the small bowel provides strength to the anastomosis [1]. The outer layer of suture closure is performed in an interrupted Lembert fashion using braided permanent suture, typically 3-0 silk suture.

Stapled Technique

Stapled anastomoses are typically faster than hand-sewn and are associated with equivalent rates of clinically evident leakage, morbidity, and post-operative mortality [8, 9]. The proximal and distal segments of bowel are aligned in a side-to-side fashion and two silk sutures are placed, one at the staple line and the other more distally, to temporarily secure the two segments in proper alignment (Fig. 19.2). Small enterotomies are then made on the anti-mesenteric side of each segment near the resection edges. A linear stapling device (e.g. GIA stapler) of either 60 or 80 mm is then inserted with one arm through each enterotomy (Fig. 19.3). After confirming that the mesenteries of the bowel segments are outside of the stapling device, it is closed and fired creating a large enteroenterostomy. The stapler is removed and an Army Navy retractor can be used to inspect the luminal staple line for hemostasis. If the patient is on therapeutic anticoagulation, a running monofilament absorbable suture can be placed along the luminal staple line to reinforce the area and assure hemostasis (Fig. 19.4). The common channel enterotomy can then be closed using a hand-sewn technique as

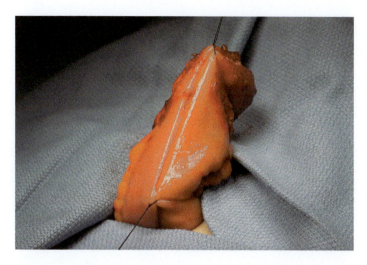

FIGURE 19.2 Silk stay sutures are placed at the proximal and distal aspects of our side-to-side small bowel anastomosis to assist in maintaining alignment during stapler placement

above or by firing across the enterotomy with a stapler (either a TA or GIA stapler) (Fig. 19.5). Some surgeons choose to oversew the staple lines with interrupted Lembert braided permanent sutures to create a second layer (Fig. 19.6). Most surgeons place one or more braided sutures distally to reinforce the end of the staple line where the two bowel segments diverge. Depending on its size, the mesenteric defect can then be closed using either running or interrupted braided absorbable sutures, taking care not to injure the blood vessels running through the mesentery (Fig. 19.7).

Laparoscopic Small Bowel Resection

A small bowel resection and anastomosis can be safely and effectively performed laparoscopically with improved post-operative recovery of activity and diet, shorter length of stay, and improved pain control [10, 11]. Compared with laparotomy, the laparoscopic approach is associated with formation

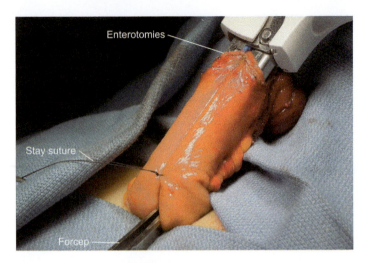

Enterotomies

Stay suture

Forcep

FIGURE 19.3 Small enterotomies are made on the antimesenteric side of each small bowel limb. The arms of a GIA stapler are then passed into the enterotomies and the stapler is advanced as shown with the tips pointed downwards. The silk stay suture is used to pull the small bowel upwards toward the handle of the stapler. A debakey forcep is used to retract downward on the mesentery in between the two stapler arms to ensure that the mesentery is not caught within the staple line

of significantly fewer peritoneal adhesions, as well as decreased morbidity and mortality [12, 13]. Laparoscopic small bowel resection can be performed either with a lap-assisted technique with an extra-corporeal anastomosis or totally laparoscopically with a double stapled technique. A minimum of four ports are typically required, and at least one port must be 12 or 15 mm to accommodate the laparoscopic stapling device if an intracorporeal stapling technique is used. Port placement varies depending on the location and extent of bowel to be resected. Abdominal entry is obtained by either the Hassan technique or a Veress needle. After the ports have been placed and a 30° camera introduced into the abdomen, atraumatic graspers can be used to examine the small bowel and run its length from the ligament of Treitz to the ileocecal valve. Adhesiolysis can be completed using a laparoscopic scissors,

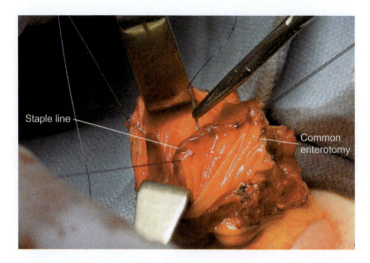

Staple line

Common enterotomy

FIGURE 19.4 Army Navy retractors are used to expose the mucosal aspect of the staple line to assess for bleeding. If hemorrhage is noted or the patient is on systemic anticoagulation, the staple line be oversewn with a running PDS suture as shown

hook cautery device, or an energy device such as the LigaSure™ or Harmonic Ultrasonic© scalpel. If a lap-assisted approach is used, the selected portion of small bowel is exteriorized through a slightly enlarged umbilical incision using a wound protector. Once the bowel has been delivered, resection and anastomosis can be completed using any of the techniques described above. If an intra-corporeal anastomotic technique is used, a linear stapling device is introduced to divide the desired segment of bowel. The mesentery can then be divided using an energy device. Metal clips, monopolar or bipolar cautery, and laparoscopic loop sutures can be used to assist in safely dividing the mesenteric vasculature. The resected portion of bowel is removed through the umbilical port using a laparoscopic specimen pouch. The anti-mesenteric sides of the proximal and distal bowel segments are then aligned and braided stay sutures are placed using either curved needle sutures cut to a short length or an endoscopic suturing device. Small enterotomies are made in each limb and the two arms of a linear stapler are introduced through

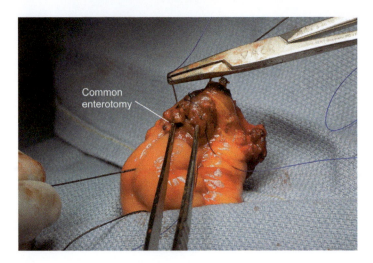

FIGURE 19.5 The common enterotomy is then closed with a Connell stitch using 3-0 PDS. Care must be taken to take full thickness bites with each pass of the needle. The Connell stitch provides hemostasis as well as inverting the bowel wall inwards so that the serosal edges are approximated. The common enterotomy can also be closed with a running stitch or a stapling device

the enterotomies, taking care that the angle of the bowel distal to the end of the stapler is straight to avoid perforation. The common enterotomy is then sealed with an additional fire of the laparoscopic stapler. The mesenteric defect can be closed with a running braided suture using either a suture on a curved needle or an endoscopic suturing device. Larger port sites and the enlarged umbilical port site should be closed at the fascial layer with absorbable monofilament suture. Smaller port sites can be closed with skin stitches only.

Post-operative Care

The length of time to return of bowel function is highly variable and depends on multiple patient factors. Close attention should be paid to electrolyte and fluid imbalances. A foley

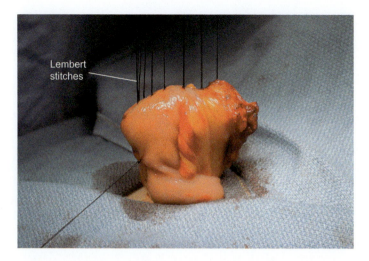

FIGURE 19.6 Interrupted silk sutures are then placed in the Lembert fashion to create the second layer of a double layer anastomosis. Lembert sutures are often also placed along the staple line laterally and a final silk suture is placed at the most distal aspect of the staple line to reduce tension on that area

catheter can be used to monitor urine output and gauge intravascular fluid resuscitation. If the patient is hemodynamically unstable, septic, or there is gross intra-abdominal contamination, a nasogastric tube is often kept in place for decompression of the stomach and proximal small bowel. When the volume of the nasogastric tube has decreased to less than 150 cc per 8 h shift, we begin clamping trials and remove the tube if residual output is low. Oral intake can be started at the surgeon's discretion, but traditionally is held until the patient is passing flatus. There is some evidence that early initiation of enteral feeding can reduce the overall risk of infection and decrease length of hospital stays [14, 15]. Oral pain medication can be started with the initiation of a diet. Multimodal postoperative analgesia should be administered and narcotics minimized as much as possible to reduce opioid-associated delayed gastrointestinal recovery [16]. Post-operative antibiotics are generally not indicated as prolonged dosing increases

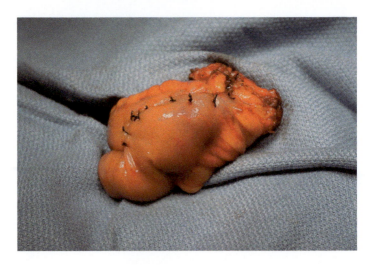

FIGURE 19.7 The completed anastomosis. The size and patency of the anastomosis can be assessed by placing the thumb and forefinger on either side of the completed anastomosis and gently pinching them together

the risk of Clostridium difficile and the development of resistant bacteria [3]. The patient can be discharged home when they are tolerating a general diet, ambulating without difficulty, and have good pain control on oral medications.

References

1. Chen C. The art of bowel anastomosis. Scand J Surg. 2012;101: 238–40.
2. Tanner J, Norrie P, Melen K. Preoperative hair removal to reduce surgical site infection. Cochrane Database Syst Rev. 2011;11:1–49.
3. Nelson RL, Gladman E, Barbateskovic M. Antimicrobial prophylaxis for colorectal surgery. Cochrane Database Syst Rev. 2014;5:1–262.
4. Yildiz BD. Where are we at with short bowel syndrome and small bowel transplant? World J Transpl. 2012;2(6):95–103.

5. Burlew CC, Moore EE, Cuschieri J, Jurkovich GJ, Codner P, Crowell K, Nirula R, Haan J, Rowell SE, Kato CM, MacNew H, Ochsner MG, Harrison PB, Fusco C, Sauaia A, Kaups KL, The WTA Study Group. Sew it up! a western trauma association multi-institutional study of enteric injury management in the postinjury open abdomen. J Trauma. 2011;70:273–7.

6. Burch JM, Franciose RJ, Moore EE, Biffl WL, Offner PJ. Single-layer continuous versus two-layer interrupted intestinal anastomosis: a prospective randomized trial. Ann Surg. 2000;231(6): 832–7.

7. Shikata S, Yamagishi H, Taji Y, Shimada T, Noguchi Y. Single- versus two- layer intestinal anastomosis: a meta-analysis of randomized controlled trials. BMC Surg. 2006;6:2.

8. Witzke JD, Kraatz JJ, Morken JM, Ney AL, West MA, Van Camp JM, Zera RT, Rodriguez JL. Stapled versus hand sewn anastomoses in patients with small bowel injury: a changing perspective. J Trauma. 2000;49:660–6.

9. Docherty JG, McGregor JR, Akyol AM, Murray GD, Galloway DJ. Comparison of manually constructed and stapled anastomoses in colorectal surgery. West of Scotland and Highland anastomosis study group. Ann Surg. 1995;221:176–84.

10. Milsom JW, Hammerhofer KA, Bohm B, Marcello P, Elson P, Fazio VW. Prospective, randomized trial comparing laparoscopic vs. conventional surgery for refractory ileocolic Crohn's disease. Dis Colon Rectum. 2001;44(1):1–8.

11. Duepree HJ, Senagore AJ, Delaney CP, Brady KM, Fazio VW. Advantages of laparoscopic resection for ileocolic Crohn's disease. Dis Colon Rectum. 2002;45(5):605–10.

12. Arung W, Meurisse M, Detry O. Pathophysiology and prevention of postoperative peritoneal adhesions. World J Gastroenterol. 2011;17(41):4545–53.

13. Daly SC, Popoff AM, Fogg L, Francescatti AB, Myers JA, Millikan KW, Deziel DJ, Luu MB. Minimally invasive technique leads to decreased morbidity and mortality in small bowel resections compared to an open technique: an ACS-NSQIP identified target for improvement. J Gastrointest Surg. 2014;18:1171–5.

14. Lewis SJ, Egger M, Sylvester PA, Thomas S. Early enteral feeding versus "nil by mouth" after gastrointestinal surgery: systematic review and meta-analysis of controlled trials. BMJ. 2001;323:1–5.

15. Andersen HK, Lewis SJ, Thomas S. Early enteral nutrition within 24 h of colorectal surgery versus later commencement of

feeding for postoperative complications. Cochrane Database Syst Rev. 2006;4:1–31.
16. Beard TL, Leslie JB, Nemeth J. The opioid component of delayed gastrointestinal recovery after bowel resection. J Gastrointest Surg. 2011;15:1259–68.

Chapter 20
Laparoscopic Splenectomy

Jason T. Wiseman and Luke M. Funk

Abstract First performed in 1991, laparoscopic splenectomy is now considered the gold standard surgical approach for elective splenectomy. Laparoscopic splenectomy can be safely performed in most cases where splenectomy is indicated, including massive splenomegaly. As compared to open splenectomy, laparoscopic splenectomy is associated with decreased 30-day mortality, decreased need for intraoperative transfusion, decreased post-operative pain and decreased length of stay. Yet despite the advantages of laparoscopy, open splenectomy remains the mainstay for emergent splenectomies, particularly for patients who are hemodynamically unstable and have high-grade splenic injuries.

J.T. Wiseman, MD, MSPH
Department of Surgery, University of Wisconsin School of Medicine and Public Health, Madison, WI, USA

L.M. Funk, MD, MPH (✉)
Department of Surgery, University of Wisconsin School of Medicine and Public Health, Madison, WI, USA

Department of Surgery, University of Wisconsin Hospitals and Clinics, 600 Highland Ave, Madison, WI 53792, USA
e-mail: funk@surgery.wisc.edu

H. Chen (ed.), *Illustrative Handbook of General Surgery*,
DOI 10.1007/978-3-319-24557-7_20,
© Springer International Publishing Switzerland 2016

Keywords Splenomegaly • Idiopathic thrombocytopenic purpura • Splenic malignancy

Indications

Most splenic pathologies are amenable to a laparoscopic approach including benign or malignant hematologic diseases and secondary hypersplenism [1–5]. Immune thrombocytopenia purpura (ITP) is the most common indication for elective splenectomy [6]. Splenectomy is usually recommended when the disease process is refractory to medical management or in attempt to avoid the side effects of long-term steroid use. Laparoscopic splenectomy may also be indicated in other benign conditions such as thrombotic thrombocytopenic purpura, hereditary spherocytosis, thalassemia with secondary hypersplenism or severe anemia, sickle cell disease, and refractory autoimmune hemolytic anemia [6]. Laparoscopic splenectomy also has a role in select malignant diseases of the spleen for which it can be used for diagnostic or therapeutic reasons. Indications include myeloproliferative disorders, lymphoproliferative diseases, hairy cell leukemia, Hodgkin and non-Hodgkin lymphoma, malignant vascular tumors, malignant lymphomas, and lymphangiosarcomas [6]. Contraindications to performing laparoscopic splenectomy include uncorrected coagulopathies, severe portal hypertension, hemodynamic instability or inability to tolerate pneumoperitoneum [7].

Preoperative Preparation

All patients should receive preoperative vaccinations against the following encapsulated bacteria: Neisseria meningitidis, Streptococcus pneumoniae, and Haemophilus influenzae type B [8]. Immunizations should be given at least 1-week prior to the operation although at least 3-weeks prior is preferable [9]. Standard hematological laboratories including hematocrit and type & screen should be obtained and corrected accordingly [10]. Preoperative splenic artery embolization is occasionally utilized for massive splenomegaly to reduce intraoperative blood loss.

Positioning and Anesthesia

Four different positions may be used when performing a laparoscopic splenectomy: supine, lithotomy, right lateral decubitus, and anterolateral (i.e. partial right lateral decubitus, right "lazy" decubitus). We prefer a right "lazy" decubitus position using a surgical bean bag because it allows gravity to assist in the dissection of the splenic attachments (as opposed to the supine position) and it leaves the abdomen readily accessible if a quick conversion to a laparotomy is required (as opposed to a formal right lateral decubitus position) (Fig. 20.1). Supine and lithotomy positions are preferred by some surgeons for children or patients who have massive splenomegaly or are undergoing additional abdominal procedures [11].

General endotracheal anesthesia is required. Deep vein thrombosis prophylaxis is administered (typically 40 mg enoxaparin subcutaneously) and sequential compression devices are applied prior to induction. A Foley catheter is placed to monitor fluid status in select patients. An orogastric tube is placed to decompress the stomach and minimize the likelihood of gastric injury; this is particularly important because we access the abdomen using a Veress technique in the left upper quadrant. Patients also receive preoperative antibiotic prophylaxis.

Description of Procedure

Abdominal Access

Entry into the abdomen is performed using a Veress needle in the left upper quadrant (Fig. 20.2). We prefer a Veress approach due to the relatively high frequency of obesity in

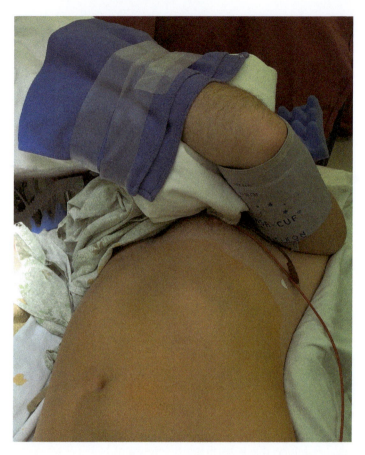

FIGURE 20.1 Patient positioning during a laparoscopic splenectomy. The patient is placed on the operating room table in the right "lazy" decubitus position using a bean bag with the right arm abducted and the left arm adducted anterior and superior. This positioning allows gravity to assist in the dissection of the splenic attachments and it leaves the abdomen readily accessible if a quick conversion to a laparotomy is required

our patient population. Intra-abdominal positioning of the needle is confirmed by aspiration and a negative saline drop test. Pneumoperitoneum is then established by insufflating

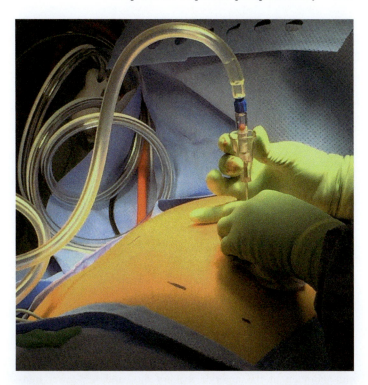

FIGURE 20.2 Entry into the abdomen with Veress needle technique. A Veress needle is placed 3 cm below the left subcostal border in the midclavicular line. Intra-abdominal positioning of the needle is confirmed by aspiration and a negative saline drop test

the abdomen to a pressure of 15 mmHg with carbon dioxide. A 5 mm port is placed into the abdomen either through the Veress incision or via an adjacent incision in the left upper quadrant.

Alternatively, using the Hasson technique, a 1 cm upper midline vertical incision is made approximately 15 cm inferior to the xiphoid process. The fascia is elevated and incised, and entry into the intra-abdominal cavity is confirmed by direct visualization. Two figure-of-eight absorbable sutures are placed in the fascia and the Hasson cannula is inserted under direct visualization.

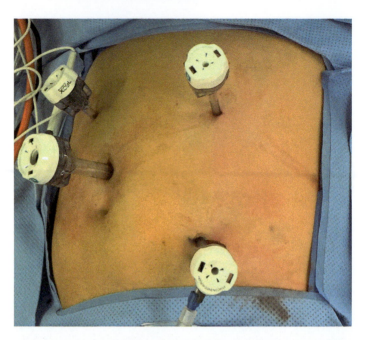

FIGURE 20.3 Trocar placement for laparoscopic splenectomy. Ports are inserted at the supra-umbilical position, right upper midline, left mid-abdomen at the anterior axillary line, and left lower mid-abdomen at the mid-clavicular line. After inspection of the abdomen, the left lower mid-abdominal 5 mm trocar (shown) was upsized to a 12 mm port to accommodate passage of the endo-GIA stapler. These trocar positions may vary if a patient has splenomegaly or other anatomical limitation

Either a 5 mm or 10 mm, 30° laparoscope is then inserted through the first trocar and the intra-abdominal cavity is inspected for any injury or pathology. Additional ports are inserted at the supra-umbilical position, right upper midline, left mid-abdomen at the anterior axillary line, and left lower mid-abdomen at the mid-clavicular line. The left lower mid-abdominal port at the mid-clavicular line is typically a 12 mm port, which allows passage of an endo-GIA stapler. To avoid direct trocar injuries to the spleen, these trocar positions may vary if a patient has splenomegaly (Fig. 20.3).

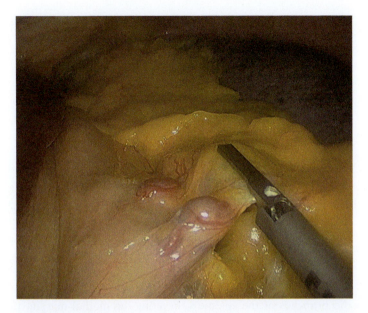

FIGURE 20.4 Mobilization of the stomach. The short gastric vessels are divided with the bipolar coagulating device, mobilizing the stomach from the spleen

Division of the Short Gastrics

The greater curve of the stomach at the level of the inferior margin of the spleen is grasped and retracted anteriorly and to the patient's right. The adjacent omentum is retracted in the opposite direction. The short gastric vessels are then divided with the bipolar coagulating device and the lesser sac is entered (Fig. 20.4). There are typically two layers of attachments that need to be transected and often a posterior layer of short gastrics. Division is complete once the left crus of the diaphragm is visualized.

Division of the Splenic Artery

Division of the short gastrics allows entry into the lesser sac and visualization of the anterior surface of the pancreas. The splenic artery can usually be identified inferior and anterior to

366 J.T. Wiseman and L.M. Funk

the splenic vein. After circumferential exposure, the splenic artery is transected with an endoscopic vascular linear stapler (Fig. 20.5). The pancreas is inspected to ensure that no injury occurred. If there is concern about possible pancreatic injury, a 15 Fr Blake drain is placed in the splenic bed to both identify and manage a possible pancreatic fistula. If it is not possible to isolate the splenic artery at this location, the arterial and venous splenic branches will be transected at the hilum.

Division of the Splenic Vein Branches

The splenic flexure of the colon is mobilized inferiorly. The splenocolic ligament is then exposed and divided using a bipolar coagulating device. Once the splenic flexure is mobilized away from the spleen, dissection continues starting at the inferior pole of the spleen and proceeds toward the upper pole of the spleen. A grasper should easily pass posterior to the branches of the splenic vein along the medial margin of the spleen (Fig. 20.6). Multiple firings of the endo-GIA vascular load 60 mm stapler are performed. The stapler should slide smoothly with each passage (Fig. 20.7). This completes division of the blood supply to the spleen.

Mobilization of the Lateral Splenic Attachments

The posterior peritoneal and diaphragmatic attachments of the spleen are subsequently divided using the bipolar coagulating device and blunt dissection.

Splenic Removal

Once the spleen is completely detached it is placed into an endoscopic retrieval bag (Fig. 20.8). Under direct visualization, the bag is brought close to the largest trocar site (typically a 15 mm port) and the spleen is morcellated with a ring forceps. It is then removed in a piecemeal fashion through the trocar and the retrieval bag is withdrawn. Care must be taken during

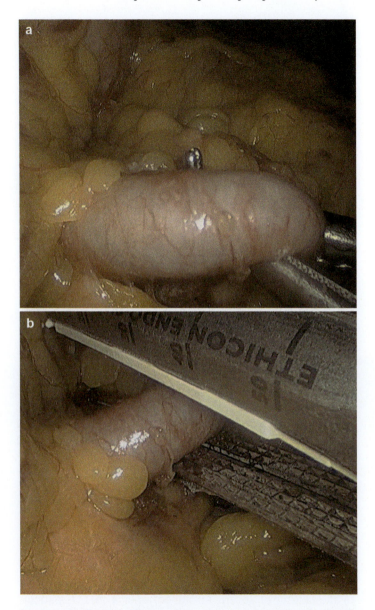

FIGURE 20.5 Division of the splenic artery. At the hilum, the splenic artery is exposed circumferentially (panel **a**) and then transected with an endoscopic vascular linear stapler (panel **b**)

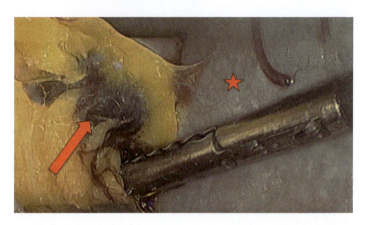

FIGURE 20.6 Preparation for division of the splenic vein branches. A grasper is easily passed posterior to the branches of the splenic vein along the medial margin of the spleen. *Red arrow marks* a splenic vein. *Red star marks* the spleen

morcellation as small bowel or other viscera can fall into the bag and inadvertently be included in the morcellation.

Inspection and Closure

The laparoscope is then re-introduced into the abdomen and the surgical field is thoroughly inspected for signs of bleeding, bowel injury or evidence of any accessory spleens. The field is then irrigated and suctioned. Trocars are removed under direct visualization, followed by the camera trocar. The abdomen is desufflated. All trocar sites with a fascial defect greater than 5 mm are closed. The skin is closed with subcuticular sutures and then with either steri-strips or topical skin adhesive (Fig. 20.9).

Special Considerations

In the setting of severe thrombocytopenia in ITP patients, platelet transfusion can be considered around the time of splenic vasculature clamping and division; we do not commonly

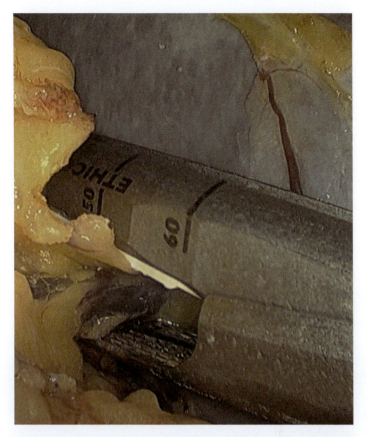

FIGURE 20.7 Division of the splenic vein branches. The endo-GIA stapler is slid smoothly around a splenic vein branch, followed by firing with a vascular load 60 mm cartridge

do this as laparoscopic splenectomy has been shown to be safe without transfusion for patients who otherwise have a normal prothrombin time and absence of preoperative bleeding or coagulopathy [12].

Hematologic changes occurring after splenectomy include granulocystosis followed by lymphocytosis and monocytosis. Additionally, thrombocytosis may arise. An antiplatelet agent,

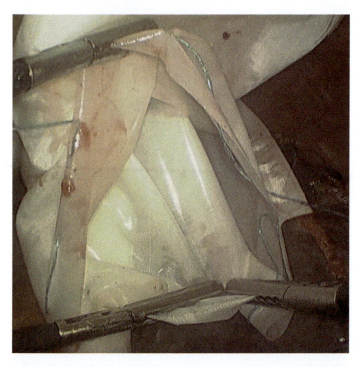

FIGURE 20.8 Preparation for splenic removal. An endoscopic retrieval bag is placed intra-abdominally and prepared for spleen removal. Once completely in the bag, the spleen is morcellated with a ring forceps and removed in a piecemeal fashion through the trocar and the retrieval bag is withdrawn

such as aspirin, is generally recommended when platelet counts are greater than 1,000,000/µL.

A known complication after laparoscopic splenectomy is splenic vein or portal vein thrombosis. Post-operative screening duplex ultrasound may be obtained to confirm the patency of these vessels although we do not routinely obtain this study. Prolonged postoperative anticoagulant prophylaxis can be considered in patients who are considered high risk for this complication, including those who have myeloproliferative disorders or hereditary hemolytic anemias [13].

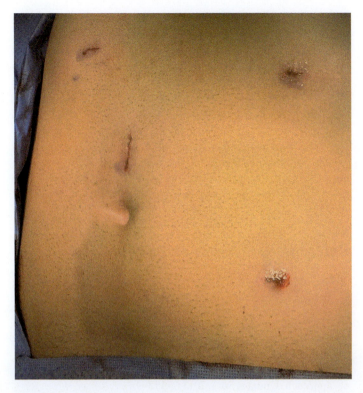

FIGURE 20.9 Skin closure. The skin is closed with subcuticular sutures followed by topical skin adhesive

Overwhelming post-splenectomy infection (OPSI), is a rare but potentially fatal infection occurring in individuals following splenectomy. OPSI is a result of the absence of splenic macrophages, which normally remove encapsulated bacteria bounded by immunoglobulins and complement. OPSI occurs in approximately 0.1 % of patients after splenectomy and has a mortality rate of nearly 50 %. The incidence is greatest within 2 years after splenectomy and is most common in patients who undergo splenectomy for hematologic abnormalities rather than traumatic injuries [5, 14]. Patients who do not receive their vaccinations for encapsulated bacteria prior to their splenectomy should receive them within the first few weeks after surgery (after the patient has recovered) [9].

In the setting of massive splenomegaly, a hand-assisted laparoscopic splenectomy (HALS) can be performed. This technique combines both laparoscopic and open approaches and has been reported to be particularly effective for spleens greater than 25 cm in the largest dimension. In HALS, a hand-port device is placed through the abdominal wall allowing hand and forearm placement into the intra-abdominal cavity. This enables tactile feedback during dissection and can help the surgeon manipulate the spleen to a greater degree than the laparoscopic instruments alone [15].

References

1. Gigot JF, Lengele B, Gianello P, Etienne J, Claeys N. Present status of laparoscopic splenectomy for hematologic diseases: certitudes and unresolved issues. Semin Laparosc Surg. 1998; 5:147–67.
2. Marte G, Scuderi V, Rocca A, Surfaro G, Migliaccio C, Ceriello A. Laparoscopic splenectomy: a single center experience. Unusual cases and expanded inclusion criteria for laparoscopic approach. Updates Surg. 2013;65:115–9.
3. Delaitre B, Maignien B. Splenectomy by the laparoscopic approach. Report of a case. Press Med. 1991;20(44):2263.
4. Musallam KM, Khalife M, Sfeir PM, Faraj W, Safadi B, Abi Saad GS, et al. Postoperative outcomes after laparoscopic splenectomy compared with open splenectomy. Ann Surg. 2013; 257(6):1116–23.
5. Gamme G, Birch D, Karmali S. Minimally invasive splenectomy: an update and review. Can J Surg. 2013;56:280–5.
6. Habermalz B, Sauerland S, Decker G, Delaitre B, Gigot J-F, Leandros E, et al. Laparoscopic splenectomy: the clinical practice guidelines of the European Association for Endoscopic Surgery (EAES). Surg Endosc. 2008;22(4):821–48.
7. Feldman LS. Laparoscopic splenectomy: standardized approach. World J Surg. 2011;35:1487–95.
8. Coignard-Biehler H, Lanternier F, Hot A, Salmon D, Berger A, de Montalembert M, et al. Adherence to preventive measures

after splenectomy in the hospital setting and in the community. J Infect Public Health (King Saud Bin Abdulaziz University for Health Sciences). 2011;4(4):187–94.

9. Holzheimer R, Mannick J, Uranus S, Sill H. Splenectomy for hematological disorders. In: Surgical Treatment: Evidence-Based and Problem-Oriented. Munich: Zuckschwerdt; 2001.

10. Pachter H, Edye M, Guth A. Concepts in splenic surgery. In: Chassin's operative strategy in general surgery. New York: Springer Science and Business Media; 2014. p. 861–5.

11. Petelin J. Patient positioning and operating room setup: splenectomy. In: The sages manual. New York: Springer Science and Business Media; 2006.

12. Wu Z, Zhou J, Li J, Zhu Y. The feasibility of laparoscopic splenectomy for ITP patients without preoperative platelet transfusion. Hepatogastroenterology. 2012;59(113):81–5.

13. Krauth M-T, Lechner K, Neugebauer EAM, Pabinger I. The postoperative splenic/portal vein thrombosis after splenectomy and its prevention – an unresolved issue. Haematologica. 2008;93(8):1227–32.

14. Brigden M. Overwhelming postsplenectomy infection still a problem. West J Med. 1992;157:440–3.

15. Yeo C, McFadden D, Pemberton J, Peters J, Matthews J. Shackelford's surgery of the alimentary tract. Philadelphia: Elsevier Health Sciences; 2012.

Chapter 21
Appendectomy

Jason T. Wiseman and Luke M. Funk

Abstract Approximately 7 % of individuals will develop acute appendicitis during their lifetime. Appendectomy is the most common emergent surgical procedure performed worldwide and in 2010, more than 300,000 appendectomies were performed in the United States. The two operative approaches for performing an appendectomy are open and laparoscopic. Laparoscopic appendectomy is performed in approximately two-thirds of the cases and results in lower overall morbidity in selected patients.

J.T. Wiseman, MD, MSPH
Department of Surgery, University of Wisconsin School of Medicine and Public Health, Madison, WI, USA

L.M. Funk, MD, MPH (✉)
Department of Surgery, University of Wisconsin School of Medicine and Public Health, Madison, WI, USA

Department of Surgery, University of Wisconsin Hospitals and Clinics, 600 Highland Ave, Madison, WI, USA, 53792
e-mail: funk@surgery.wisc.edu

H. Chen (ed.), *Illustrative Handbook of General Surgery*,
DOI 10.1007/978-3-319-24557-7_21,
© Springer International Publishing Switzerland 2016

Keywords Appendectomy • Laparoscopic Appendectomy
• Open Appendectomy • Appendicitis • Complicated
Appendicitis

Indications

The primary indication for an appendectomy is the presentation
of acute appendicitis [1, 2]. An appendectomy is also indicated for
incidental imaging findings of a mass within the appendix or as an
interval appendectomy following ruptured appendicitis, although
there is some debate as to whether this is indicated.

Evaluation

The first step in diagnosing acute appendicitis is taking a
thorough history and physical examination. Patients with
appendicitis usually present with complaints of vague peri-
umbilical pain that migrates to the right lower quadrant.
This discomfort is often associated with fever, anorexia,
nausea and vomiting. Within 24 h from the initial onset of
symptoms, the area over McBurney's point (i.e. the point
approximately two-thirds the distance between the umbilicus and the right anterior superior iliac spine) will be tender on exam. The patient may also have rebound tenderness
and involuntary guarding. If the appendix is retroperitoneal and adjacent to the iliopsoas muscle, the patient may
have a positive psoas sign (pain produced by passively
extending the thigh of a patient lying on his/her side with
knees extended). If the inflamed appendix is adjacent to
the obturator internus muscle, the patient may have a positive obturator sign (pain produced by internally rotating
and flexing the hip of a patient lying on his/her back with
hip and knee flexed). A pelvic exam should also be performed when there is a reasonable consideration for gynecological pathology such as pelvic inflammatory disease or
ovarian torsion.

Laboratories

A complete blood count should be performed for all cases of suspected appendicitis. Results may reveal a mild elevation in the white blood cell count with an associated left shift of neutrophils to greater than 70 % (elevation of the white blood cell count has a sensitivity >80 %) [3]. A routine chemistry ("chem 7") may also be obtained to assess electrolytes and renal status. A pregnancy test should be performed for women of childbearing age to rule out a uterine or ectopic pregnancy.

Imaging

If the patient is male, then the preceding constellation of history and exam findings may be enough information to proceed to the operating room for appendectomy. If there is uncertainty regarding the diagnosis or there is concern regarding a gynecological pathology, additional imaging such as an abdominal computerized tomography (CT) scan is often helpful. Imaging is advantageous because it has the potential to confirm the suspicion of appendicitis or detect another pathology that may be causing the patient's symptoms. In adults, a CT scan is more sensitive and specific than an ultrasound [4]; CT has a sensitivity of approximately 95 % and specificity of at least 95 % while ultrasound is typically closer to 90 % and is user-dependent [5]. Ultrasound is preferable, however, in children given the desire to avoid radiation. Magnetic resonance imaging (MRI) is also useful if avoidance of radiation is a high priority. The most common indication for using MRI in this setting is suspected appendicitis in a pregnant patient.

Choice of Surgical Approach

Traditionally, open appendectomy has been the standard of care. However with the evolution of minimally invasive techniques, laparoscopic appendectomy has become the surgical modality of choice for most surgeons due to its association with quicker recoveries and less pain [6]. Although there are a few clinical scenarios that may force the surgeon to choose one method over the other, the choice of approach is ultimately dictated by surgeon preference.

Laparoscopic Appendectomy

One advantage of performing the procedure laparoscopically is that it provides excellent visualization of the peritoneal cavity. This is particularly beneficial in females where the laparoscopic approach may allow identification of ovarian or uterine abnormalities [7]. Laparoscopy also provides an optimal visualization in obese patients and is the preferred approach.

Laparoscopic appendectomy can also be safely performed in cases of perforated appendicitis [6, 8]. Compared to open appendectomy, the laparoscopic approach has a marginally longer operative time, but is associated with decreased post-operative length of stay and less postoperative pain. Additionally, patients experience an earlier return to baseline functional activity, decreased incidence of wound infection, and an overall decrease in morbidity and mortality [9–12].

Open Appendectomy

An open approach may be preferable if there is a contraindication to laparoscopy such as refractory coagulopathy, inability to tolerate pneumoperitoneum, or generalized peritonitis with hemodynamic compromise [13]. If the patient is pregnant, obtaining laparoscopic access may be difficult with limited exposure of the appendix, potentially influencing a surgeon to take an open approach.

Non-Operative Management

Complicated appendicitis, including a presentation of a periappendiceal abscess or an abscess in the right lower quadrant occurs in approximately 2–7 % of patients. The preferred approach for these patients with an intra-abdominal abscess on CT scan is percutaneous drainage and IV-antibiotic administration, followed by an interval appendectomy [14]. There is emerging evidence that antibiotics alone may be sufficient for cases of uncomplicated appendicitis, however this data is not conclusive and we do not recommend this treatment pathway [15, 16].

Preoperative Preparation

Once the diagnosis of appendicitis has been made, the patient should be taken to the operating room in an expedited manner as the incidence of rupture increases by approximately 5 % for each ensuing 12-h period beyond the initial 36 h [17]. IV-antibiotics with gram-negative and anaerobic coverage should be initiated. Patients with delayed presentation or perforated appendicitis may need aggressive fluid resuscitation and electrolyte replacement prior to surgery.

Positioning and Anesthesia

The patient should be placed in the supine position on the operating table. For laparoscopic surgery, the patient's right arm is abducted to facilitate IV-access and the left arm tucked along the patient's side to allow the surgeon and assistant to stand on the patient's left side (Fig. 21.1). In an open appendectomy, both arms are abducted to allow the surgeon and the assistant room to stand on either side.

General endotracheal anesthesia is the preferred method of anesthesia. Deep vein thrombosis prophylaxis should be administered prior to induction as either sequential compression devices, unfractionated heparin, or low molecular weight heparin [18]. A Foley catheter may be placed to monitor fluid status and an orogastric tube may be placed to decompress the stomach. This is particularly important if we access the abdomen using a Veress needle in the left upper quadrant because it allows decompression of the stomach and minimizes the likelihood of gastric injury.

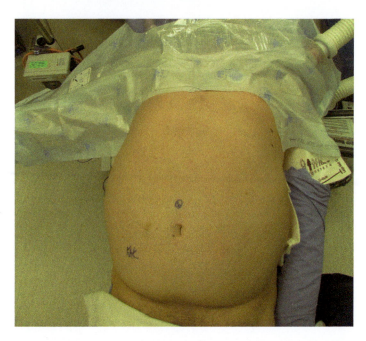

FIGURE 21.1 Patient positioning during a laparoscopic appendectomy. The patient is placed on the operating room table in the supine position with the right arm abducted to facilitate intravenous axis and the left arm tucked against the body to allow room for the surgeon and assistant to stand

Open Appendectomy: Procedure Description

Abdominal Access

A 2–6 cm incision is made at McBurney's point; a Rocky-Davis (i.e. transverse) or a McBurney (i.e. parallel to the external oblique muscle) incision can be used. The location of the incision may be made at a slightly different point depending on location of maximum tenderness on palpation prior to anesthesia or if there is a palpable mass. An alternative and less commonly performed incision is a lower midline, which may facilitate exposure if the patient is obese or assist in exploration of the pelvis if the operating surgeon suspects underlying pelvic pathology.

Identification of Appendix

The incision is carried down to the external oblique which is incised parallel to its fibers. The internal oblique is then bluntly separated exposing the transversus abdominus and underlying transversalis fascia, which is then divided. The peritoneum is exposed, lifted and incised, opening a window into the peritoneal cavity. The appendix and cecum are identified and mobilized anteriorly toward the wound. To do this, it is often necessary to sharply or bluntly mobilize the cecum and terminal ileum away from their retroperitoneal attachments. If the appendix cannot be located, the surgeon can identify the taenia coli of the cecum and track them down to the base of the appendix.

Ligation of Mesoappendix

The mesoappendix is usually ligated first to avoid appendiceal artery injury during excision of the appendix. The mesoappendix and adjoining appendiceal artery may be ligated with a non-absorbable suture and then divided, or alternatively transected with a GIA or TA stapler.

Ligation of Appendix

We prefer to resect the appendix by initially crushing it at the base with a clamp followed by a suture ligature. A purse-string suture is then placed in the cecum surrounding the base of the appendix. The appendix is divided just beyond the suture ligature. Electrocautery may be used to cauterize the appendix with the intention of preventing a mucoceole. The appendiceal stump is inverted into the cecum and the purse-string suture secured to invert the appendiceal base. An alternative to using a suture ligature to remove the appendix is to transect the appendix with a GIA or TA stapler.

Inspection and Closure

Once the appendix and mesoappendix are removed from the operative field, hemostasis is ensured and the right lower quadrant inspected. If spillage is present, the area is aspirated and irrigated with several liters of normal saline. The peritoneum and transversalis fascia are closed with a running suture followed by closure of the internal oblique with another running suture. The external oblique fascia is closed with a running suture. The subcutaneous tissue is closed with interrupted sutures. The skin is closed with subcuticular sutures and then with either steri-strips or topical skin adhesive. The skin is typically left open if the appendix is perforated.

Laparoscopic Appendectomy: Procedure Description

Abdominal Access

There are numerous ways to gain access into the intraperitoneal cavity. In a non-obese patient, we prefer to access the intra-abdominal cavity by the Hasson technique. A transverse curvilinear incision is made below the umbilicus followed by blunt dissection to the midline fascia and umbilical stalk. The umbilical stalk is then grasped at its base and elevated. An approximately 1-cm vertical incision is made with a scalpel entering the peritoneal cavity taking care not to injure underlying bowel or blood vessels. A finger is placed within this opening to ensure entrance into the intraperitoneal cavity. A suture is then placed into the fascia to secure the Hasson port and also for eventual closure. A 12 mm Hasson trocar is then secured in place.

If the patient is obese, a Veress needle is initially placed into the left upper quadrant. Intra-abdominal positioning of

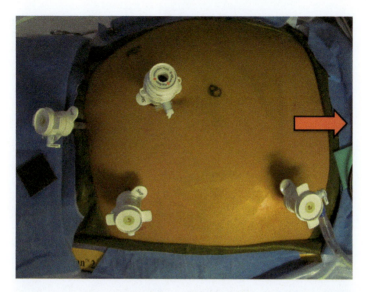

FIGURE 21.2 Trocar placement for laparoscopic appendectomy. One 12 mm trocar is placed below the umbilicus; one 5 mm trocar is placed in the left lower quadrant lateral to the rectus muscle; one 5 mm trocar is placed in the suprapubic position. One 5 mm trocar may be placed in the left upper quadrant if a Veress needle is used for access at this same point (optional). *Red arrow* marks the head of the patient

the needle can be confirmed by aspiration and a negative saline drop test. Pneumoperitoneum is then established by insufflating the abdomen to a pressure of 15 mmHg with carbon dioxide. A 5 mm port is then placed into the left upper quadrant.

A 30° laparoscopic camera is then introduced and all four quadrants of the abdomen are visually inspected. If the Veress needle is used for access in the left upper quadrant, an additional 12 mm trocar is inserted inferior to the umbilicus. This is the primary camera port during the case and also allows for passage of the endo-GIA linear stapler. Two 5 mm trocars are subsequently placed under direct visualization: one in the left lower quadrant lateral to the left rectus muscle and the other in the suprapubic position (Fig. 21.2). This is performed with attention not to injure the bladder or inferior

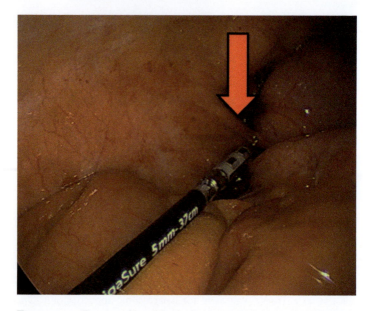

FIGURE 21.3 Retroperitoneal attachments of the cecum and terminal ileum. Access to the base of the appendix and mesoappendix may be difficult when there are robust retroperitoneal attachments between the cecum and the abdominal wall. *Red arrow* marks a retroperitoneal attachment

epigastric vessels. The patient is then placed in the Trendelenburg position with the right side up to facilitate visualization of the appendix.

Identification of Appendix

The cecum and terminal ileum are mobilized away from the retroperitoneum with scissors or electrocautery allowing improved access to the base of the appendix and mesoappendix (Figs. 21.3 and 21.4). This step is critical in being able to identify the appendiceal base. The tip of the appendix is grasped and retracted medially and anteriorly providing complete exposure.

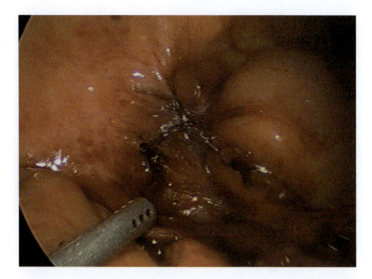

FIGURE 21.4 Dissection of retroperitoneal attachments. Mobilization of the cecum and terminal ileum away from retroperitoneal attachments is performed allowing improved access to the base of the appendix and mesoappendix; this step is critical in being able to identify the appendiceal base

Ligation of Mesoappendix

Our preferred approach is to transect the mesoappendix with a bipolar vessel sealing system (Figs. 21.5 and 21.6). This method avoids the need to create a mesoappendiceal window, decreasing the chance of appendiceal artery injury. Alternatively, a window can be created in the base of the mesoappendix adjacent to the appendix. This maneuver can be performed with a Maryland or blunt grasper. Once the window is complete, the mesoappendix and associated appendiceal artery can be divided using a bipolar vessel sealing system, ultrasonic sheers or a linear stapler with a vascular load. If the stapler is used, due to its size, the 10 mm laparoscopic camera is exchanged for a 5 mm camera and moved to the left lower quadrant 5 mm port, allowing placement of the stapler into the abdomen via the periumbilical 12 mm port.

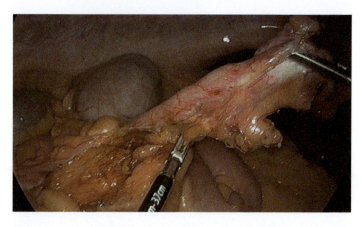

FIGURE 21.5 Ligation of mesoappendix. The mesoappendix is transected with a bipolar vessel sealing system while the appendix is retracted

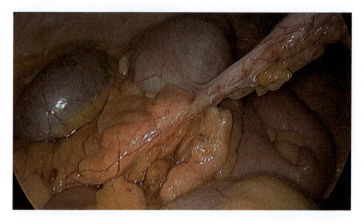

FIGURE 21.6 Visualization of the appendiceal base. The mesoappendix is completely transected allowing complete visualization of the appendiceal base

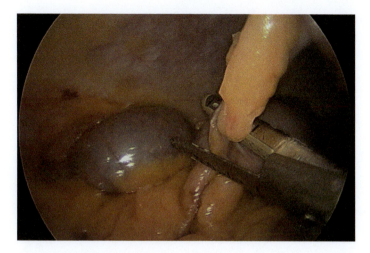

FIGURE 21.7 Transection of the appendix. The appendix is divided with an endo-GIA stapler

Transection of Appendix

The appendix is then divided with an endo-GIA stapler paying careful attention to locate the stapler at the appendiceal base (Fig. 21.7). A 30 or 45 mm stapler is typically adequate. An alternative method for dividing the appendix is using a pre-tied endoscopic ligature. Once resected, the appendix is placed into an endoscopic retrieval bag and brought out through the 12 mm umbilical port or port site.

Inspection and Closure

The staple line is closely inspected for staple malformation or ongoing bleeding (Fig. 21.8). The right lower quadrant, pelvis, and right subdiaphragmatic space are inspected for any contamination and irrigated if desired. The 5 mm trocars are then removed under direct visualization followed

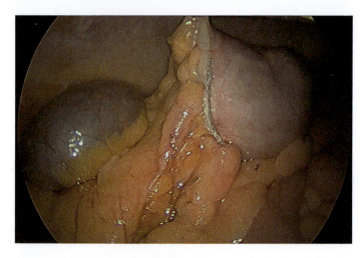

FIGURE 21.8 Inspection of staple line and other transected areas. The staple line and other transected areas are closely inspected for staple failures or inadequate hemostasis

by the 12 mm trocar. The abdomen is desufflated and the fascial defect at the umbilical trocar site is closed with an absorbable figure-of-eight suture. The skin is closed with subcuticular sutures and either steri-strips or topical skin adhesive (Fig. 21.9).

Special Postoperative Considerations

Antibiotics should be discontinued immediately after surgery in uncomplicated cases. In complicated cases or cases where the appendix is perforated, antibiotics may be given for 5–7 days, however this is controversial [19]. If the patient's clinical parameters do not normalize within the first 24–48 h after surgery (i.e. vital signs, pain, fevers/chills, leukocytosis) the surgeon should have a heightened suspicion for a surgical complication including an abscess, leak or hematoma.

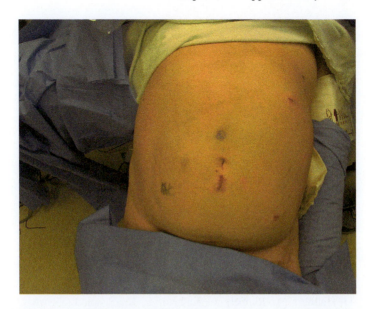

FIGURE 21.9 Skin closure. The skin is closed with subcuticular sutures followed by topical skin adhesive

References

1. National Health Statistics Reports [Internet]. National hospital discharge survey. 2010. Available from http://www.cdc.gov/nchs/nhds/nhds_tables.htm#number.
2. Addiss DG, Shaffer N, Fowler BS, Tauxe RV. The epidemiology of appendicitis and appendectomy in the United States. Am J Epidemiol. 1990;132:910–25.
3. Dueholm S, Bagi P, Bud M. Laboratory aid in the diagnosis of acute appendicitis. A blinded, prospective trial concerning diagnostic value of leukocyte count, neutrophil differential count, and C-reactive protein. Dis Colon Rectum. 1989;32(10):855–9.
4. Van Randen A, Bipat S, Zwinderman A. Acute appendicitis: meta-analysis of diagnostic performance of CT and graded compression US related to prevalence of disease. Radiology. 2008;249(1):97–106.

5. Petroianu A. Diagnosis of acute appendicitis. Int J Surg. 2012; 10:115–9.

6. Korndorffer JR, Fellinger E, Reed W. SAGES guideline for laparoscopic appendectomy. Surg Endosc. 2010;24(4):757–61.

7. Zaninotto G, Rossi M, Anseimino M, Costantini M, Pianalto S, Baldan N, et al. Laparoscopic versus conventional surgery for suspected appendicitis in women. Surg Endosc. 1995;9:337–40.

8. Guller U, Jain N, Peterson ED, Muhlbaier LH, Eubanks S, Pietrobon R. Laparoscopic appendectomy in the elderly. Surgery. 2004;135(5):479–88.

9. Ingraham AM, Cohen ME, Bilimoria KY, Pritts TA, Ko CY, Esposito TJ. Comparison of outcomes after laparoscopic versus open appendectomy for acute appendicitis at 222 ACS NSQIP hospitals. Surgery. 2010;148:625–37.

10. Masoomi H, Mills S, Dolich MO, Ketana N, Carmichael JC, Nguyen NT, et al. Comparison of outcomes of laparoscopic versus open appendectomy in children: data from the Nationwide Inpatient Sample (NIS), 2006–2008. World J Surg. 2012;36: 573–8.

11. Hellberg A, Rudberg C, Kullman E, Enochsson L, Fenyö G, Graffner H, et al. Prospective randomized multicentre study of laparoscopic versus open appendicectomy. Br J Surg. 1999;86(1):48–53.

12. Katkhouda N, Mason RJ, Towfigh S, Gevorgyan A, Essani R. Laparoscopic versus open appendectomy: a prospective randomized double-blind study. Ann Surg. 2005;242(3):439–50.

13. Fischer J, Bland K, Callery M, editors. Mastery of surgery. 5th ed. Philadelphia: Lippincott Williams & Wilkins; 2006.

14. Kim J-K, Ryoo S, Oh H-K, Kim JS, Shin R, Choe EK, et al. Management of appendicitis presenting with abscess or mass. J Korean Soc Coloproctol. 2010;26(6):413–9.

15. Di Saverio S, Sibilio A, Giorgini E, Biscardi A, Villani S, Coccolini F, et al. The NOTA study (Non Operative Treatment for Acute Appendicitis): prospective study on the efficacy and safety of antibiotics (amoxicillin and clavulanic acid) for treating patients With right lower quadrant abdominal pain and long-term follow-up of conser. Ann Surg. 2014;260(1):109–17.

16. Minneci PC, Sulkowski JP, Nacion KM, Mahida JB, Cooper JN, Moss RL, et al. Feasibility of a nonoperative management strategy for uncomplicated acute appendicitis in children. J Am Coll Surg. 2014;219(2):272–9.

17. Bickell N, Aufses A, Rojas M, Bodian C. How time affects the risk of rupture in appendicitis. J Am Coll Surg. 2006;202(3): 401–6.

18. Levine J. Guidelines for deep venous thrombosis prophylaxis during laparoscopic surgery. Surg. Endosc. Soc Am Gastrointest Endosc Surg; 2006 p. 1–6.
19. Taylor E, Berjis A, Bosch T, Hoehne F, Ozaeta M. The efficacy of postoperative oral antibiotics in appendicitis: a randomized prospective double-blinded study. Am Surg. 2004;70(10):858–62.

Part V
Colorectal Surgery

Charles P. Heise

Chapter 22
Right Hemicolectomy

Terrah J. Paul Olson and Charles P. Heise

Abstract   Surgical resection of the right colon is performed for benign and malignant disease. Resection margins are determined by the blood supply to the right colon as well as surgical indication. Hemicolectomy can be performed open or laparoscopically. Preoperative preparation is briefly discussed. The steps for successful open right hemicolectomy are described. Similarly, both a lateral-to-medial and medial-to-lateral laparoscopic approach is explained. The technique for a side to side stapled ileocolic anastomosis is demonstrated, along with further innovations in surgical technique. Postoperative care is briefly outlined.

Keywords   Right hemicolectomy • Laparoscopic • Surgical technique • Colectomy • Colon • Anastomosis • Stapled • Colon cancer

———

T.J. Paul Olson, MD (✉)
Department of General Surgery, University of Wisconsin Hospital and Clinics, Madison, WI, USA
e-mail: tpaulolson@uwhealth.org

C.P. Heise, MD
Department of Surgery, University of Wisconsin Hospital and Clinics, Madison, WI, USA

University of Wisconsin School of Medicine and Public Health, Madison, WI, USA

H. Chen (ed.), *Illustrative Handbook of General Surgery*,
DOI 10.1007/978-3-319-24557-7_22,
© Springer International Publishing Switzerland 2016

Anatomy and Indications

The right colon extends from the cecum, which is typically fixed in the right lower quadrant to the hepatic flexure, where it transitions to the transverse colon. The arterial supply to the right colon is derived from the superior mesenteric artery. The ileocolic branch supplies the terminal ileum and cecum. In 32–63 % of the population, the right colic artery supplies the ascending colon, but a substantial proportion of the population derives arterial blood flow to the right colon from the ileocolic artery alone [1, 2]. Branches of the middle colic artery can supply the hepatic flexure. There can be collateral vessels between these branches and those from the right colic artery forming the right portion of the marginal artery. The venous drainage of the right colon mirrors the arterial supply – the ileocolic, right colic, and middle colic veins drain into the superior mesenteric vein. The lymphatic supply to the colon follows the blood supply through the mesentery.

Benign or malignant lesions of the cecum and right colon can be treated by right hemicolectomy. Indications for benign processes involving the right colon are Crohn's disease, ischemia, trauma, diverticulitis and cecal volvulus. Malignant or premalignant lesions are also appropriately managed with right hemicolectomy, including adenocarcinomas or colonoscopically unresectable adenomas. In addition, appendiceal neoplasms such as adenocarcinoma or carcinoid tumors larger than 2 cm, those not confined to the appendix, or with positive lymph nodes require right hemicolectomy [3].

The extent of resection for malignant lesions located within the cecum or ascending colon is dictated primarily by the blood supply and lymphatic drainage. Where formal oncologic resection is required, the extent of colon removed is based upon the area supplied by the ileocolic and right colic artery. If extended right hemicolectomy is warranted, removal of additional transverse colon supplied by the middle colic artery may be required.

Preoperative Preparation

Individual patient risk factors will determine what additional cardiac and pulmonary work-up is required preoperatively. Pertinent preoperative work-up is determined by the underlying diagnosis requiring right colon resection. Colonoscopy is used to identify, obtain tissue diagnosis, and permanently mark (tattoo) the location of an intra-luminal lesion. This is particularly important when a laparoscopic approach is planned. Using india ink, the endoscopist should tattoo immediately adjacent to the lesion and ideally in at least 2 quadrants, allowing intra-operative identification [4].

In cases where malignancy is proven or suspected, preoperative work-up should also include a chest x-ray and computed tomography of the abdomen and pelvis for complete oncologic staging [5]. Preoperative carcinoembryonic antigen (CEA) is obtained to facilitate postoperative surveillance. Evidence of metastatic disease does not necessarily exclude right hemicolectomy, but may alter the treatment approach and planning. Careful discussion with the patient about goals of therapy, patient preferences, and relative balance of risks and benefits is required prior to performing any operative procedure.

Preoperative patient preparation usually involves full mechanical bowel preparation with oral antibiotics. An updated Cochrane Review concluded that there is no evidence that preoperative mechanical bowel preparation alone decreases rates of anastomotic leak, mortality, peritonitis, need for reoperation, wound infection, or morbidity. Additionally, there is some suggestion that inadequate bowel preparation which leaves liquid stool within the colon may be associated with poorer outcomes [6]. However, a Veteran's Administration study noted that mechanical bowel preparation with oral antibiotics may decrease rates of surgical site infections [7]. Other preoperative considerations must include appropriate DVT prophylaxis and Surgical Care Improvement Project (SCIP) appropriate IV antibiotics [8].

Anesthesia and Positioning

General anesthesia is utilized for open and laparoscopic right hemicolectomy. In extremely high risk patients, spinal anesthesia can be considered for open procedures [9]. In open cases a thoracic epidural catheter may be utilized and can be placed preoperatively or postoperatively for pain control, and may reduce narcotic requirements and promote earlier return of bowel function [10].

The patient is positioned supine on the operating room table. Arms may be tucked at the patient's sides for a laparoscopic approach. Deep vein thrombosis prophylaxis is provided with sequential compression devices and subcutaneous unfractionated heparin given prior to beginning the case. Preoperative antibiotics with gram positive and gram negative coverage (SCIP inf-2 guidelines [8]) are given within 60 min of making incision (SCIP inf-1 [8]) and re-dosed as needed throughout the case. An indwelling urinary catheter is placed for monitoring during the procedure.

Operative Descriptions

Open Right Hemicolectomy

The decision to perform an open or laparoscopic right hemicolectomy will depend on patient factors and the surgeon's familiarity with the laparoscopic approach. We will begin with a description of the open approach.

An incision in made from just above to just below the umbilicus. The subcutaneous tissues and linea alba are divided with either the scalpel or electrocautery until the peritoneum is identified. This is elevated and entered sharply with a scalpel or Metzenbaum scissors. A self-retaining retractor is placed, and the liver, peritoneum and other organs are inspected and palpated for evidence of other pathology.

The peritoneal reflection is incised lateral to the cecum, and this incision is carried superiorly toward the hepatic

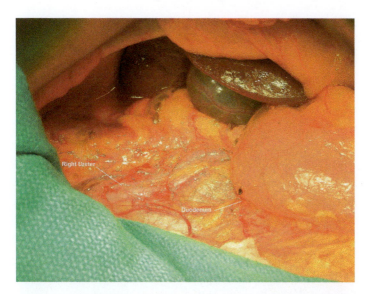

FIGURE 22.1 The right colon is retracted medial while dividing the lateral peritoneal attachments, taking care to identify and preserve the right ureter. As the dissection is carried superiorly, the duodenum must be identified and protected

flexure of the colon. The right ureter must be identified and preserved as it crosses anteriorly over the right common iliac bifurcation. The colon is further mobilized medially lifting the mesentery from the retroperitoneum. As the dissection is carried toward the hepatic flexure, the second and third portions of the duodenum must be identified and protected from injury (Fig. 22.1). The duodenum is kept posteriorly while the colon is brought anteriorly during dissection from the retroperitoneum (Fig. 22.2). The vessels in the hepatocolic ligament are ligated and divided and the lesser sac is entered mobilizing the proximal transverse colon.

The omentum is dissected free from the transverse colon at the distal resection site and divided using either the clamp and tie technique, or using a vessel sealing device (ultrasonic coagulating shears or electrothermal bipolar vessel sealers). If performing the operation for benign disease, the mesenteric

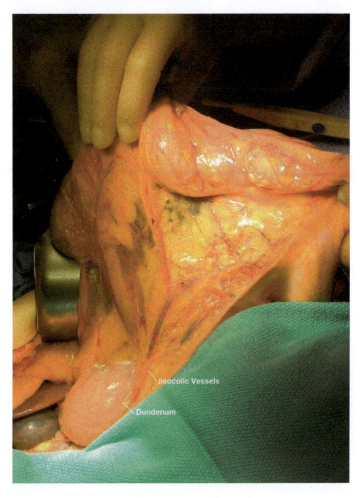

FIGURE 22.2 As the right colon is mobilized and rotated medially, the second and third portion of the duodenum should be identified and kept posterior

attachments of the right colon can be divided close to the mesenteric border of the colon. If the operation is performed for malignancy, the resection site should be chosen to ensure a luminal margin of at least 5 cm [11]. A window is created in the transverse mesocolon at the site where the colon will be

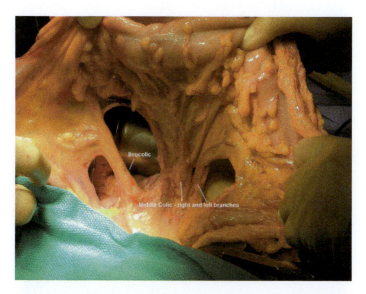

FIGURE 22.3 The mesentery of the right colon and, if necessary, the transverse colon is ligated. When malignant disease is resected, the ileocolic and right colic (if present) vessels are identified and divided near their origin to allow for adequate lymph node sampling. The right branch of the middle colic is usually divided at its bifurcation from the left branch

divided, the marginal artery of Drummond is ligated and divided, and the transverse mesocolon is divided down to the base of the mesentery to identify the middle colic vessel bifurcation. The right branch of the middle colic is ligated and divided at its origin while the left branch is preserved. If the lesion is at the hepatic flexure or proximal transverse colon, the specimen can be extended by dividing the middle colic vessels at their base. If the right colic vessels are present, these are also divided at their origin, and the mesentery is divided down to the base of the ileocolic vessels (Fig. 22.3), which are also ligated and divided. The mesentery of the terminal ileum is divided, and the proximal margin of the specimen should include 5–10 cm of small bowel [11, 12], although more can be excised for cecal tumors. The specimen is opened on the back table and inspected to ensure that it contains the

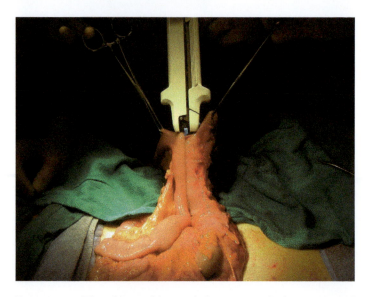

FIGURE 22.4 The side-to-side stapled anastomosis is constructed after resecting the specimen. Each half of the linear cutting stapler is passed through enterotomies in the terminal ileum (*left*) and transverse colon (*right*). Firing the stapler creates a lumen through the antimesenteric borders of the intestine

lesion of interest and margins are appropriate. It can then be passed off the table and sent to surgical pathology.

The ileocolic anastomosis can be created either in a hand-sewn or stapled fashion. We describe the side-to-side stapled approach. After initially dividing the mesentery as already described, the ileum and transverse colon are aligned side by side and enterotomies are made on the antimesenteric borders of both limbs of bowel. The two halves of a linear stapler (typically 75 or 80 mm) are passed into the lumen of both the large and small bowel (Fig. 22.4). After firing the stapler, the intraluminal staple lines are inspected for bleeding. The anterior and posterior staple lines should be slightly off-set, and a 60-mm transverse non-cutting stapler is used to close the end of the anastomosis distal to the prior enterotomies (Fig. 22.5). The bowel is divided sharply on the stapler.

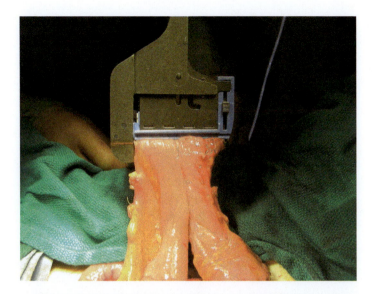

FIGURE 22.5 The common enterotomy from the side-to-side stapled anastomosis is closed using the transverse non-cutting stapler. Care is taken not to narrow the newly created lumen, and the staple line can be oversewn

This staple line can be oversewn if desired with interrupted imbricating sutures, and the mesenteric defect can be closed with a running absorbable suture to prevent risk of internal hernia. The abdomen is irrigated, inspected for bleeding, and the fascia is closed with running absorbable suture. The subcutaneous tissue is again irrigated, and the skin is closed.

Laparoscopic Assisted Right Hemicolectomy

Laparoscopic assisted right hemicolectomy can be performed under general anesthetic with similar preparation and positioning as described above. Because of the reduction of tactile sensation during the laparoscopic portion of the case, tattooing of the lesion colonoscopically takes on increased importance.

The abdomen can be entered using a Veress needle technique or the Hasson technique [13]. With the Hasson approach a 1–1.5 cm peri-umbilical incision is made and dissection is carried down until the linea alba can be identified and elevated. This is divided, and the peritoneum is sharply incised. Stay sutures are placed at the lateral edges of the fascia, and the 12 mm Hasson trocar is inserted into the abdomen. The stay sutures are used to secure the trocar in place, and the abdomen is insufflated to 15 mmHg with carbon dioxide. The laparoscope is inserted, and the abdomen is inspected for injury during insertion and for other intra-abdominal pathology which may preclude resection. In general, a 30 ° scope is utilized for this procedure. Additional 5 mm ports are placed in the supra-pubic midline and in the left lower quadrant; a third port can be placed in the left upper quadrant or in the right lower quadrant, depending on the need during dissection.

The colon may be mobilized using either a lateral to medial or medial to lateral approach. The lateral to medial approach is as follows: the patient is placed in Trendelenberg with tilt to elevate the right side. The terminal ileum is identified and retracted anteriorly, as is the appendix and cecum to allow incision of the peritoneal attachments. These are divided and dissection continues in a cephalad direction, taking care to identify the gonadal vessels and the right ureter as it passes over the right common iliac vessels and ensure that this remains posterior as the colon is mobilized anteriorly (Fig. 22.6). As the dissection approaches the hepatic flexure, the duodenum must be identified and protected (Fig. 22.7). The hepatocolic ligament and omental attachments are divided after placing the patient in a reverse Trendelenberg position. After completing the mobilization of the specimen, the terminal ileum and ascending colon are elevated to identify the ileocolic vessels at their origin (Fig. 22.8). A window is created on either side, and the vessels are divided using a vessel sealing or stapling device.

For the medial to lateral approach, after entering the abdomen, the mesentery of the terminal ileum and right

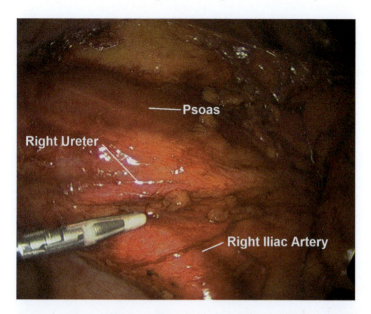

FIGURE 22.6 Laparoscopic lateral-to-medial mobilization: the right colon lateral peritoneal attachments are incised and the colon retracted medially, anteriorly, and cephalad to allow dissection from underlying retroperitoneal structures including the right ureter and gonadal vessels. The psoas muscle and right iliac vessels are also seen

colon is elevated, and the ileocolic vascular pedicle is identi-fied (Fig. 22.9). The peritoneum overlying the mesentery is incised, and windows are made on either side of the vessels at the proximal base (Fig. 22.10). The duodenum is visual-ized and swept posteriorly as the mesentery is elevated from the retroperitoneum. The ileocolic vessels are then divided with a stapler or energy sealing device (Fig. 22.11). Once they are divided, dissection can then continue, mobilizing the lateral peritoneal reflection of the colon. Care is again taken to free the hepatic flexure from the underlying duo-denum during dissection. The remainder of the operation is as described above. Advantages of the medial to lateral approach include easier mesenteric dissection as the colon

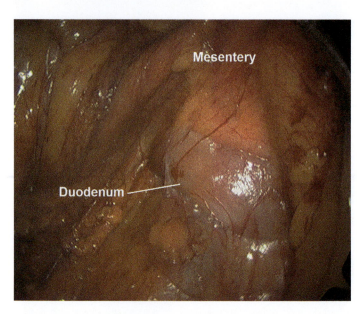

FIGURE 22.7 As with the open dissection, the right colon is lifted medially and anteriorly, allowing dissection of the third portion of the duodenum, which falls posteriorly as the retroperitoneal attachments to the colon are divided

is tethered to the abdominal wall rather than being free to move, earlier identification and preservation of the ureter and gonadal vessels, decreased bleeding from early control of vascular pedicles, and decreased manipulation of the diseased portion of colon [14].

The proximal colon or terminal ileum is secured with laparoscopic graspers and all other ports are removed to desufflate the abdomen. The peri-umbilical port site is extended if necessary to accommodate a small wound protector device (2–6 cm length). The specimen is extracted and the remaining mesentery is

FIGURE 22.9 Laparoscopic medial-to-lateral mobilization: after identifying the terminal ileum and cecum, the vascular pedicle containing the ileocolic vessels is identified and elevated

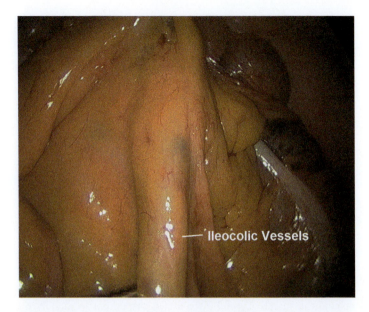

FIGURE 22.8 Lateral-to-medial mobilization: after the right colon has been mobilized laterally, the ileocolic vessels are identified by elevating the terminal ileum and cecum. This allows creation of mesenteric windows on either side of the vessels prior to division at their origin

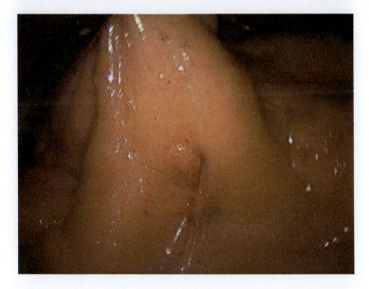

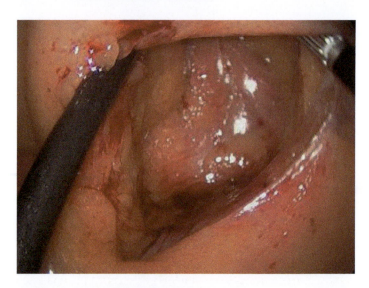

FIGURE 22.10 Medial-to-lateral mobilization: the mesentery is incised around the vessels. Careful dissection is carried out to identify the duodenum and sweep the retroperitoneal structures posterior

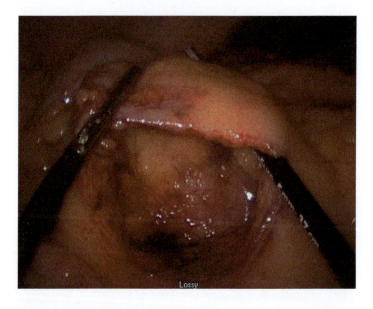

divided to the mid-transverse colon and distal ileum. The side to side stapled ileocolic anastomosis is then created as described above. Closure of the large mesenteric defect is usually not possible, and thus is left open. The anastomosis is then replaced back into the abdomen, which is irrigated and inspected for bleeding. The fascial incision is closed with absorbable suture, and the skin and remaining port sites are irrigated and closed.

Further Innovations

Laparoscopic assisted colectomy is well accepted for treatment of benign and malignant disease of the colon [15, 16]. Variations of minimally invasive surgery are also described. This has included a single incision laparoscopic right hemicolectomy. For this technique, a gel port or specially formatted port allowing insertion of multiple instruments is placed in the abdomen at the umbilicus. The case is then performed as described above. The specimen is then retrieved through the umbilicus, with the bowel exteriorized and anastomosis performed. A recent meta-analysis of nine comparative studies revealed no significant difference in postoperative outcomes or oncologic results with single incision laparoscopic right hemicolectomy compared to the standard laparoscopic approach, though prospective randomized studies are lacking [17].

Postoperative Care

Patients are admitted to the general care floor for postoperative monitoring and pain control. A nasogastric tube is not utilized. Early mobilization should be encouraged, and deep

FIGURE 22.11 Medial-to-lateral mobilization: the ileocolic vascular pedicle is isolated allowing safe division of the vessels at their mesenteric origin. Once divided, mobilization of the lateral peritoneal attachments of the right colon is performed

vein thrombosis prophylaxis should be continued. In appropriate patients, non-steroidal anti-inflammatory medications and other non-narcotic modalities of analgesia should be included to minimize narcotic requirements. A liquid diet can be started early postoperatively, and the diet advanced upon full return of bowel function. Patients can anticipate a 3–5 day hospital stay and are ready for discharge upon return of bowel function, tolerating oral intake, ambulating, and appropriate pain control. Complications include wound infection, prolonged ileus, and anastomotic leak.

References

1. Tajima Y, Ishida H, Ohsawa T, et al. Three-dimensional vascular anatomy relevant to oncologic resection of right colon cancer. Int Surg. 2011;94(4):300–4.
2. Ignjatovic D, Sund S, Stimec B, Bergamaschi R. Vascular relationships in right colectomy for cancer: clinical implications. Tech Coloproctol. 2007;11(3):247–50.
3. National Comprehensive Cancer Network Guidelines Panel. National Comprehensive Cancer Network Guidelines version 2.2014. Carcinoid tumor. http://www.nccn.org/professionals/physician_gls/pdf/neuroendocrine.pdf. Accessed 16 Oct 2014.
4. Yeung JMC, Maxwell-Armstrong C, Acheson AG. Colonic tattooing in laparoscopic surgery – making the mark? Colorectal Dis. 2009;11(5):527–30.
5. National Comprehensive Cancer Network Guidelines Panel. National Comprehensive Cancer Network Guidelines version 2.2015. Colon cancer. http://www.nccn.org/professionals/physician_gls/pdf/colon.pdf. Accessed 16 Oct 2014.
6. Güenaga KF, Matos D, Wille-Jørgense P. Mechanical bowel preparation for elective colorectal surgery. Cochrane Database Syst Rev. 2011;(9):CD001544. doi:10.1002/14651858.CD001544.pub4.
7. Cannon JA, Altom LK, Deierhoi RJ, et al. Preoperative oral antibiotics reduce surgical site infection following elective colorectal resections. Dis Colon Rectum. 2012;55:1160–6.
8. The Joint Commission. Surgical Care Improvement Project. http://www.jointcommission.org/surgical_care_improvement_project/. Accessed 16 Oct 2014.

9. Kumar CM, Corbett WA, Wilson RG. Spinal anaesthesia with a micro-catheter in high-risk patients undergoing colorectal cancer and other major abdominal surgery. Surg Oncol. 2008; 17(2):73–9.

10. Carli F, Trudel JL, Belliveau P. The effect of intraoperative thoracic epidural anesthesia and postoperative analgesia on bowel function after colorectal surgery: a prospective, randomized trial. Dis Colon Rectum. 2001;44(8):1083–9.

11. Hida J, Okuno L, Yasutomi M, et al. Optimal ligation level of the primary feeding artery and bowel resection margin in colon cancer surgery: the influence of the site of the primary feeding artery. Dis Colon Rectum. 2005;48(12):2232–7.

12. Toyota S, Ohta H, Anazawa S. Rationale for extent of lymph node dissection for right colon cancer. Dis Colon Rectum. 1995;38:705–11.

13. Hasson HM. Open laparoscopy. Biomed Bull. 1984;5(1):1–6.

14. Poon JT, Law WL, Fan JK, et al. Impact of the standardized medial-to-lateral approach on outcome of laparoscopic colorectal resection. World J Surg. 2009;33(10):2177–82.

15. Clinical Outcomes of Surgical Therapy (COST). Study group. A comparison of laparoscopically assisted and open colectomy for colon cancer. N Engl J Med. 2004;350:2050–9.

16. Kahnamoui K, Cadeddu M, Farrokhyar F, Anvari M. Laparoscopic surgery for colon cancer: a systematic review. Can J Surg. 2007;50(1):48–57.

17. Vettoretto N, Cirocchi R, Randolph J, et al. Single incision laparoscopic right hemicolectomy: a systematic review and meta-analysis. Colorectal Dis. 2014;16(4):O123–32. doi:10.1111/codi.12526.

Chapter 23
Sigmoid Colectomy

Laura E. Fischer and Charles P. Heise

Abstract Sigmoid colectomy is the removal of the sigmoid colon for any benign or malignant indication, including diverticulitis, volvulus, rectal prolapse, trauma, or malignancy. The procedure can be performed with either an open or laparoscopic approach depending on patient factors and surgeon experience. Potential advantages of a laparoscopic approach include faster recovery and a shorter hospital stay while remaining equivalent to open surgery in terms of oncologic outcomes. Currently, alternative methods including robotic and single site procedures are being further investigated.

Keywords Sigmoid • Colectomy • Anastomosis • Laparoscopy • Stapled • Diverticulitis • Volvulus • Colon cancer

L.E. Fischer, MD, MS
Department of Surgery, University of Wisconsin, Madison, WI, USA
e-mail: lfischer22@yahoo.com

C.P. Heise, MD, FACS (✉)
Department of Surgery, University of Wisconsin School of Medicine and Public Health, K4/734 Clinical Sciences Center, 600 Highland Avenue, Madison, WI 53792, USA
e-mail: Heise@surgery.wisc.edu

H. Chen (ed.), *Illustrative Handbook of General Surgery*, 413
DOI 10.1007/978-3-319-24557-7_23,
© Springer International Publishing Switzerland 2016

Indications

Sigmoid colectomy is indicated for a variety of benign and malignant conditions. More common benign indications for sigmoidectomy include diverticulitis, sigmoid volvulus, trauma, and rectal prolapse when combined with rectopexy. Sigmoid resection for colon cancer is indicated for all cancers without evidence of advanced disease.

The risk of developing diverticular disease approaches 50 % by age 60 for patients in the United States with diverticulitis occurring in 20–30 % [1]. Complicated diverticulitis is defined as diverticulitis associated with free perforation, abscess, obstruction, stricture or fistula. Extent of diverticulitis can be classified using the Hinchey system [2, 3]. Emergent surgical intervention is indicated in cases of perforated diverticulitis with peritonitis, Hinchey stages III and IV [3]. Laparoscopic surgery has been shown to be safe and feasible even for severe diverticulitis [4]. Elective surgery can be offered after recovery of multiple recurrent episodes of simple diverticulitis or a single episode of complicated diverticulitis, though patient selection and operative timing are somewhat controversial and more conservative than previous guidelines [1, 3].

Sigmoid volvulus typically affects elderly males older than 70, diabetics, and those with neuropsychiatric disorders and has a high overall mortality approaching 10 %. Management often begins with colonoscopic decompression followed by surgical resection during the hospital stay [5]. Sigmoid resection has historically been combined with rectopexy using an anterior approach to treat rectal prolapse. This may be performed when a very redundant sigmoid colon is encountered or severe constipation symptoms coexist [6].

Sigmoid colectomy is indicated for most cases of malignancy where widespread disease is not evident. However, with isolated, resectable liver metastasis, resection of a colonic primary adenocarcinoma along with hepatectomy can significantly improve 5-year survival up to 64 % [7]. As with any oncologic colectomy, appropriate en bloc mesenteric resection is required to adequately sample lymph nodes for staging purposes.

Laparoscopic sigmoid colectomy for both benign and malignant disease is associated with significantly shorter hospital stay, lower hospital cost, lower re-admission rate, and fewer complications [8]. The rate of recurrence after oncologic resection is similar for laparoscopic and open surgery [9]. In carefully selected patients with BMI 20–30, single incision laparoscopic (SILS) colectomy is safe and feasible with low morbidity (12 %) and good oncologic outcome. Most surgeons report that SILS is more difficult than conventional laparoscopy with longer operative times and equivalent post-operative outcomes [10].

Preoperative Preparation

Pre-operative imaging and endoscopic evaluation should be completed as needed to thoroughly evaluate the condition prior to the operation. A bowel preparation is usually ordered and administered at home the day prior to surgery. Standard preparations include polyethylene glycol or magnesium citrate combined with erythromycin, neomycin, or metronidazole. The use of oral antibiotics with a mechanical bowel preparation alone does not reduce surgical site infections, but is effective when combined with systemic peri-operative antibiotics [11]. Bowel preparation reduces the rate of abscess formation after anastomotic leak, but does not reduce the rate of leak itself [12]. However, the routine use of bowel preparation has been questioned as an updated review failed to demonstrate significant differences in infectious complications [13]. The patient should then be made "nil per os" 12 h prior to the procedure. An epidural may be considered for post-operative pain control after open procedures, though its effect on return of bowel function and length of hospital stay is uncertain [14].

Positioning and Anesthesia

The patient receives general anesthesia with endotracheal intubation. Sequential compression devices should be placed on the lower legs bilaterally and subcutaneous heparin should be administered for deep vein thrombosis prophylaxis prior to induction. A foley catheter should be placed for urinary drainage and monitoring. The patient is placed in a modified low lithotomy position with ample padding to protect the patient's lower legs, with particular attention paid to the lateral leg to avoid compression of the peroneal nerve again the head of the fibula. It is important that the hips have minimal flexion for laparoscopic procedures to maximize the surgeon's range of motion during dissection. The legs should be abducted sufficiently to allow exposure to the anus. The arms can be secured either on padded arm boards at a 90° angle to the body's axis for an open procedure or the right arm or both can be tucked for laparoscopic procedures. An orogastric tube should be placed to decompress the stomach during the procedure. The skin of the abdomen and perineum should be widely prepped. A single dose of antibiotics is administered within 60 min of incision as per the Surgical Care Improvement Program guidelines (SCIP inf-1). The choice of antibiotic is based on SCIP inf-2 recommendations, often a second generation cephalosporin or a combination of ciprofloxacin and metronidazole. These should be appropriately re-dosed according to pharmaceutical guidelines as needed during the procedure [15].

Description of the Procedure

Open Sigmoid Colectomy

An open procedure begins with a lower midline laparotomy from the umbilicus to the pubic symphysis. A scalpel is used to incise the skin and cautery used to dissect through the subcutaneous fat. The fascia can then be incised sharply with either a scalpel or scissors. Cautery can be used to divide the fascia superiorly and inferiorly with two fingers placed beneath to protect the bowel. The peritoneum and pre-peritoneal fat can also be divided in this fashion, taking care to avoid the bladder inferiorly by incising the peritoneum in a lateral direction as the incision nears the pubic symphysis. The incision can be

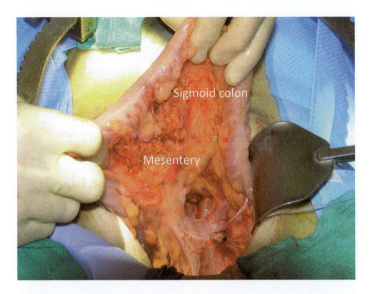

FIGURE 23.1 Mobilization of the sigmoid colon can be performed in a lateral to medial fashion by incising the white line of Toldt and separating the sigmoid mesentery from the retroperitoneum. Here is the sigmoid colon after complete mobilization

taken superior to the umbilicus if additional exposure is needed. After the incision has been enlarged to the desired size, a self-retaining retractor is placed to secure exposure of the surgical site. The abdomen is first explored and the small bowel is gently packed out of the surgical field by placing damp laparotomy pads over the small bowel loops and gently securing them in place superiorly with a self-retaining retractor. Additional damp laparotomy pads can be placed as needed to expose the surgical field.

Mobilization of the sigmoid colon then begins by incising the lateral peritoneal attachments, along the white line of Toldt usually using cautery. Care is taken to stay anterior to the retroperitoneal fascia to avoid iatrogenic injury of retroperitoneal structures, including the ureter and iliac vessels. The mobilization is taken both superiorly to the splenic flexure and inferiorly to the pelvic brim (Fig. 23.1). As the left

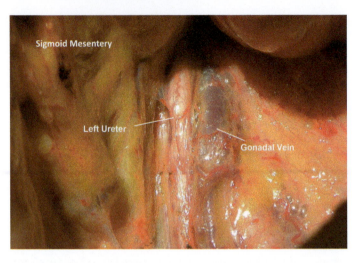

FIGURE 23.2 Care should be taken to avoid injuring the structures in the retroperitoneum during mobilization, in particular the ureter and the gonadal vessels

colon is mobilized medially, the left ureter and gonadal vessels can be identified in the retroperitoneum (Fig. 23.2). If it appears during medialization of the left colon that additional length will be needed to complete the anastomosis after resection, the splenocolic ligament can be divided and the splenic flexure carefully dissected free. It is important to gently gauge the amount of pressure exerted on the ligamentous attachments to the spleen in order to avoid iatrogenic injury. The omentum can be removed from the distal transverse colon if necessary to increase mobility.

The bowel can then be divided proximally using a linear stapling device or sharply with a scalpel between two noncrushing bowel clamps. The distal bowel is divided at the rectosigmoid junction (or more distal if necessary to achieve adequate margins) using either a non-cutting or a linear stapler. The mesentery is then divided using a bipolar energy device, such as the LigaSure™ (Covidien, Mansfield MA). Alternatively, sections of mesentery can be clamped and sharply divided between absorbable ties for vascular ligation.

If the resection is being performed for malignancy, the mesenteric resection should occur proximally at the root of the mesentery where the inferior mesenteric artery (IMA) and vein (IMV) are identified. The peritoneum is scored on either side of the IMA and the vessel completely dissected to allow safe transection. A LigaSure™ device (Covidien, Mansfield MA) or suture ligation can be used to ligate this vessel. The IMV is identified lateral to the IMA, near the ligament of Treitz and is divided separately. After completion of the sigmoid resection, the specimen should be opened off the field to ensure the presence of the expected lesion and confirm margins.

The bowel anastomosis is generally performed using a stapled technique, which is faster than hand-sewn and associated with equivalent rates of clinically evident leakage, morbidity, and post-operative mortality [16]. The proximal bowel is elevated and a purse-string suture is placed circumferentially. The bowel is then opened and the anvil of an end-to-end circular stapler is placed inside the bowel lumen. The purse-string suture is closed tightly around the shaft of the anvil and tied. It is important to ensure good apposition of the bowel to the anvil shaft circumferentially. Care should also be taken to exclude epiploica, colonic fat, or diverticula from the surface of the anvil at the chosen anastomotic location as these can inhibit the creation of an intact staple line. One of the operating surgeons then inserts an end-to-end circular stapler trans-anally and gently maneuvers it in place so that the spike is deployed near the center of the distal staple line. The shaft of the anvil is secured to the circular stapler spike and the stapler is then closed and fired. The proper alignment of the descending colon and the absence of tension should be confirmed prior to completing the anastomosis. The stapler is then opened and slowly removed using small twisting movements, until the luminal anvil has traversed the new anastomosis. The anastomotic rings are inspected on the back table to ensure a full circumferential anastomosis. We typically perform a leak test to inspect our anastomosis. The proximal colon is digitally occluded, the anastomosis submerged with warm normal saline irrigation, and the rectum and distal colon insufflated with air using a rigid proctoscope. The anastomosis is carefully observed for any evidence of air bubbles. With the anastomosis complete, the abdomen is then inspected for hemostasis, warm irrigation can be performed, and the retractors removed. All laparotomy pads are removed and a count confirmed prior to closure. The fascia is closed using a running monofilament absorbable suture and the skin closed.

Laparoscopic-Assisted Sigmoid Colectomy

A sigmoid colectomy can be safely and effectively performed laparoscopically with improved post-operative recovery, length of stay, and pain control [8]. We perform sigmoid colectomies with a lap-assisted technique using a small lower midline, transverse Pfannenstiel or vertical peri-umbilical incision to extract the specimen and exteriorize the proximal bowel limb for anvil placement. Hand-assisted techniques also exist for sigmoid colectomy. Entry to the abdomen is obtained by either the Hassan technique or a Veress needle at the umbilicus. Two additional ports are placed, often in the suprapubic (5 mm) and right lower quadrant (12 mm) locations. A fourth port can be placed as needed to aid retraction either in the left lower quadrant or the right upper quadrant, depending on patient habitus and anatomy (Fig. 23.3). After the ports are placed, a 30° camera is introduced into the abdomen and the bowel underlying the ports is examined for iatrogenic injury.

There are two approaches for a laparoscopic sigmoid colectomy: lateral-to-medial and medial-to-lateral dissection. In the lateral-to-medial approach, atraumatic graspers are used to retract the sigmoid colon medially and a scissors cautery or LigaSure™ (Covidien, Mansfield MA) device are used to take down the lateral peritoneal attachments (Fig. 23.4). The left ureter and gonadal vessels are identified and preserved lateral to the dissection plane. The dissection proceeds superiorly as described previously and the splenic flexure attachments mobilized if necessary (Fig. 23.5). Once the colon has

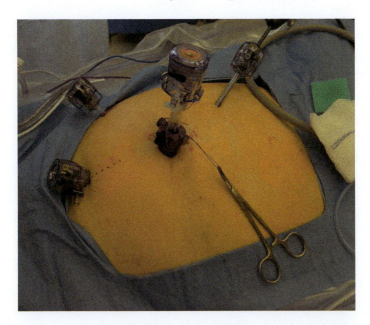

FIGURE 23.3 Port placement for a laparoscopic sigmoid colectomy. In this case, we chose use the Hassan technique to enter the abdomen at the umbilicus. Three additional 5 mm ports are placed in the suprapubic midline, the right lower quadrant and the right upper quadrant. We have additionally marked the patient's lower midline prior to insufflation

been sufficiently mobilized, the IMA is identified near its take-off from the aorta and the mesenteric peritoneum scored on either side of the vessel. The IMA is then ligated using a linear stapling device with a vascular load or the LigaSure™ (Covidien, Mansfield MA) bipolar device. If additional security is desired, metal clips can be placed on the proximal IMA prior to transection. The IMV is then identified laterally and also transected. The mesentery is then sequentially divided inferiorly toward the rectosigmoid junction. In the medial-to-lateral approach, the IMA and IMV are identified and transected prior to mobilization of the colon. With the mesentery divided, the rectosigmoid or

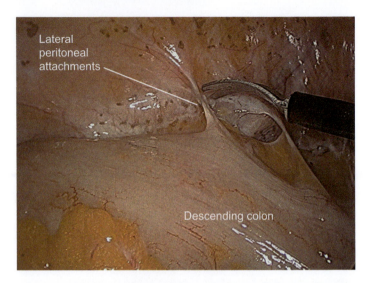

FIGURE 23.4 The lateral-to-medial dissection begins laparoscopically with division of the lateral peritoneal attachments of the descending colon to the left lateral abdominal wall

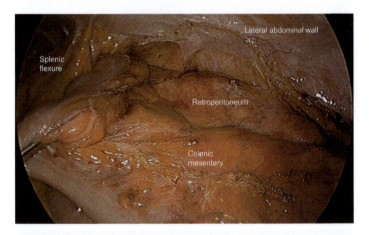

FIGURE 23.5 The descending colon is completely mobilized medially as the plane between the colonic mesentery and the retroperitoneum is developed. The splenic flexure can be mobilized as needed to gain additional length on the remaining colon in order to complete the anastomosis

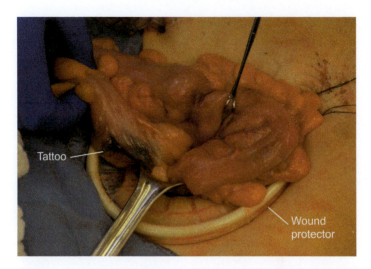

FIGURE 23.6 The sigmoid colon is exteriorized through a small lower midline or Pfannenstiel incision. A wound protector is placed to minimize the risk of surgical site infection. In this case, the lesion had been previously tattooed during colonoscopy to allow for proper identification during surgery

proximal rectum is divided intra-corporeally with an endo-GIA stapler placed via the right lower quadrant port.

A small access incision can now be made in either a transverse or vertical midline suprapubic or peri-umbilical location. A small wound protector is placed and the sigmoid specimen delivered from the abdomen (Fig. 23.6). The proximal colon is divided with a linear cutting stapler or transected after placing a non-crushing bowel clamp followed by purse string suture and anvil placement (Fig. 23.7). If the distal anastomosis is not divided intra-corporeally, it can be transected via the suprapubic incision with a non-cutting stapler (Fig. 23.8). The specimen is again examined off the field to confirm lesion location and margins. The anastomosis can now be completed as described above (Figs. 23.9, 23.10, and 23.11) or by placing the colon back into the abdomen with re-insufflation. A stapled intra-corporeal anastomosis is then

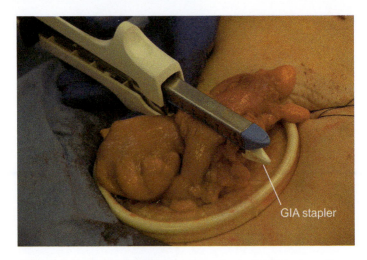

FIGURE 23.7 The proximal descending colon is divided using a linear cutting stapler via the extraction site

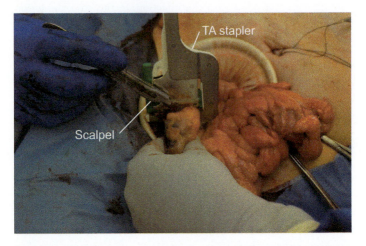

FIGURE 23.8 Dividing the specimen at the desired distal location completes the resection. This can be done with a non-cutting stapler (open). This device only staples, so the surgeon must cut the specimen using a scalpel after the stapler has been fired. This portion of the procedure can be done laparoscopically as well using a cutting stapler

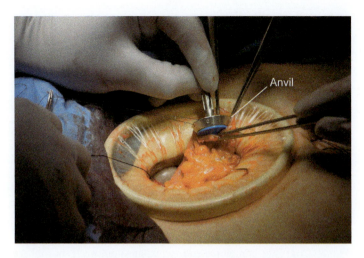

FIGURE 23.9 After the staple line has been sharply divided from the proximal colon, the anvil is carefully placed inside the lumen

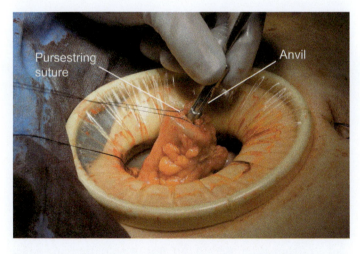

FIGURE 23.10 The purse-string suture is then tightly closed to circumferentially secure the bowel edges around the shaft of the anvil. It is critical to ensure that the bowel wall encircling the anvil is clear of diverticuli or fatty deposits. A second purse-string can be placed as needed to ensure a successful anastomosis

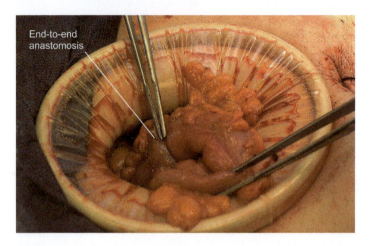

FIGURE 23.11 The completed end-to-end anastomosis is shown here. An additional layer of silk Lembert interrupted sutures can be placed to reinforce the anastomosis if desired

performed with the circular end-to-end anastomosis stapler. The abdomen is inspected for hemostasis and irrigated as needed. The access incision is closed with a running absorbable monofilament suture as is the 12 mm port site using an endo-close needle technique. The skin of all port sites and the access incision can be closed with subcuticular absorbable sutures.

Post-operative Care

The length of time to return of bowel function depends on multiple patient factors and is highly variable. Close attention should be paid to electrolyte and fluid imbalances and a foley catheter should be used to monitor urine output and gauge intravascular fluid resuscitation. Oral intake can be started at the surgeon's discretion. Existing evidence suggests that early initiation of enteral feeding can reduce the overall risk of infection and decrease length of hospital stay without increasing re-admissions [17, 18]. Oral pain medication can be started with the initiation of a diet. Multimodal post-operative analgesia should be administered and narcotics minimized as much as possible to reduce opioid-associated delayed gastrointestinal recovery [19]. Post-operative antibiotics are generally not indicated as prolonged dosing increases the risk of Clostridium difficile and the development of resistant bacteria [15]. The patient can be discharged home when they are tolerating a general diet, ambulating without difficulty, and have good pain control on oral medications.

References

1. Bordeianou L, Hodin R. Controversies in the surgical management of sigmoid diverticulitis. J Gastrointest Surg. 2007;11:542–8.
2. Hinchey EJ, Schaal PGH, Richards GK. Treatment of perforated diverticular disease of the colon. Adv Surg. 1978;12:85–109.
3. Feingold D, Steele SR, Lee S, Kaiser A, Boushey R, Buie WD, Rafferty JF. Practice parameters for the treatment of sigmoid diverticulitis. Dis Colon Rectum. 2014;57:284–94.
4. De Magistris L, Azagra JS, Georgen M, De Blasi V, Arru L, Facy O. Laparoscopic sigmoidectomy in moderate and severe diverticulitis: analysis of short-term outcomes in a continuous series of 121 patients. Surg Endosc. 2013;27:1766–71.
5. Halabi WJ, Jafari MD, Kang CY, Nguyen VQ, Carmichael JC, Mills S, Pigazzi A, Stamos MJ. Colonic volvulus in the United States: trends, outcomes, and predictors of mortality. Ann Surg. 2014;259:293–301.
6. Bordeianou L, Hicks CW, Kaiser AM, Alavi K, Sudan R, Wise PE. Rectal prolapse: an overview of clinical features, diagnosis, and patient-specific management strategies. J Gastrointest Surg. 2014;18:1059–69.
7. Rees M, Tekkis P, Welsh FKS, O'Rourke T, John TG. Evaluation of long-term survival after hepatic resection for metastatic colorectal cancer: a multifactorial model of 929 patients. Ann Surg. 2008;247(1):125–35.
8. Hinojosa MW, Murrell ZA, Konyalian VR, Mills S, Nguyen NT, Stamos MJ. Comparison of laparoscopic vs open sigmoid colectomy for benign and malignant disease at academic medical centers. J Gastrointest Surg. 2007;11:1423–30.

9. Liang JT, Huang KC, Lai HS, Lee PH, Jeng YM. Oncologic results of laparoscopic versus conventional open surgery for stage II and III left-sided colon cancers: a randomized controlled trial. Ann Surg Oncol. 2007;14(1):109–17.

10. Makino T, Milsom JW, Lee SW. Feasibility and safety of a single-incision laparoscopic colectomy: a systematic review. Ann Surg. 2012;255(4):667–76.

11. Fry DE. Colon preparation and surgical site infection. Am J Surg. 2011;202:225–32.

12. Contant CM, Hop WC, van't Sant HP, Oostvogel HJ, Smeets HJ, Stassen LP, Neijenhuis PA, Idenburg FJ, Dijkhuis CM, Heres P, van Tets WF, Gerritsen JJ, Weidema WF. Mechanical bowel preparation for elective colorectal surgery: a multicentre randomised trial. Lancet. 2007;370:2112–7.

13. Guenaga KF, Matos D, Wille-Jorgensen P. Mechanical bowel preparation for elective colorectal surgery. Cochrane Database Syst Rev. 2011;9:1–56.

14. Halabi WJ, Jafari MD, Nguyen VQ, Carmichael JC, Mills S, Stamos MJ, Pigazzi A. A nationwide analysis of the use and outcomes of epidural analgesia in open colorectal surgery. J Gastrointest Surg. 2013;17:1130–7.

15. Nelson RL, Gladman E, Barbateskovic M. Antimicrobial prophylaxis for colorectal surgery. Cochrane Database Syst Rev. 2014;5:1–262.

16. Docherty JG, McGregor JR, Akyol AM, Murray GD, Galloway DJ. Comparison of manually constructed and stapled anastomoses in colorectal surgery. West of Scotland and Highland Anastomosis Study Group. Ann Surg. 1995;221:176–84.

17. Lewis SJ, Egger M, Sylvester PA, Thomas S. Early enteral feeding versus "nil by mouth" after gastrointestinal surgery: systematic review and meta-analysis of controlled trials. BMJ. 2001;323:1–5.

18. Andersen HK, Lewis SJ, Thomas S. Early enteral nutrition within 24h of colorectal surgery versus later commencement of feeding for postoperative complications. Cochrane Database Syst Rev. 2006;4:1–31.

19. Beard TL, Leslie JB, Nemeth J. The opioid component of delayed gastrointestinal recovery after bowel resection. J Gastrointest Surg. 2011;15:1259–68.

Chapter 24
Low Anterior Resection and Abdominoperineal Resection

Laura E. Fischer and Charles P. Heise

Abstract Low anterior resection (LAR) and abdomino-perineal resection (APR) are the primary surgical interventions for rectal cancer. Proctectomy with an ultra-low or colo-anal anastomosis can also be performed as part of the surgical treatment for benign diseases, such as ulcerative colitis and familial adenomatous polyposis. The procedures are performed both open and laparoscopically, depending on various patient factors, disease pathophysiology, and surgeon preference. Robotic LAR or APR may also be performed with similar outcomes depending on surgeon experience.

L.E. Fischer, MD, MS
Department of Surgery, University of Wisconsin, Madison, WI, USA
e-mail: lfischer22@yahoo.com

C.P. Heise, MD, FACS (✉)
Department of Surgery, University of Wisconsin School of Medicine and Public Health, K4/734 CSC 600 Highland Avenue, Madison, WI 53792, USA
e-mail: heise@surgery.wisc.edu

H. Chen (ed.), *Illustrative Handbook of General Surgery*,   429
DOI 10.1007/978-3-319-24557-7_24,
© Springer International Publishing Switzerland 2016

Keywords Rectal cancer • Low Anterior Resection • Abdominoperineal Resection • Colectomy • Laparoscopy • Colostomy • Ileostomy

Indications

Low anterior resection (LAR) and abdominoperineal resection (APR) are the primary surgical interventions for rectal cancer, which is any malignant lesion within 12–15 cm of the anal verge. Low anterior resection with a 5 cm distal margin is typically performed for lesions in the upper rectum. For low or mid rectal lesions, an LAR can be performed if a 1–2 cm margin can be obtained without compromising anal sphincter function along with a complete mesorectal excision. If an appropriate margin cannot be obtained, the lesion invades the anal sphincter complex or the levator musculature, or the patient has significant pre-operative incontinence, an abdominoperineal resection is performed. This involves the en bloc resection of the rectum, anus, mesorectum, and perianal soft tissues, as well as the creation of a permanent end colostomy. Select small, early stage rectal cancers (e.g. Tis and T1) can be treated with a transanal approach, including transanal endoscopic microsurgery, however, this is controversial as the risk of local recurrence is higher (13.2 % versus 2.7 %, respectively) and disease specific survival lower than with radical surgical excision [1, 2].

The hallmark of an appropriate oncologic resection for rectal cancer is a total mesorectal excision: the complete resection of the mesorectum including the vasculature, lymphatic structures, fatty tissue, and intact mesorectal fascia. A successful mesorectal excision removes tissues which contain early lymphatic spread of cancer and can significantly lower the local recurrence rate in node-positive rectal cancers [3, 4]. The circumferential resection margin has significant prognostic importance: tumor located within 1 mm of this margin is considered positive. The circumferential margin, especially when less than 2 mm, is a strong predictor of both local recurrence and overall survival [5].

The current standard of care is to offer neoadjuvant chemotherapy and radiotherapy to patients who have clinical stage II or III rectal cancer, as determined by endorectal ultrasound or pelvic MRI. Pre-operative chemoradiotherapy is associated with a reduction in local recurrence and similar overall survival when compared with post-operative treatment [6]. Chemotherapy, when combined with radiation, increases the chance of pathologic complete response and improves local control when compared to radiation alone [7]. Pre-operative treatment also increases the chance of preserving the sphincter complex and reduces potential post-operative radiation damage to other intraabdominal organs, such as the small bowel. Twenty percent of patients undergoing neoadjuvant therapy will have a pathologic complete response which confers a significant survival advantage compared to moderate or non-responders [8]. This has led some groups to take up a "wait and see" non-surgical management policy for complete responders, as based on imaging and endoscopy, with good initial results [9].

The surgical procedures can be performed both open and laparoscopically, depending on various patient factors, disease pathophysiology, and surgeon preference and experience. Robotic LAR or APR is also being performed at some centers.

Preoperative Preparation

Pre-operative imaging and procedures, such as endorectal ultrasound, pelvic MRI, and computed tomography of the chest, abdomen, and pelvis with IV and oral contrast should be completed as needed to thoroughly stage the patient prior to an operation. All patients diagnosed with rectal cancer should undergo a complete colonoscopy to evaluate for synchronous lesions and rule out other pathology prior to consideration for resection. If sphincter preservation (LAR) is planned, consideration should also be given to current continence status as well, since this may influence final procedural decision making. A bowel preparation consisting of magnesium citrate or polyethylene glycol combined with erythromycin, neomycin, or metronidazole is administered the evening prior to surgery. There is some conflicting data regarding the efficacy of a mechanical bowel preparation in preventing surgical site infection and anastomotic complications [10–12], so its use is ultimately determined by the surgeon. The patient should then be made "nil per os" 12 h prior to the procedure. An epidural can be considered for post-operative pain control for open procedures.

Positioning and Anesthesia

The patient should undergo induction of general anesthesia with endotracheal intubation. Sequential compression devices should be placed on the lower legs bilaterally and subcutaneous heparin should be administered for deep vein thrombosis prophylaxis prior to induction, unless there is a documented contraindication. A foley catheter should be placed for urinary drainage and monitoring of urine. The patient should be placed in a modified low lithotomy position as described in the prior chapter with sterile leg covers in place to allow for intra-operative adjustment to access the perineum. Care should be taken to ensure that the patient's perineum is located at the break of the table to allow access during the perineal dissection (APR) or passage of the circular stapler (LAR). The arms can be secured either on padded arm boards at a 90° angle to the body's axis for an open procedure or the right arm can be tucked for laparoscopic procedures. An orogastric or nasogastric tube should be placed to decompress the stomach and proximal small bowel during the procedure. The skin of the abdomen and perineum is widely prepped and the rectum irrigated with a flexible rubber catheter and betadine solution. A single dose of antibiotics which covers gram negative, gram positive, and anaerobic bacteria should be administered (SCIP INF-2) within 60 min of incision (SCIP INF-1) [13], often a second generation cephalosporin or a combination of ciprofloxacin and metronidazole. These should be appropriately re-dosed according to pharmaceutical guidelines as needed during the case [14]. A digital rectal exam should always be performed prior to draping the patient to confirm tumor location and planned level of resection.

Description of the Procedure

Low Anterior Resection

The open procedure begins with a lower midline laparotomy from the umbilicus to the pubic symphysis. Care should be taken to avoid the bladder inferiorly by incising the peritoneum in a lateral direction as the incision nears the pubic symphysis. If the operation is being performed for a malignancy, the abdomen should be examined for metastases, particularly the liver and omentum. A self-retaining retractor is placed and the small bowel packed out of the field using damp laparotomy pads. The patient can be placed in Trendelenburg position to facilitate the pelvic dissection.

Mobilization of the sigmoid colon then begins by incising the lateral peritoneal attachments, starting with the white line of Toldt, using cautery. Care is taken to stay anterior to the retroperitoneal fascia to avoid iatrogenic injury of retroperitoneal structures, including the ureter and iliac vessels. The mobilization is taken both superiorly to the splenic flexure (which may be taken down as needed) and inferiorly to the pelvic brim. As the left colon is mobilized medially, the left ureter and gonadal vessels are identified in the retroperitoneum.

The bowel can then be divided at an appropriate location in the sigmoid or descending colon using a linear stapling device. This allows for improved mobility of the distal bowel segment to aid in the pelvic dissection. The mesentery may be divided using an energy device, such as the LigaSure™ (Covidien, Mansfield MA) or clamps and absorbable ties. The inferior mesenteric artery (IMA) and vein are identified by palpation. The peritoneum is scored on either side of the IMA and the vessel should be completely dissected to allow safe transection (Fig. 24.1). A LigaSure™ device or suture ligation can be used to ligate the vessel at its take-off from the aorta ("high ligation"). The hypogastric nerves should be visualized and swept posteriorly, to avoid inadvertent injury. The LigaSure™ can then be used to further divide the mesentery inferiorly toward the rectosigmoid junction.

A total mesorectal excision is then performed by retracting the distal sigmoid colon and rectum anteriorly and finding the avascular plane behind the mesorectum (Fig. 24.2). The peritoneum is first scored on either side of the rectum down to its anterior reflection which is also incised. Then electrocautery is used to dissect the areolar tissues posteriorly and laterally down to the level of the pelvic floor, keeping the mesorectal envelope intact (Fig. 24.3). Care should be

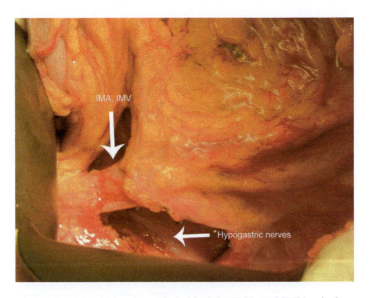

FIGURE 24.1 A window is made behind the IMA and IMV to isolate these structures prior to transection. The hypogastric nerves are identified and swept posteriorly to avoid injury

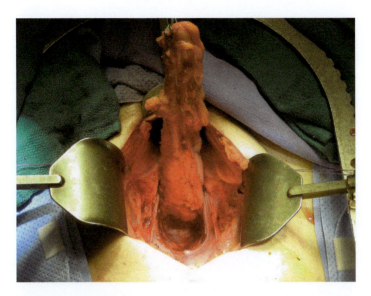

FIGURE 24.2 The divided colon is retracted anteriorly to visualize the posterior, avascular, retro-rectal dissection plane

taken to avoid the hypogastric nerves which course along the pelvic sidewalls bilaterally. Injury to these nerves can result in sexual and urinary dysfunction. Anteriorly, the dissection follows closely along the rectum and care is taken to avoid injury to the seminal vesicles and prostate gland in the male and the posterior vaginal wall in the female (Fig. 24.4). Preservation of the fascia propria which envelops the rectum is a key maneuver that has been shown to reduce local tumor recurrence [3, 4]. The dissection continues distally until the levator muscles have been identified circumferentially at the pelvic floor, and the mesorectum has ended.

For upper third rectal tumors, a general margin of approximately 5 cm is suggested. In these cases the mesorectum may be divided perpendicular to the rectum. For middle or lower third rectal tumors, a complete mesorectal excision is necessary and a distal margin of 2 cm is customary, although a smaller margin may be acceptable in certain patient populations where preservation of the sphincter complex is possible,

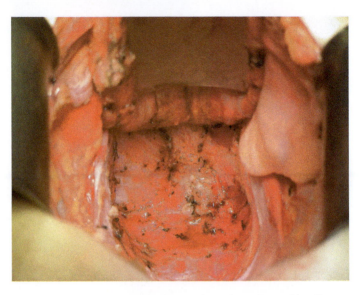

FIGURE 24.3 The total mesorectal excision is performed by dissecting in the avascular plane posterior to the mesorectum and anterior
to the sacrum. The dissection continues down to the levator muscles
bilaterally. Identification and preservation of the hypogastric nerves
is maintained throughout the dissection

especially after neo-adjuvant treatment [15]. The rectum is
divided distal to the tumor with an appropriate margin with
a thoracoabdominal (TA) linear stapler and a scalpel
(Fig. 24.5). A digital rectal exam should be performed after
the TA has been positioned to confirm appropriate location
prior to completion of the resection. The specimen should be
opened on the back table and subsequently sent to pathology
to confirm negative margins. An anvil is then secured within
the lumen of the proximal colon using a purse-string suture.
Care should also be taken to exclude epiploica, colonic fat, or
diverticula from the surface of the anvil as these can compromise the integrity of the staple line. The end-to-end circular
stapler is then inserted transanally and gently maneuvered
into place so that the spike is deployed in the center of the
distal staple line (Fig. 24.6). The anvil is secured to the circu-

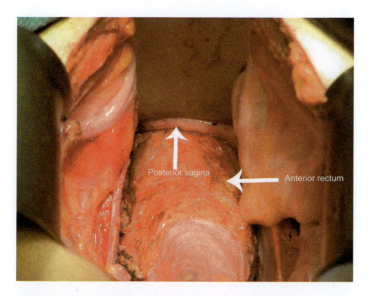

FIGURE 24.4 In females, the dissection continues between the anterior rectum and posterior vaginal wall, leaving the anterior mesorectum intact. In males, care should be taken to avoid injuring the prostatic urethra

lar stapler spike and the stapler is then closed and fired. The alignment of the descending colon should be confirmed to be in a straight line with no tension and all small bowel loops cleared from the surgical area prior to completing to anastomosis. The stapler is then slowly removed until the luminal anvil has traversed the new anastomosis. The anastomotic rings are inspected on the back table to ensure a full circumferential anastomosis and sent to pathology for evaluation. A leak test is typically performed.

Alternatively, for extremely low-lying rectal tumors, a colo-anal anastomosis can be performed with a colonic J-pouch in either a hand-sewn or stapled fashion. Colonic J-pouches may confer some advantages, such as reduced fecal incontinence, reduce frequency of bowel movements and urgency [16]. The J-pouch is configured by folding the distal colon back upon itself approximately 5–6 cm (Fig. 24.7). A

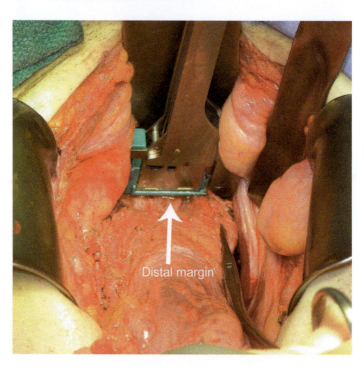

FIGURE 24.5 When performing an LAR, at the completion of the mesorectal mobilization, the rectum is transected at least 1 cm beyond the level of the tumor utilizing a transverse, non-cutting stapler

colotomy is made at the base of the fold with cautery. A linear GIA stapler is then inserted through the colotomy with each arm passing into a separate lumen and fired, creating a common pouch. An anvil is then placed through this colotomy and a secured in place. The anastomosis is completed as previously described. A hand-sewn colo-anal anastomosis is typically performed when the rectum must be sharply divided without closure, rather than using a stapler, in order to obtain a distal margin. A retractor is placed at the anal opening to view the dental line and the proximal resection margin. The segment of proximal colon is then brought down into the

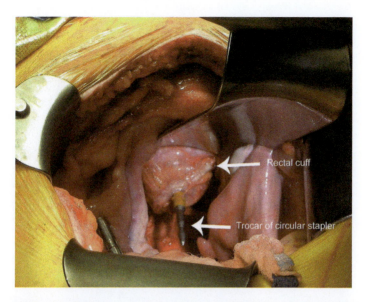

FIGURE 24.6 An assistant then inserts the circular stapler through the anus and into the rectal pouch. The spike is advanced until it is visualized penetrating the center of the rectal cuff staple line. It is then fully deployed prior to attaching the anvil component and completing the anastomosis

surgical field and full-thickness interrupted absorbable sutures are used to circumferentially sew the colon to the anal canal.

In most LAR cases, especially post-chemoradiation therapy, a diverting loop ileostomy (see Stoma section) is performed to reduce the morbidity associated with anastomotic leak.

Abdominoperineal Resection

APR is indicated for low-lying rectal cancers which are close to or involve the anal sphincter complex, in patients who require a rectal resection and have fecal incontinence at

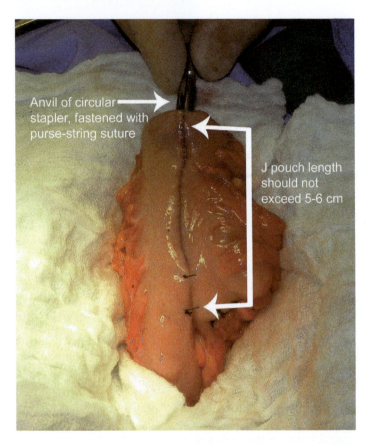

FIGURE 24.7 A colonic J-pouch is illustrated. The colon is folded over on itself and a side-to-side J-pouch is constructed with a linear cutting stapler. The J-pouch length should not exceed 5–6 cm in order to optimize post-operative function. The anvil of the circular stapler is placed at the apex and secured with a purse-string suture

baseline, or those with severe peri-anal inflammatory bowel disease in whom a distal anastomosis is not advised. The procedure involves the en bloc removal of the rectum, mesorectum, and anus.

The abdominal portion of the APR is identical to the LAR. After complete mobilization of the rectum and mesorectum, the perineal dissection begins. The patient's legs can be adjusted as needed to a high lithotomy position to expose the perineum. The anus is then exposed with a self-retaining retractor. An elliptical incision is made sharply around the anus and includes the entire anal sphincter complex (Fig. 24.8). Dissection continues posteriorly until the coccyx is encountered. The anococcygeal ligament is divided and blunt dissection is used to enter the presacral space just anterior to the coccyx that had been previously dissected transabdominally (Fig. 24.9). A finger can then be placed deep to the levator muscles laterally on either side to act as a guide for division bilaterally with cautery. Dissection then continues to the anterior aspect of the anal canal and distal rectum. This portion of the dissection can be quite challenging in males as the

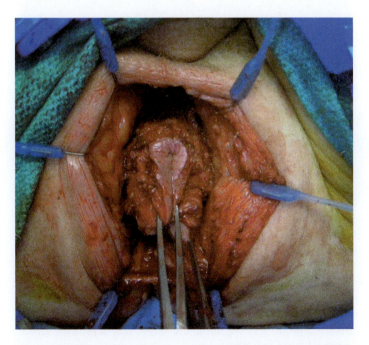

FIGURE 24.8 The perineal portion of the APR begins with an elliptical skin incision, including the anus and sphincter complex. Dissection continues circumferentially through the ischiorectal fat

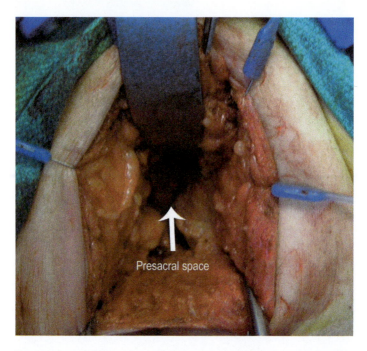

FIGURE 24.9 The anus is retracted anteriorly and the posterior dissection continues to the level of the coccyx. The anococcygeal ligament is divided and the presacral space can then be entered

membranous portion of the prostatic urethra is just anterior to this plane and can be easily damaged. In females, retraction of the vagina can facilitate separation of the anterior rectum and posterior vaginal wall. Eversion of the specimen through the perineal opening can also assist in completing the anterior dissection plane (Fig. 24.10). Once the specimen has been completely dissected circumferentially, it is removed from the perineal opening and sent to pathology for permanent section (Fig. 24.11). The perineal incision in then closed in multiple layers in an anterior-posterior fashion using absorbable suture. We typically close the skin with nylon suture (Fig. 24.12). After the perineum has been closed, attention is then turned to the creation of an end colostomy, which is described in the Stoma section. Much of the abdominal and

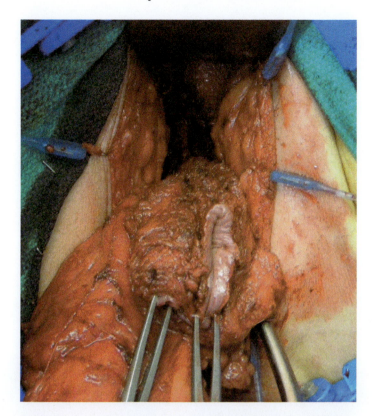

FIGURE 24.10 With the posterior and lateral dissection complete, the specimen can be exteriorized posteriorly through the perineal incision to facilitate dissection of the anterior plane

perineal portions of the APR procedure can be done simultaneously by two operating surgeons.

Laparoscopic and Robotic LAR and APR

Laparoscopic LAR may be performed safely and effectively with similar 10-year oncologic outcomes and improved short-term post-operative recovery [17]. We typically use a lap-

444   L.E. Fischer and C.P. Heise

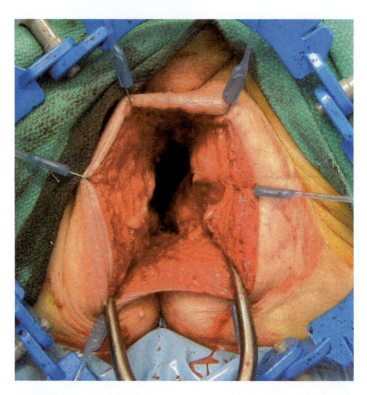

FIGURE 24.11 After the dissection and excision is complete, the specimen is removed and the perineal wound is in direct communication with the pelvis

assisted technique and with a small lower midline or Pfannenstiel incision to remove the resected specimen and place the anvil prior to anastomosis. Alternatively, the site of the diverting loop ileostomy can be used to remove the specimen and access the bowel, thus decreasing the number of larger incisions on the abdominal wall. The technique is the same as that described in the prior sigmoid chapter using a medial to lateral approach, though the mesorectal excision is then performed laparoscopically followed by intra (endo-GIA) or extracorporeal (TA) stapling.

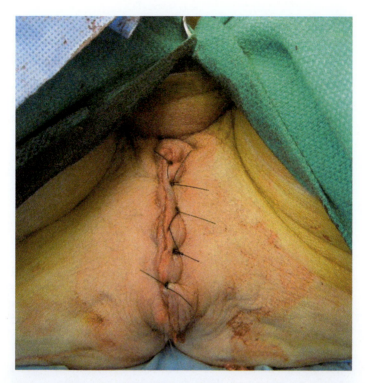

FIGURE 24.12 The perineal wound is closed in multiple layers with absorbable suture to prevent dehiscence. We typically approximate the skin with vertical mattress sutures to accommodate wound drainage. Care must be taken in the post-operative period to avoid unnecessary pressure on the perineal wound from sitting

Robotic APR has been shown to be safe and feasible with comparable short-term oncologic outcomes, however, more studies are needed to elucidate improved outcomes in order to justify the higher cost [18]. The technique begins with the placement of four robotic trocars across the lower mid-abdomen, as well as one or two laparoscopic-assisted trocars in the right upper quadrant. The sigmoid colon is dissected laparoscopically in a medial to lateral fashion with a high ligation of the IMA as previously described. The proximal colon is then divided with a linear GIA stapler and the robot is subsequently docked. The TME is then performed with the robot using three arms to aid in retraction and dissection. The levators can be divided circumferentially to the level of the ischial fat with this technique, allowing a much easier and faster perineal dissection. Once the robotic dissection has been completed, the perineal dissection and end colostomy formation are performed as usual. The use of the robot has been suggested to provide superior visualization of pelvic structures allowing a more precise dissection [19].

Post-operative Care

In the immediate post-operative period, a foley catheter is maintained to monitor urine output and to avoid voiding difficulties with the extended pelvic dissection. Initiation of oral intake can be started at the surgeon's discretion, but patients are often able to advance quickly due to the presence of a diverting or end ostomy. Oral pain medication can be started with the initiation of a diet. In LAR patients, per rectum medications should be strictly avoided to reduce the risk of anastomotic injury. In APR patients, the perineal wound should be examined daily for evidence of breakdown or infection. The patient can be discharged home when they are tolerating a general diet, ambulating without difficulty, and have good pain control on oral medications.

References

1. Nash GM, Weiser MR, Guillem JG, Temple LK, Shia J, Gonen M, Wong WD, Paty PB. Long-term survival after transanal excision of T1 rectal cancer. Dis Colon Rectum. 2009;52(4):577–82.
2. Heidary B, Phang TP, Raval MJ, Brown CJ. Transanal endoscopic microsurgery: a review. Can J Surg. 2014;57(2):127–38.
3. Heald RJ, Husband EM, Ryall RD. The mesorectum in rectal cancer surgery–the clue to pelvic recurrence? Br J Surg. 1982;69(10):613–6.

4. Cecil TD, Sexton R, Moran BJ, Heald RJ. Total mesorectal excision results in low recurrence rates in lymph node-positive rectal cancer. Dis Colon Rectum. 2004;47(7):1145–9.
5. Bernstein TE, Endreseth BH, Romundstad P, Wibe A, Norwegian Colorectal Cancer Group. Circumferential resection margin as a prognostic factor in rectal cancer. Br J Surg. 2009;96:1348–57.
6. Sauer R, Becker H, Hohenberger W, Rodel C, Wittekind C, Fietkau R, Martus P, Tschmelitsch J, Hager E, Hess CF, Karstens JH, Liersch T, Schmidberger H, Raab R, German Rectal Cancer Study Group. Preoperative versus postoperative chemoradiotherapy for rectal cancer. N Engl J Med. 2004;351(17):1731–40.
7. DeCaluwe L, Van Nieuwenhove Y, Ceelen WP. Preoperative chemoradiation versus radiation alone for stage II and III resectable rectal cancer. Cochrane Database Syst Rev. 2013;2, CD006041.
8. Janjan NA, Crane C, Feig BW, Cleary K, Dubrow R, Curley S, Vauthey JN, Lynch P, Ellis LM, Wolff R, Lenzi R, Abbruzzese J, Pazdur R, Hoff PM, Allen P, Brown T, Skibber J. Improved overall survival among responders to preoperative chemoradiation for locally advanced rectal cancer. Am J Clin Oncol. 2001;24(2):107–12.
9. Maas M, Beets-Tan RG, Lambregts DM, Lammering G, Nelemans PJ, Engelen SM, van Dam RM, Jansen RL, Sosef M, Leijtens JW, Hulsewe KW, Buijsen J, Beets GL. Wait-and-see policy for clinical complete responders after chemoradiation for rectal cancer. J Clin Oncol. 2011;29(35):4633–40.
10. Contant CM, Hop WC, van't Sant HP, Oostvogel HJ, Smeets HJ, Stassen LP, Neijenhuis PA, Idenburg FJ, Dijkhuis CM, Heres P, Vantets WF, Gerritsen JJ, Weidema WF. Mechanical bowel preparation for elective colorectal surgery: a multicentre randomised trial. Lancet 2007;22:370(9605):2112–7.
11. Fry DE. Colon preparation and surgical site infection. Am J Surg. 2011;202:225–32.
12. Guenaga KF, Matos D, Wille-Jorgensen P. Mechanical bowel preparation for elective colorectal surgery. Cochrane Database Syst Rev. 2011;9:1–56.
13. The Joint Commission. Surgical Care Improvement Project. http://www.jointcommission.org/surgical_care_improvement_project/. Accessed 16 Oct 2014.
14. Nelson RL, Gladman E, Barbateskovic M. Antimicrobial prophylaxis for colorectal surgery. Cochrane Database Syst Rev. 2014;5:1–262.
15. Moore HG, Riedel E, Minsky BD, Saitz L, Paty P, Wong D, Cohen AM, Guillem JG. Adequacy of 1-cm distal margin after

restorative rectal cancer resection with sharp mesorectal excision and preoperative combined-modality therapy. Ann Surg Oncol. 2003;10(1):80–5.

16. Hallbook O, Pahlman L, Krog M, Wexner SD, Sjodahl R. Randomized comparison of straight and colonic J pouch anastomosis after low anterior resection. Ann Surg. 1996;224(1):58–65.

17. Vennix S, Pelzers L, Bouvy N, Beets GL, Pierie JP, Wiggers T, Breukink S. Laparoscopic versus open total mesorectal excision for rectal cancer. Cochrane Database Syst Rev. 2014;4:CD005200.

18. Mak TW, Lee JF, Futaba K, Hon SS, Ngo DK, Ng SS. Robotic surgery for rectal cancer: a systematic review of current practice. World J Gastrointest Oncol. 2014;6(6):184–93.

19. Kang CY, Carmichael JC, Friesen J, Stamos MJ, Mills S, Pigazzi A. Robotic-assisted extralevator abdominoperineal resection in the lithotomy position: technique and early outcomes. Am Surg. 2012;78(10):1033–7.

Chapter 25
Stomas (Colostomy and Ileostomy)

Sarah E. Tevis and Charles P. Heise

Abstract Small bowel and colon stomas are used to divert bowel contents for healing of a new anastomosis, in the setting of abnormal gastrointestinal function, or in patients with incontinence or a low rectal cancer. Patients should undergo preoperative counseling regarding living with an ostomy, as well as preoperative stoma site marking. Important concepts in stoma creation include avoidance of stoma creation in the setting of infection, ensuring adequate blood supply to the stoma, and preventing tension in the underlying bowel. Postoperative care consists of patient education on stoma care and avoidance of dehydration due to high ostomy output.

S.E. Tevis, MD (✉)
Department of General Surgery, University of Wisconsin,
650 Highland Ave, Madison, WI 53792, USA
e-mail: stevis@uwhealth.org

C.P. Heise, MD
Department of Surgery,
University of Wisconsin Hospital and Clinics,
K4/734 Clinical Science Center, 600 Highland Ave, Madison, WI 53792, USA
University of Wisconsin School of Medicine and Public Health, Madison, WI USA

H. Chen (ed.), *Illustrative Handbook of General Surgery*,
DOI 10.1007/978-3-319-24557-7_25,
© Springer International Publishing Switzerland 2016

449

Keywords   Stoma • Ileostomy • Colostomy • Bowel diversion • Loop ileostomy

Indications

The terms stoma or ostomy refer to surgically created openings in the gastrointestinal tract that allows for diversion of the fecal stream. In the setting of abdominal surgery, the small bowel or colon may be used. The procedure is named for the segment of intestine used. For example, a stoma created from colon is called a colostomy, while the use of the ileum creates an ileostomy. An intact loop of intestine can be used creating a loop colostomy or ileostomy, however if the bowel is completely transected and brought out of the abdomen it is termed an end colostomy or ileostomy.

Stomas are formed to divert gastrointestinal contents to allow for healing and prevent contamination of the abdominal cavity [1]. Indications for stoma formation include intestinal perforation or obstruction secondary to neoplasm, inflammatory bowel disease, or diverticulitis. An ostomy may also be indicated to divert enteric transit from a new intestinal anastomosis following bowel resection. Diverting ostomies have been demonstrated to decrease complication rates following low pelvic anastomoses [2]. Stomas are typically temporary and a second operation is required to restore bowel continuity. A permanent ostomy may be indicated when the muscles controlling elimination are ineffective or when normal intestinal function is impaired. The most common indications for permanent ostomies are low rectal cancers and inflammatory bowel disease.

Preoperative Preparation

Pre-operative patient counseling is necessary to prepare patients for caring for and living with an ostomy. While patients have varying responses to ostomy formation, creation of a stoma is associated with many psychosocial issues and can dramatically affect patients' quality of life [3]. Patients who receive ostomy specific pre-operative teaching have been found to have shorter length of hospital stay, become proficient in ostomy care more quickly, and have fewer post-operative interventions in the community [4].

Pre-operative stoma site marking is essential to ensure a proper stoma site and good overall function. The location of the ostomy plays an important part in its overall function and pre-operative marking has been found to be associated with decreased complication rates and improved patient quality of life [4]. Often this is performed by an enterostomal therapist or ostomy nurse. The following variables should be taken into consideration when marking a potential stoma site: abdominal wall contour while sitting and standing, accessibility of site to patient, relation to belt line, segment of bowel to be utilized, and abdominal girth. Due to concerns about ostomy appliance placement, skin folds and pannus should be avoided. End colostomies are typically located on the patient's left side in the left lower quadrant, while ileostomies are often in the right lower quadrant. The ostomy should be created through the rectus muscle to provide additional support. Most commonly, the ostomy is placed on the imaginary line from the umbilicus to the anterior superior iliac spine, through the rectus muscle, in either the right or left lower quadrant. However, if the belt line, skin folds, or pannus prevent easy access by the patient in this location, alternative sites may be chosen. In elective operations, it may be helpful to have the patient wear an adhesive ostomy appliance for a few days prior to the procedure to ensure optimal placement.

Positioning and Anesthesia

The patient may be placed in the supine or low lithotomy position depending on the procedure. Patients who are having a bowel resection with a planned rectal anastomosis should be placed in low lithotomy, while patients with more proximal bowel pathology can be positioned in the supine position. The abdominal incision and exposure is dictated by the indication for the operation and the segment of bowel to be mobilized.

Procedure Description

Ostomy creation is typically the final step in the operation. First, an adequate length of the chosen segment of bowel is mobilized to the abdominal wall by freeing attachments of the peritoneum and lengthening the mesentery. Adequate blood supply, lack of tension, and avoidance of pre-existing infection are key principles in stoma construction [5, 6]. Special care should be taken in patients with morbid obesity or with a shortened, inflamed mesentery.

A circular skin incision is made measuring 2–4 cm in diameter at the pre-marked site (Fig. 25.1), while holding pressure on the undersurface of the rectus with the opposite hand to protect the underlying viscera. A disk of skin is excised with electrocautery, taking care to leave some subcutaneous fat behind to support the bowel at the abdominal wall. Blunt retraction is used to expose the underlying anterior rectus sheath (Fig. 25.2). The fascia is divided either vertically or with a cruciate incision (Fig. 25.3). Simple retraction is used to separate the rectus muscle parallel to its fibers, exposing the posterior sheath.

Electrocautery is then used to divide the posterior fascia and peritoneum, taking care to protect the underlying viscera. The defect in the fascia should admit two fingerbreadths to allow adequate space for the bowel without vascular compromise. Large fascial defects should be avoided as they are associated with a high rate of parastomal hernia formation [7, 8].

The bowel segment is gently retrieved from the peritoneal cavity with a Babcock clamp placed through the hole in the skin, while taking care to avoid pulling the intestine or tearing the mesentery. For loop stomas, gentle traction can be applied by passing a penrose drain adjacent to the bowel wall (Fig. 25.4). The bowel should protrude 2–4 cm from the skin.

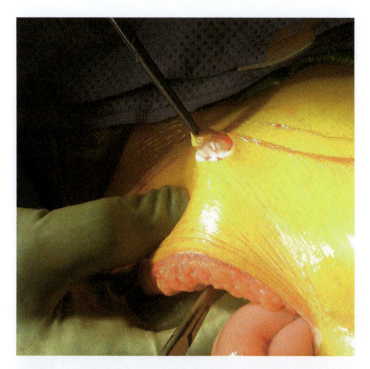

FIGURE 25.1 Excision of the circular skin disk while applying pressure beneath the abdominal wall protects the underlying bowel

The abdominal incision is then closed to avoid contamination when the bowel is reopened for stoma maturation.

First described by Brooke, the stoma is matured by everting the bowel edges [9]. This step allows for the ostomy to easily empty into the appliance away from the skin, protecting the skin and preventing leakage around the appliance. This is especially important for high volume stomas, such as ileostomies. This also prevents stricture formation of the distal bowel. The bowel is then opened by excision the previous staple line in the setting of an end ostomy or opening the bowel on the antimesenteric border for a loop ostomy.

In the case of an end ostomy, 3–4 seromuscular absorbable sutures are placed circumferentially around the bowel lumen

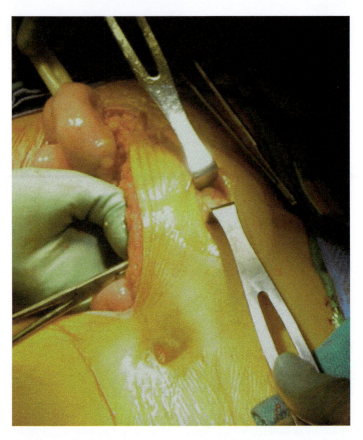

FIGURE 25.2 Exposure of the anterior rectus sheath using blunt dis-section

to evert the edges. Each suture is passed from inside to out-side through the lumen of the bowel including the mucosa and serosa. The next bite is seromuscular at the bowel wall where the abdominal skin and protruding bowel meet. The final bite is through the dermis and each suture is tagged with a hemostat. To evert the edge, the blunt end of a forceps is placed along the bowel wall, and tucked under the stitch. The suture is gently pulled tight and tied as the bowel everts over the forceps and slightly intussuscepts (Fig. 25.5). Once the

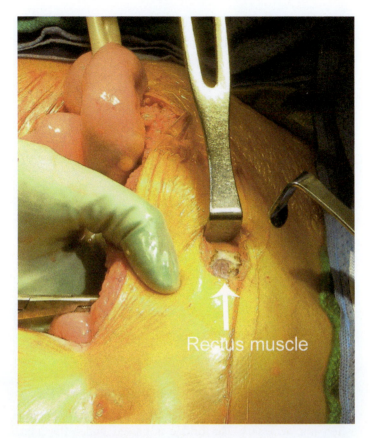

FIGURE 25.3 Division of the anterior rectus sheath exposing the rectus muscle. The muscle fibers are separated bluntly, but are not divided

corners are secure, simple interrupted sutures are placed evenly around the lumen, starting inside-out through the entire thickness of the bowel and into the dermis. A clear stoma appliance is then placed over the everted bowel.

Maturation of a loop ostomy follows similar principles, although it requires securing two bowel lumens to the abdominal wall instead of one. In addition, since the bowel is only partially transected, the posterior bowel wall remains intact. In order to prevent this portion from retracting, a bridge of a

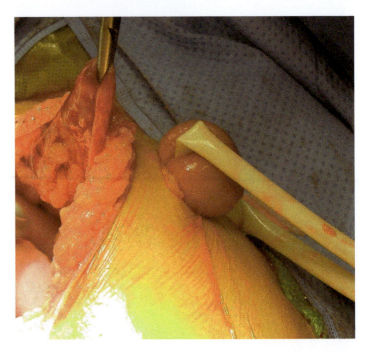

FIGURE 25.4 Gentle retraction of the bowel through the fascial defect with a penrose drain

short segment of plastic or rubber catheter may be used but is often not necessary. The bridge is passed under the intact bowel wall and secured in place with permanent suture to further support the bowel (Fig. 25.5). It is important to take care during loop colostomy formation to not occlude the marginal artery when placing a bridge. The bridge is typically removed within 5 days of ostomy formation. The completed loop ostomy after bridge removal is pictured in Fig. 25.6.

Postoperative Care

A clear ostomy appliance is applied post-operatively to facilitate inspection of the bowel for viability. Ostomy output is directly related to the segment of intestine used. Left colon or

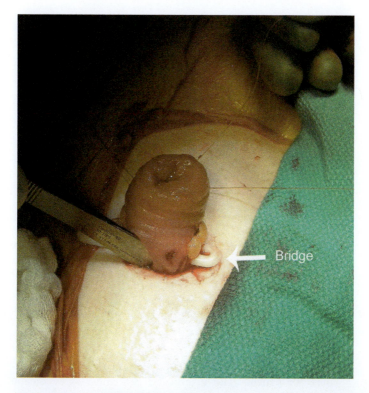

FIGURE 25.5 Circumferential placement of sutures around the stoma incorporating full thickness bowel wall, serosa, and dermis. Placement of a bridge to temporarily support the loop ostomy is optional (*white arrow*)

sigmoid colostomies produce formed stool, whereas more proximal colostomies and ileostomies have a thin and higher volume output. It is not uncommon for ileostomy output to average 1–1.5 L/day, especially in the perioperative period [5]. Patients should be carefully monitored for dehydration and fluid resuscitated both during the post-operative hospital stay as well as after discharge. Skin complications and dehydration are common post-operative complications and dehydration is the most common reason for readmission in this patient population [10, 11]. Patients should complete all education and should be carefully assessed prior to hospital discharge.

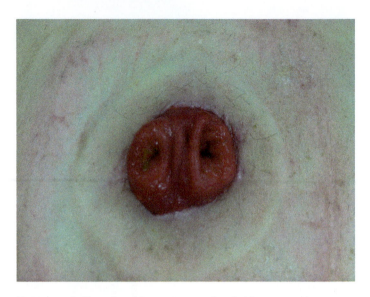

FIGURE 25.6 Completed loop ostomy after bridge removal

References

1. Salem L, Flum DR. Primary anastomosis or Hartmann's procedure for patients with diverticular peritonitis? A systematic review. Dis Colon Rectum. 2004;47(11):1953–64.
2. Matthiessen P, Hallbook O, Rutegard J, et al. Defunctioning stoma reduces symptomatic anastomotic leakage after low anterior resection of the rectum for cancer: a randomized multicenter trial. Ann Surg. 2007;246(2):207–14.
3. McLeod RS, Lavery IC, Leatherman JR, et al. Patient evaluation of the conventional ileostomy. Dis Colon Rectum. 1985;28(3):152–4.
4. Zimnicki KM. Preoperative stoma site marking in the general surgery population. J Wound Ostomy Continence Nurs. 2013;40(5):501–5.
5. Williams JG. "Intestinal Stomas." ACS Surgery, Principles and Practice. Eds. Souba WW, Fink MP, Jurkovich GJ, Kaiser LR, Pearce WH, Pemberton JH, Soper NG. WebMD Publishing, New York, 2005, Chapter 31.
6. Orkin BA, Cataldo PA. "Intestinal Stomas." ASCRS Textbook of Colon and Rectal Surgery. Eds. Wolff BG, Fleshman JW, Beck BE, Pemberton JH, Wexner SD. Springer, New York, 2007. Chapter 44.

7. Cheung MT, Chia NH, Chiu WY. Surgical treatment of parastomal hernia complicating sigmoid colostomies. Dis Colon Rectum. 2001;44(2):266–70.
8. Carne PW, Robertson GM, Frizelle FA. Parastomal hernia. Br J Surg. 2003;90(7):784–93.
9. Brooke BN. The management of an ileostomy, including its complications. Lancet. 1952;2(6725):102–4.
10. Paquette IM, Solan P, Rafferty JF, et al. Readmission for dehydration or renal failure after ileostomy creation. Dis Colon Rectum. 2013;56(8):974–9.
11. Phatak UR, Kao LS, You YN, et al. Impact of ileostomy-related complications on the multidisciplinary treatment of rectal cancer. Ann Surg Oncol. 2014;21(2):507–12.

Part VI
Anorectal Surgery

Gregory D. Kennedy

Chapter 26
Cryptoglandular Disease

Christina M. Papageorge and Gregory D. Kennedy

Abstract Cryptoglandular disease encompasses two related entities: anorectal abscess and fistula-in-ano. Anorectal abscess is an infection of the perianal or perirectal region arising most commonly from obstruction of the anal ducts. The various types of anorectal abscess (perianal, ischioanal, intersphincteric, and supralevator) are defined based on their anatomic location. Treatment typically requires incision and drainage of the abscess cavity, which can be performed either at the bedside or in the operating room depending on complexity and extent of the abscess. Approximately one-third to half of patients with anorectal abscess will go on to develop a persistent inflammatory tract between the anal canal and the perianal skin, known as fistula-in-ano. There are multiple surgical options for treatment of fistula-in-ano, all with the general underlying principle that the internal opening must be obliterated to facilitate healing of the tract.

C.M. Papageorge, MD (✉)
Department of Surgery,
University of Wisconsin Hospital and Clinics,
H4/785A Clinical Science Center, 600 Highland Avenue,
Madison, WI 53792-7375, USA
e-mail: cpapageorge@uwhealth.org

G.D. Kennedy, MD, PhD
Department of Surgery, University of Alabama at Birmingham,
Birmingham, AL, USA

H. Chen (ed.), *Illustrative Handbook of General Surgery*, 463
DOI 10.1007/978-3-319-24557-7_26,
© Springer International Publishing Switzerland 2016

Fistulotomy is the traditional and most effective technique for achieving fistula closure, however it is only appropriate for those fistulae with minimal sphincter complex involvement. Alternatives to fistulotomy include setons (either cutting or draining), endorectal advancement flap, anal fistula plug, fibrin glue, and ligation of the intersphincteric fistula tract (LIFT) procedure.

Keywords Anorectal abscess • Perianal abscess • Perirectal abscess • Incision and drainage • Fistulotomy • Seton • Endorectal advancement flap • Fistula plug • Fibrin glue • Ligation of the intersphincteric fistula tract (LIFT) procedure

Anorectal Abscess

Indications

Anorectal abscesses typically arise from obstruction of the anal ducts, which drain the anal glands into anal crypts located at the dentate line of the anal canal. The resulting infection begins in the space between the internal and external sphincters where the anal glands originate, and can spread through the perianal spaces, forming pockets of purulent material. Locations of anorectal abscesses include (in order of frequency): (1) perianal (2) ischioanal (3) intersphincteric (4) supralevator [1–3] (Figs. 26.1 and 26.2). Patients typically present with pain, palpable mass, fever, urinary retention, or sepsis. Predisposing factors may include diarrhea, trauma, or underlying inflammatory bowel disease, particularly Crohn's disease. Physical exam almost universally reveals a tender, swollen, erythematous, fluctuant mass in the setting of perianal or ischioanal abscess, however intersphincteric and supralevator abscesses may present with minimal external exam findings discordant with patient discomfort [4].

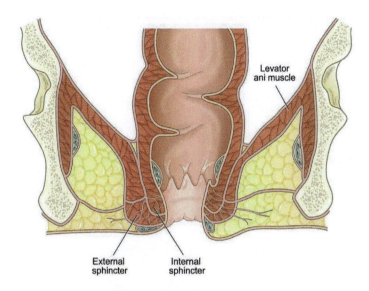

FIGURE 26.1 Normal anorectal anatomy

Anorectal abscess must be differentiated from other inflammatory processes of the perineum such as hidradenitis suppurativa, or other infectious diseases such as HSV, HIV, TB, syphilis, and actinomycosis. Once the diagnosis has been established, usually based on history and physical exam alone, drainage of the abscess cavity must occur expediently in order to minimize progressive symptoms and infectious complications.

Perioperative Care

Preoperative Preparation

Preoperative imaging is not routinely recommended. CT, MRI, or endoanal ultrasound studies may be used to clarify the anatomic location of complex, recurrent, or atypical presentations, or to differentiate isolated Crohn's-associated rectal inflammation from true abscess or fistula, but may be

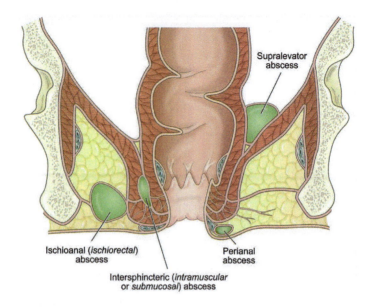

FIGURE 26.2 Location of anorectal abscesses

deferred in typical cases. Examination under anesthesia is usually the most efficient means to both confirm a questionable diagnosis and provide definitive treatment. Pre-procedure antibiotics are indicated for prosthetic valves, history of infective endocarditis, some forms of congenital heart disease, and heart transplant recipients with valve disease [5].

Positioning and Anesthesia

The choice of positioning and anesthesia depends on the location and extent of the abscess. Perianal abscesses are often palpable at the anal verge, and may be effectively drained at the bedside in the lateral decubitus position under local anesthesia. However, ischioanal, intersphincteric, and supralevator abscesses can be large and require examination under anesthesia to confirm location and extent. Therefore, these abscesses should be drained in the operating room in either lithotomy or prone jackknife position. Regional, local with monitored anesthesia care, or general endotracheal anesthesia may be utilized as long as the patient is sufficiently relaxed to facilitate anoscopy and complete examination. The legs must be adequately padded while in lithotomy stirrups, and sequential compression devices should be used.

Description of Procedure

Anorectal Abscess Drainage

Candidates for bedside drainage include patients *without* (1) signs/symptoms of sepsis, including hypotension, high fever, and leukocytosis, (2) evidence of fistula or fissure on physical exam, (3) history of IBD, (4) history of prior complex cryptoglandular disease, (5) history of recent abscess drainage or fistula procedure, (6) history of recent abdominal or pelvic operation, or (7) CT evidence of complex disease, including supralevator, intersphincteric, or horseshoe type configuration. All patients should be initially examined in the lateral decubitus position for an area of fluctuance in the perianal skin, generally with overlying erythema and occasional drainage. Once identified, those patients who are candidates for bedside drainage should have the area cleansed with chlorhexidine scrub. Lidocaine with epinephrine is infiltrated to provide local anesthesia to the overlying skin and surrounding tissue, and IV or PO narcotics may be administered for pain relief. An 18-gauge needle may be used to determine the location of the underlying purulent fluid. A generous cruciate incision is then made over the area of fluctuance using an 11-blade scalpel, and the corners of skin are removed. Removing the corners of skin prevents early closure of the cavity and recollection of the abscess. Alternatively, an elliptical incision may be utilized. Care should be taken to make the incision close to the sphincter muscles in order to minimize the formation of complex fistulas with long tracts. Drainage of the cavity is facilitated by digital manipulation or lysis of intraluminal loculations with a Kelly clamp as needed.

The cavity is then copiously irrigated with normal saline and explored to ensure no further areas of fluctuance requiring drainage. Sterile packing tape is used to lightly pack the cavity, which is then covered using sterile gauze.

Patients with any of the features concerning for complex abscess listed above should be brought to the operating room for examination under anesthesia and abscess drainage. Following induction of anesthesia, the patient is placed in either high lithotomy or prone jackknife position based on surgeon preference. The perineum is prepped and draped in sterile fashion. Digital rectal examination is performed to evaluate for palpable mass, fissure, fistula opening, or other abnormality. An anoscope is then inserted, and visual examination for fissure or fistula is carefully performed. The location of the abscess cavity is determined relative to the sphincter complex and the pelvic floor muscles.

- *Perianal abscess*: identified by bulging of perianal skin. A cruciate or elliptical incision should be made over the area of maximal fluctuance and the abscess cavity drained and irrigated as described above.
- *Ischioanal abscess*: identified by bulging over the ilioanal fossa. The incision should be made as medially as possible, close to the sphincter complex, to reduce the risk of large/complex transsphincteric fistula formation. A horseshoe abscess is identified by bulging in the posterior and lateral anal canal and is drained via a longitudinal incision between the coccyx and the anal canal. This exposes the anococcygeal ligament, which is then incised along its fibers to facilitate entry into the deep postanal space and subsequent abscess drainage. Counter-incisions may be required over the ischioanal spaces on either side of the rectum. As described above, these incisions should be made lateral and as close to the sphincter complexes as possible.
- *Intersphincteric abscess*: identified by bulging in the posterior (most commonly) or lateral anal canal within the sphincter complex but with minimal or absent external

exam findings. An incision is made through the anal mucosa dividing the internal sphincter and may require widening to facilitate complete drainage, while preserving as much sphincter mass as possible. A mushroom tip catheter is left in the cavity and secured with suture to prevent the sphincter muscles from contracting and thereby preventing adequate drainage [6].

- *Supralevator abscess*: identified by palpation of a tender mass on posterior or lateral rectum above the anorectal ring. Drainage route is determined by associated pathology:

  - If associated with ischioanal abscess, drain through cruciate incision on the perianal skin near the sphincter complex to avoid formation of extrasphincteric fistula.
  - If associated with intersphincteric abscess, drain through rectum to avoid formation of complex suprasphincteric fistula.
  - If associated with intraabdominal abscess, use imaging to guide choice of incision.

Additional Operative Considerations

Large cavities may require placement of a small mushroom tip catheter to serve as a drain and maintain patency of the external tract. The external component of this drain should be kept relatively short (2–3 cm) and sutured in place to prevent dislodgement. Postoperatively, the patient should be taught how to flush the drain with sterile saline and perform a gentle irrigation twice daily. The drain can be downsized once per week as tolerated until the cavity is small and manageable with local wound care.

There has been debate in the literature regarding whether or not to perform a fistulotomy at the time of initial incision and drainage of anorectal abscess. The main reason cited for deferring primary fistulotomy is that it exposes patients to the risk of sphincter compromise when they may not have gone on to develop a persistent fistula-in-ano. However, the proposed advantage is reduced recurrence of abscess and avoidance of a second operation for fistulotomy. A 2010 Cochrane review addressed this question, and meta-analysis of six randomized controlled trials including 479 patients concluded that in the setting of perianal abscess associated with low anal fistula, primary fistulotomy significantly reduces the risk of persistent abscess, fistula, and need for repeat surgery, without significantly compromising continence [7]. Regardless, the decision to perform primary fistulotomy should be made on an individualized basis.

Special Postoperative Considerations

All patients should begin sitz baths two times per day on postoperative day number two. Such a regimen ensures perianal hygiene and improves comfort of the area. Fiber or other bulk-producing agents should be added to a regular diet to prevent diarrhea and improve hygiene. There is no role for postoperative antibiotic therapy in most cases. Antibiotics may be considered in patients with significant associated cellulitis, systemic sepsis, valvular heart disease, mechanical valve, diabetes, or immunosuppression [3, 4]. Close follow-up is necessary as there is approximately 30% risk of recurrent anorectal sepsis and 30–50% risk of fistula formation requiring future intervention [4, 6].

Fistula-in-Ano

Indications

In approximately one-third to half of patients who experience a cryptoglandular abscess, an inflammatory tract develops and persists between an internal opening at the dentate line and an external opening on the perianal skin, defined as a fistula-in-ano [1, 2, 4]. The location and course of the fistula directly reflects the location of the original abscess and is classified anatomically in relation to the sphincter muscles: (1) intersphincteric (2) transsphincteric (3) suprasphincteric (4) extrasphincteric [8] (Fig. 26.3). Patients present with persistent purulent drainage from the internal and/or external openings, either spontaneously or following I&D procedures for abscess. Differential diagnosis considerations include pilonidal sinus, hidradenitis suppurativa, infected perianal cysts, diverticular disease, IBD, malignancy, or radiation injury. In general, the location of a fistula tract and its internal opening follows Goodsall's rule. This rule suggests that when the external opening is located within 3 cm of the anal verge and is anterior to a transverse line through the anus, then the tract travels radially in a straight line to the anal canal. Alternatively, when the external opening is located within 3 cm of the anus and posteriorly, the tract follows a curvilinear path terminating in the posterior midline of the anal canal.

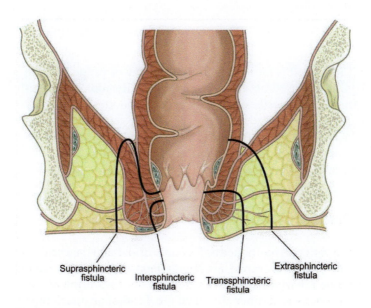

FIGURE 26.3 Location of fistula-in-ano

Perioperative Care

Preoperative Preparation

Although most fistulae-in-ano represent sequelae of spontaneous or surgical drainage of anorectal abscess, risk factors
for underlying malignancy and inflammatory bowel disease
must prompt consideration of a colonoscopy prior to operation. As a general rule, fistulizing Crohn's disease should be
managed with aggressive medical rather than surgical therapy [1]. Techniques for identifying tract location include digital palpation or imaging techniques such as endoanal
ultrasound and MRI, with or without injection of dilute
hydrogen peroxide. In one cohort, these methods successfully
identified 61, 81, and 90% of fistulous tracts, respectively [9].
If local inflammation is minimal, enemas should be given the
night before the procedure; complete bowel preparation is
not necessary. Preoperative antibiotics should be given prior
to incision.

Positioning and Anesthesia

The patient is placed in either lithotomy or prone jackknife
position based on surgeon preference. Regional, local with
monitored anesthesia care, or general endotracheal anesthesia may be utilized, but must adequately relax the patient to
facilitate anoscopy. Care should be taken to ensure adequate
padding of the legs and other pressure points, and sequential
compression devices should be placed on all patients.

Description of Procedure

The patient is positioned as described above and the perineum
is prepped and draped in sterile fashion. Digital rectal examination is performed to evaluate for mass, fissure, internal fistula opening, or other abnormalities. In addition, the depth of
the fistula tract relative to the external sphincter is assessed

in order to select the appropriate procedure: if less than 50 % of the posterior or lateral external sphincter or less than 30 % of the anterior external sphincter is superficial to the tract, a one-stage fistulotomy may be considered. However, if a greater portion of the external sphincter is involved, staged repair with initial seton placement is recommended to minimize the risk of incontinence and stricture [10]. Other criteria state that if the internal opening is above the dentate line, the deep external sphincter is involved, and thus a staged repair should be considered [11].

Gentle dilation is performed to allow introduction of the anoscope, and complete examination of the anal canal is performed to localize the internal opening. This may be enhanced by injection of hydrogen peroxide or methylene blue into the external opening, or by gentle introduction of a probe through the external opening. Care must be taken not to force a new tract or opening, thus creating a more complex fistula.

Fistulotomy

Fistulotomy is only appropriate for the treatment of intersphincteric and low transsphincteric fistulae given risk for incontinence when more of the sphincter complex is involved. After gently passing a probe down the tract through the external opening (Fig. 26.4), an incision is made on the probe using a scalpel or electrocautery through the perianal skin and rectal mucosa to lay open the tract (Fig. 26.5). The fistula tract is then cleaned with a curette to remove any granulation tissue. The surgeon must continually assess for sphincter musculature involvement and aim to avoid division of such muscle. Complicated tracts may require a stepwise approach where the incision is extended only as far as the probe can be safely passed; once the tract has been partially opened, the probe is advanced accordingly as the direction of the tract becomes apparent. At the completion of the procedure, light packing tape may be placed in the fistula tract, and an InStat (petroleum jelly on gauze) dressing placed in the rectum (Fig. 26.6).

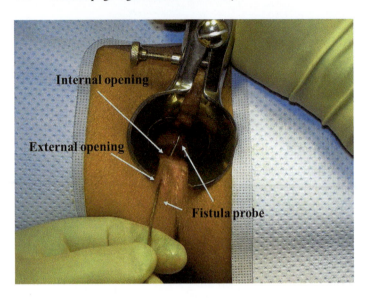

FIGURE 26.4 Locating the fistula tract. The probe is carefully inserted through the external opening, and allowed to follow the tract until it exits through the internal opening. This will serve as a guide for either subsequent fistulotomy or seton placement

Seton Placement

In the setting of significant sphincter complex involvement or risk factors for incontinence, such as diminished preoperative sphincter function, chronic diarrhea, or anterior fistula, it is safer to proceed with a staged procedure starting with seton placement rather than fistulotomy. The skin and mucosa overlying the fistula tract is opened with electrocautery or scalpel until the sphincter musculature is encountered, thus partially opening the fistula tract. At this point, the tract and openings are curetted and prepped for seton placement. Selection of type of seton is dependent on the goal of the operation:

1. *Cutting setons* will gradually cut through the sphincter muscle via pressure necrosis, with formation of fibrosis behind the seton preventing sphincter retraction and

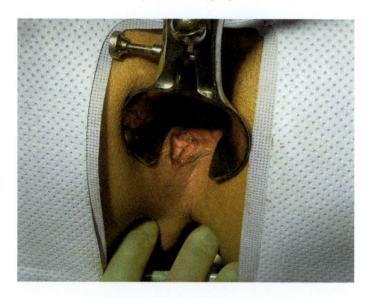

FIGURE 26.5 Fistulotomy. After carefully opening along the probe, granulation tissue at the base of the tract is removed with a curette. Note that the edges are clean and are not undermined

incontinence. A large Ethibond or other braided suture is placed through the internal and external openings of the fistula tract and tied down onto the sphincter complex. The seton will then be "advanced" over the course of the next several weeks until the fistula tract is completely incised. Advancement of a cutting seton can be performed in the outpatient surgery clinic or in the operating room. However, care must be taken to not advance the seton too quickly, as the patient will experience a tremendous amount of pain as well as suffer a complication of sphincter division. Complete division of the external sphincter and fistula tract usually takes 1–6 weeks and is apparent when the seton falls out [6].

2. *Draining setons* will keep the fistula tract open, allowing for abscess drainage and tract maturation, therefore facilitating a future fistulotomy or other advanced fistula closure technique. A vessel loop or large Ethibond suture is passed

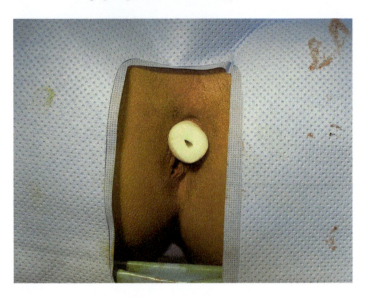

FIGURE 26.6 InStat placement. At the end of the procedure, the perineum should be cleaned and an InStat dressing placed in the anal canal. Patients should be instructed to keep this light packing in place using a temporary mesh undergarment until it falls out with the first postoperative bowel movement

through the internal and external openings of the fistula tract and tied loosely around the sphincter complex (Fig. 26.7). Indications for use of a draining seton include: (1) complex anorectal fistula extensively involving the external sphincter, with the goal of staged fistulotomy; (2) complex anorectal fistula in the setting of sepsis; (3) anterior high transsphincteric fistula in a female patient; (4) high transsphincteric fistula in a patient with AIDS; (5) long-term fistula treatment in a patient with active IBD; and (6) concern for fistulotomy leading to fecal incontinence [10].

Repeat examination should be performed in 6–8 weeks, with either fistulotomy, seton replacement, or alternative approach to fistula closure as described below.

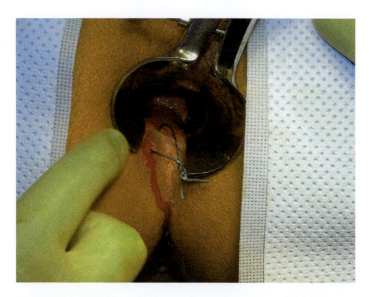

FIGURE 26.7 Draining seton placement. The seton is placed through the external and internal fistula openings and tied loosely to maintain drainage. Here, a vessel loop is used, but Ethibond suture may be substituted

Endorectal Advancement Flap

For patients with high or complex anal fistula, particularly in locations threatening to produce incontinence with traditional fistulotomy, the endorectal advancement flap can provide definitive treatment by occluding the internal opening. This elimination of the drainage source allows the fistula tract and external opening to close over time.

Granulation tissue is cleaned from the fistula tract and the internal opening using a curette. A trapezoidal flap is elevated distal to the internal fistula opening using electrocautery, initially remaining in the submucosal plane, but transitioning to full-thickness as the flap is developed in the cephalad direction. Once adequately elevated with good hemostasis, the internal opening is closed in a transverse fashion using interrupted 4-0 chromic sutures. The area is cleaned with gentle irrigation. Finally, using gentle traction, the flap is advanced distally, and sutured to the underlying mucosa using interrupted 2-0 vicryl sutures, progressing from proximal to distal. Care should be taken to space the sutures sufficiently to achieve a tension-free repair. When the flap has been laid down and confirmed to extend beyond the internal opening, sutures may be placed in the anoderm as well. If needed, Bacitracin and Gelfoam may be applied with light pressure to achieve hemostasis at the completion of the flap procedure. Any open external portion should be dressed with wet-to-dry gauze dressing overnight. Alternatively, a deep cavity can be drained with a mushroom tip catheter left in place for several days. The patient should be admitted for postoperative observation and pain management.

Healing time is estimated at 6 weeks. Incidence of recurrent fistula after endorectal advancement flap has been reported to be 3 % in a series of 164 patients [12].

Alternative Surgical Approaches

Patients who are not candidates for primary fistulotomy present a surgical challenge. The treatment of choice is not clear and is surgeon-dependent. Many surgeons prefer to proceed with an endorectal advancement flap as described above, however there are several alternative sphincter-sparing approaches.

Anal Fistula Plug

The anal fistula plug is a bioabsorbable plug that is inserted into the fistula tract and serves as a scaffold for the ingrowth of the patient's own tissue. It may be employed in patients with fistulae otherwise requiring seton placement. Reported success rates of the anal fistula plug vary widely in the literature, however a recent systematic review that pooled data from 530 patients suggested a success rate of approximately 54 % in both Crohn's and non-Crohn's-related fistulas, a plug extrusion rate of 8.7 %, and no reported cases of continence impairment [13].

Prior to fistula plug placement, the patient should have undergone an examination under anesthesia and had a draining seton placed. The seton allows the tract to mature and remain open while anorectal sepsis resolves. After approximately 6 weeks, the patient is brought back to the operating room for fistula plug placement.

The patient is positioned as previously described and the perineum prepped and draped in sterile fashion. Following digital rectal examination, the tract is identified, and any granulation tissue at the internal or external openings is gently debrided with a curette. The anal fistula plug is then brought onto the field and reconstituted in saline. A fistula probe is passed through the opening, and the fistula plug is secured to the probe to facilitate advancement. The plug is then carefully pulled through the fistula tract from the internal opening to the external opening, just flush with the opening and the internal sphincter. The internal portion of the plug is trimmed, and 2 figure-of-eight sutures are placed through the plug, submucosa, and internal sphincter muscle to secure and cover the plug. The plug is secured to one side of the external opening of the tract using a single 3–0 vicryl suture. Alternatively, an endorectal advancement flap may also be utilized to cover the internal opening with the plug in place. Bacitracin ointment is applied to the external portion, and an InStat dressing left in the rectum.

Fibrin Glue

Fibrin glue may be used as an alternative means of obliterating the fistula tract. The patient is positioned and the perineum prepped and draped in sterile fashion. Following digital rectal examination, the tract is identified, and any granulation tissue at the internal or external openings is gently debrided with a curette. The internal opening is closed, either primarily or in combination with an endorectal advancement flap. Fibrin glue or other similar sealant is then gently injected through the external opening until the tract is full. An external dressing is applied, and an InStat dressing left in the rectum.

Success with this technique is highly variable, with reported success rates of 25–85 % depending on the type of fistula and duration of follow-up [14]. Despite inconsistent results, this technique can be used to avoid a large operation in high risk patients and has minimal associated morbidity.

Ligation of the Intersphincteric Fistula Tract (LIFT) Procedure

The LIFT procedure is a new technique, described in 2007, for treating complex anorectal fistulae [15]. As the name suggests, this technique involves division of the fistula tract in the intersphincteric plane, in order to isolate the internal opening from the remainder of the fistula tract. This procedure has been described both as an initial intervention for the treatment of anorectal fistula, or a staged procedure following insertion of a draining seton for 6–8 weeks [15, 16]. The patient is positioned, prepped, and draped, and the fistula tract is identified with a fistula probe. A curvilinear skin incision is made at the intersphincteric groove in order to enter the intersphincteric plane. The fistula tract is then identified where it traverses the intersphincteric space, and this is dissected free from surrounding tissue, taking care not to injure the sphincter muscles. The tract is ligated with an absorbable suture adjacent to the internal sphincter and then divided distal to the point of ligation. The origin of the distal portion of the tract is oversewn in figure-of-8 fashion at the level of the external sphincter. The perianal skin incision is reapproximated with 4-0 absorbable suture in interrupted fashion. Granulation tissue at the external opening is debrided with a curette. Finally, the wounds are dressed with sterile gauze.

Long-term data for this technique is currently limited; however, a pooled analysis of 1,110 patients undergoing the LIFT procedure with a mean follow up time of 10 months demonstrated a success rate of 76 % with no major associated impact on continence [17].

Special Postoperative Considerations

Warm sitz baths may be used for comfort, and fiber or other bulk-producing agents should be introduced to reduce diarrhea. Patients undergoing seton placement should be reminded that drainage will continue postoperatively and to return for evaluation if the drainage increases, changes in quality, or is accompanied by increased pain or fever.

References

1. Cosman BC, Morris AM, Nivatvongs S, Madoff RD. Anorectal disorders. In: Doherty GM, Mulholland MW, Maier RV, Lillemoe KD, Simeone DM, Upchurch Jr GR, editors. Greenfield's surgery: scientific principles & practice. 5th ed. Philadelphia: Lippincott Williams & Wilkins; 2010. p. 1130–58.
2. Bullard KM, Rothenberger DA. Colon, rectum, and anus. In: Brunicardi FC, Anderson DK, Billiar TR, Dunn DL, Hunter JG, Pollock RE, editors. Schwartz's manual of surgery. 8th ed. New York: The McGraw-Hill Companies, Inc.; 2006. p. 732–83.
3. Vasilevsky C-A. Anorectal abscess and fistula. In: Beck DE, Roberts PL, Saclarides TJ, Senagore AJ, Stamos MJ, Wexner SD, editors. The ASCRS textbook of colon and rectal surgery. 2nd ed. New York: Springer Publishing Company; 2011. p. 219–44.
4. Steele SR, Kumar R, Feingold DL, Rafferty JL, Buie WD. Practice parameters for the management of perianal abscess and fistula-in-ano. Dis Colon Rectum. 2011;54(12):1465–74. doi:10.1097/DCR.0b013e31823122b3.
5. Wilson W, Taubert KA, Gewitz M, Lockhart PB, Baddour LM, Levison M, Bolger A, Cabell CH, Takahashi M, Baltimore RS, Newburger JW, Strom BL, Tani LY, Gerber M, Bonow RO, Pallasch T, Shulman ST, Rowley AH, Burns JC, Ferrieri P, Gardner T, Goff D, Durack DT. Prevention of infective endocarditis: guidelines from the American Heart Association: a guideline from the American Heart Association Rheumatic Fever, Endocarditis, and Kawasaki Disease Committee, Council on Cardiovascular Disease in the Young, and the Council on Clinical Cardiology, Council on Cardiovascular Surgery and Anesthesia, and the Quality of Care and Outcomes Research Interdisciplinary Working Group. Circulation. 2007;116(15):1736–54. doi:10.1161/circulationaha.106.183095.

6. Keighley MRB. Anorectal disorders. In: Fischer JE, Jones DB, Pomposelli FB, et al., editors. Fischer's mastery of surgery. 6th ed. Philadelphia: Lippincott Williams & Wilkins; 2011.

7. Malik AI, Nelson RL, Tou S. Incision and drainage of perianal abscess with or without treatment of anal fistula. Cochrane Database Syst Rev. 2010;7:Cd006827. doi:10.1002/14651858. CD006827.pub2.

8. Parks AG, Gordon PH, Hardcastle JD. A classification of fistula-in-ano. Br J Surg. 1976;63(1):1–12.

9. Buchanan GN, Halligan S, Bartram CI, Williams AB, Tarroni D, Cohen CR. Clinical examination, endosonography, and MR imaging in preoperative assessment of fistula in ano: comparison with outcome-based reference standard. Radiology. 2004;233(3):674–81. doi:10.1148/radiol.2333031724.

10. Pearl RK, Andrews JR, Orsay CP, Weisman RI, Prasad ML, Nelson RL, Cintron JR, Abcarian H. Role of the seton in the management of anorectal fistulas. Dis Colon Rectum. 1993;36(6):573–7; discussion 577–9.

11. Zollinger Jr RM, Ellison EC. Zollinger's atlas of surgical operations. 9th ed. New York: The McGraw-Hill Companies, Inc.; 2010.

12. Golub RW, Wise Jr WE, Kerner BA, Khanduja KS, Aguilar PS. Endorectal mucosal advancement flap: the preferred method for complex cryptoglandular fistula-in-ano. J Gastrointest Surg. 1997;1(5):487–91.

13. O'Riordan JM, Datta I, Johnston C, Baxter NN. A systematic review of the anal fistula plug for patients with Crohn's and non-Crohn's related fistula-in-ano. Dis Colon Rectum. 2012;55(3):351–8. doi:10.1097/DCR.0b013e318239d1e4.

14. Maralcan G, Baskonus I, Gokalp A, Borazan E, Balk A. Long-term results in the treatment of fistula-in-ano with fibrin glue: a prospective study. J Kor Surg Soc. 2011;81(3):169–75. doi:10.4174/jkss.2011.81.3.169.

15. Rojanasakul A, Pattanaarun J, Sahakitrungruang C, Tantiphlachiva K. Total anal sphincter saving technique for fistula-in-ano; the ligation of intersphincteric fistula tract. J Med Assoc Thai. 2007;90(3):581–6.

16. Shanwani A, Nor AM, Amri N. Ligation of the intersphincteric fistula tract (LIFT): a sphincter-saving technique for fistula-in-ano. Dis Colon Rectum. 2010;53(1):39–42. doi:10.1007/DCR.0b013e3181c160c4.

17. Hong KD, Kang S, Kalaskar S, Wexner SD. Ligation of intersphincteric fistula tract (LIFT) to treat anal fistula: systematic review and meta-analysis. Tech Coloproctol. 2014;18(8):685–91. doi:10.1007/s10151-014-1183-3.

Chapter 27
Pilonidal Disease

Christina W. Lee and Gregory D. Kennedy

Abstract Pilonidal disease is a common acquired condition characterized by occluded hair within small midline pits superior to the intergluteal cleft. Varying presentations are possible which include an acute abscess, simple pilonidal cyst or complicated, recurrent sinus. Pre-operative preparations should include resolution of an acute abscess and appropriate preparation in positioning in addition to antibiotics. Many surgical options exist for the treatment of pilonidal disease including, incision and curettage, marsupialization, excision and primary closure, cleft closure, Z-plasty, V-Y advancement flap, rhomboid flap, and gluteus maximus myocutaneous flap. Time to healing remains variable from 3 to 4 weeks on average. Recurrence rates following surgical therapy may be as high as 40 % with simple drainage of the abscess to as low as 1 % with advancement flap procedures. This chapter presents a myriad of common surgical approaches to the treatment of pilonidal disease, complete with descriptive illustrative figures.

———
C.W. Lee, MD (✉)
Department of Surgery, University of Wisconsin School of
Medicine and Public Health,
600 Highland Avenue, Madison, WI 53792, USA
e-mail: clee6@uwhealth.org

G.D. Kennedy, MD, PhD
Department of Surgery, University of Alabama at Birmingham,
Birmingham, AL, USA

H. Chen (ed.), *Illustrative Handbook of General Surgery*,   483
DOI 10.1007/978-3-319-24557-7_27,
© Springer International Publishing Switzerland 2016

Keywords Pilonidal disease • Pilonidal cyst • Pilonidal abscess • Cleft closure • Advancement flap • Local excision • Fistulotomy • Marsupialization

Indications

Pilonidal sinus is associated with small midline pits over the sacrum and coccyx along the intergluteal cleft. These midline pits often contain hair. This condition commonly affects young adults following puberty, and is more common in men than women. Caucasians are principally affected, and is rare among African Americans and Asians [1]. The incidence of pilonidal disease is approximately 0.7 % in young adults and is commonly accepted to be an acquired condition caused by embedded hairs in the intergluteal cleft, which subsequently become suppurative secondary to infection by skin flora [2]. Pilonidal disease may spontaneously resolve with age, however common presentations include, an acute abscess, a simple pilonidal cyst, or a complicated or recurrent sinus. Primary midline openings or pits may be seen in the gluteal cleft approximately 5 cm cephalad to the anus [2]. Acute abscesses present as warm, tender and fluctuant swellings which often exudes purulent discharge through the midline at the apex. Management at this stage is by incision and drainage. Chronic sinus tracts become lined with squamous epithelium, and treatment may be approached by various procedures described below. Recurrence rates vary depending on the study and procedure (Table 27.1).

Perioperative Care

Preoperative Preparation

Acute infection should be resolved prior to definitive operation. Abscesses should be drained and cellulitis treated with antibiotics. Most patients are under the age of 40; therefore, minimal preoperative testing is required. Smoking cessation should be encouraged to assist wound healing.

TABLE 27.1 Comparison of treatment methods for pilonidal disease [1]

Method	IP or OP treatment	Dressing changes required	Weeks to healing (average)	Recurrence (%)
Abscess drainage/Shaving	OP	Yes	3–4	25–40
Excision	OP	No	3	16
Fistulotomy	OP	Yes	4–6	1–19
Marsupialization	OP	Yes	6	8
Wide local excision only	OP	Yes	8	Up to 38
Wide local excision, primary closure	OP	No	4–8	Up to 38
Excision, advancement flap	IP	No	3–4	6–20
Karydakis advancement flap	IP	No	3	1.3
Cleft closure	OP	No	3	3.3

Positioning and Anesthesia

After general anesthesia is induced, the patient is placed in the prone jack-knife position. Tape to spread the gluteus facilitates full visualization of the cleft. Hair is clipped in the affected area. Patients are administered intravenous antibiotics prior to surgical incision.

Description of Procedures

Many operations have been described for the treatment of pilonidal disease. Few have been studied in a randomized controlled fashion. Therefore, recommendations on operative approach are difficult to make. However, we prefer to start with the simplest operation and advance our interventions to the more complex as necessary. Below we describe the operative approaches employed at our institution.

Incision and Curettage

Sinus tracts are identified with a probe and opened longitudinally using a knife or bovie cautery. The wound base is then curetted, and the skin edges are excised in order to expose the open granulating wound. The wound heals by secondary intention, and must be kept clean and free of hair. The patients are then advised to partake in BID postoperative wound care to allow for adequate healing. Alternatively, a wound vacuum can be employed to assist in wound care and shorten the length of healing.

Marsupialization

If a sinus is infected at the time of excision, primary closure should be avoided. Marsupialization is a technique by which the surrounding skin edges of a defect are sutured down to the presacral fascia [1]. Sinus tracts are identified and typically excised but can be unroofed. The wound base is curetted and all hair is removed. The defect that remains is often large and requires significant dressing changes. Therefore, the skin edges are sewn to the fibrotic wound base or presacral fascia using interrupted 3-0 vicryl suture (Fig. 27.1). This decreases the size of the wound significantly and anecdotally shortens healing time. Figures 27.2, 27.3, 27.4, 27.5, and 27.6 demonstrate this operative technique in a patient with recurrent pilonidal disease.

Excision and Primary Closure

This operation by definition, requires excision of the entire sinus tract. This includes wide excision of the pilonidal region,

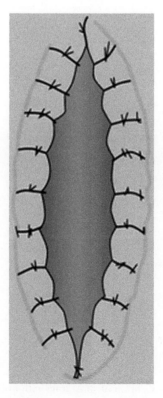

FIGURE 27.1 Marsupialization

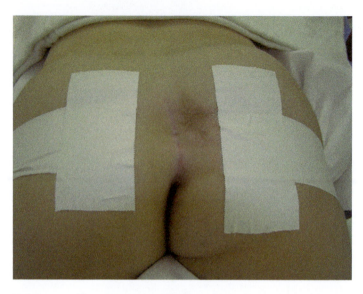

FIGURE 27.2 Preoperative positioning in this patient with recurrent pilonidal disease

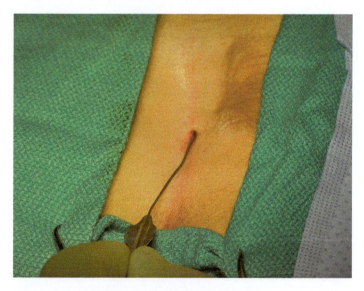

FIGURE 27.3 Identification of sinus tract with probe

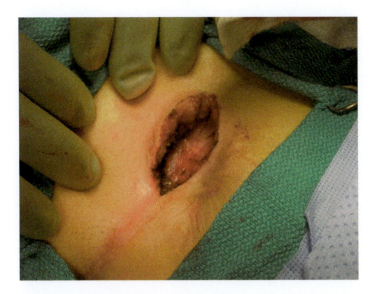

FIGURE 27.4 Debridement to the sacral fascia

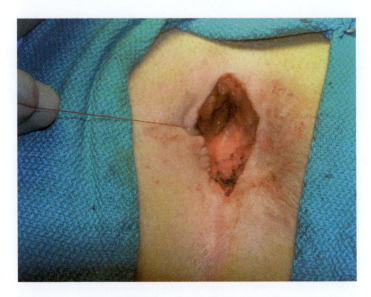

FIGURE 27.5 Marsupialization with interrupted suture

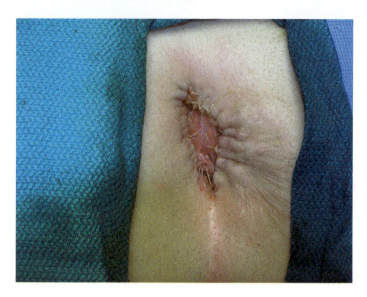

FIGURE 27.6 Completed marsupialization

including the skin and entirety of the tract involving the sub-cutaneous issues down to the presacral fascia. Excision is completed by a midline incision, and left open or closed primarily. Due to shearing forces around the buttock region, as seen in young and active adults, skin breakdown and delayed healing in common. This is avoided by an off-midline incision as in the Karydakis modified the operation. The sinus is excised elliptically and the wound is closed off of the midline (Fig. 27.7). To accomplish this, a thick flap is created and advanced across the midline.

Cleft Closure

Full thickness skin flaps are raised bilaterally (Fig. 27.8). The wound is debrided. Gluteal fat is apposed with absorbable suture. Excess skin is removed and the wound is closed with 4-0 nylon interrupted suture.

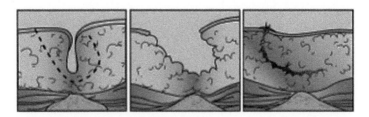

FIGURE 27.7 Primary excision and closure

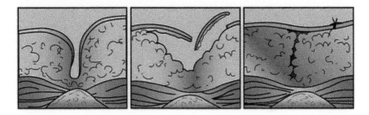

FIGURE 27.8 Cleft closure

Z-Plasty

The sinus tract is excised in the midline which becomes the central limb of the Z (Fig. 27.9). For the classic Z-plasty, wide excision is performed around the pilonidal region, as previously described, so as to include the entire tract, the limbs are incised at 60° angles to the central limb. The length gain of a Z-plasty varies based on the angle incised (Table 27.2). All limbs are of equal length. Subcutaneous skin flaps are created under 'a' and 'b' so as to allow mobilization without tension, then transposed as shown. The resulting central limb will be perpendicular to the original central limb. The skin is closed with 4-0 nylon interrupted suture.

V-Y Advancement Flap

These flaps can be unilateral or bilateral (Fig. 27.10). A unilateral flap is capable of covering 8–10 cm defects while a

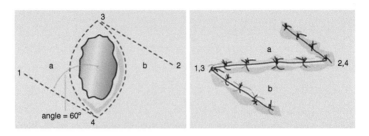

FIGURE 27.9 Z-plasty

TABLE 27.2 Length gain after Z-plasty

Angles of Z-plasty (degrees)	Theoretical gain in length (%)
30–30	25
45–45	50
60–60	75
75–75	100
90–90	120

bilateral flaps are needed to cover >10 cm defects [3]. The sinus tracts are excised in the midline and the base of the V points laterally. The triangular flap is made 1.5–2× as long as the defect in the direction of the advancement. However, some authors have reported flaps up to 3x as long as the defect, and should be personalized to the dimensions so as to avoid making acute angles at corners [3]. The base of the triangle is made equal to the perpendicular diameter of the defect. The skin flap is undermined at the medial edge while fascia is undermined as little as necessary at the lateral edge (Fig. 27.11). Skin hooks are used to pull the leading edge of the flap to the far edge of the defect. The lateral aspect of the harvest site is re-approximated making the stem of a Y. The inferior and superior edges of the Y are closed with 3-0 vicryl deep dermal interrupted sutures and 4-0 nylon interrupted sutures for skin.

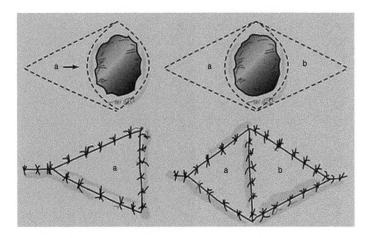

FIGURE 27.10 V-Y advancement flap

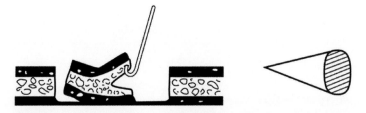

FIGURE 27.11 V-Y advancement flap cross sectional view

Rhomboid Flap

The sinus tract is excised from the midline, enclosed within the shape of a rhomboid. This flap depends on the looseness of the adjacent tissue. The rhomboid has two opposite 60° angles and two opposite 120° angles. Each side of the rhomboid is equal to the short axis 2–4. This axis is extended by its own length to point 5. The 3–4 line and 6–5 line are parallel. A flap is created down to the muscular fascia and rotated as shown (Fig. 27.12). The flap is secured with 4-0 nylon interrupted suture. Four flaps are available for any rhomboid defect (Fig. 27.13).

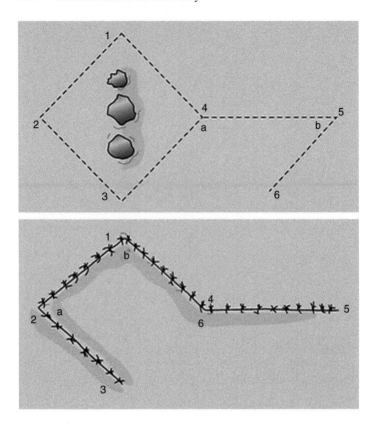

FIGURE 27.12 Rhomboid flap

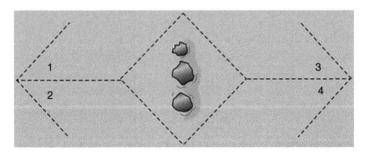

FIGURE 27.13 Rhomboid flaps available for a defect

Gluteus Maximus Myocutaneous Flap

This rotational flap is capable of covering large defects. To avoid functional deficits, only one half of the muscle is used. For pilonidal disease, the superior aspect of the gluteus muscle is typically used to create a flap. A sterile Doppler is utilized to locate the perforators to be included in the flap, and may be used continuously throughout the dissection. The superior gluteal muscle vessels exit above the piriformis muscle and just lateral to the sacrum. The sciatic nerve exits below the piriformis muscle, as do the inferior gluteal vessels and should be avoided. The defect is excised down to presacral fascia removing all prior scar tissue. A circular flap is created and the upper portion of the gluteus maximus is transected down to the gluteus medius and piriformis muscles. The base of the flap should be four to five times the length of the defect. After flap rotation, a suction drain is placed. The wound is closed in layers and skin edges are secured with 4-0 nylon interrupted suture (Fig. 27.14). The patient should not lie flat for several days, although variation amongst surgeons may permit patients to lie on the operated area at time intervals that are no longer than one hour at a time. A short course of oral antibiotics, such as a first generation cephalosporin, is usually recommended.

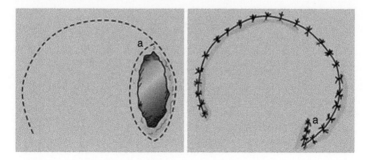

FIGURE 27.14 Gluteus maximus myocutaneous flap

References

1. Cameron JL. Current surgical therapy. 9th ed. St. Louis: Mosby; 2007.
2. Charles T, Grabb WC, Beasley RW. Grabb and Smith's plastic surgery, vol. 1. 6th ed. Philadelphia: Lippincott Williams & Wilkins; 2006. p. 929.
3. Sahasrabudhe P, Panse N, Waghmare C, et al. V-Y Advancement flap technique in resurfacing postexcisional defect in cases with pilonidal sinus disease-study of 25 cases. Indian J Surg. 2012; 74(5):364–70.

Chapter 28
Anal Fissure

Sarah E. Tevis and Gregory D. Kennedy

Abstract Fissure in ano is characterized by severe pain with defecation. Conservative treatment involves increasing dietary fiber intake and topical administration of smooth muscle relaxants. When these conservative options fail, surgery may be indicated. Closed and open lateral internal sphincterotomy will be discussed in detail in this chapter.

Keywords Fissure • Sphincterotomy • Hypertrophied anal papilla

Etiology and Diagnosis

Anal fissure, or fissure-in-ano, is described as a tear in the anoderm distal to the dentate line. Anal fissures occur in 10 % of patients and are more common in women [1].

S.E. Tevis, MD (✉)
Department of General Surgery, University of Wisconsin,
650 Highland Avenue, 53792 Madison, WI, USA
e-mail: stevis@uwhealth.org

G.D. Kennedy, MD, PhD
Department of Surgery, University of Alabama at Birmingham,
Birmingham, AL, USA

H. Chen (ed.), *Illustrative Handbook of General Surgery*,
DOI 10.1007/978-3-319-24557-7_28,
© Springer International Publishing Switzerland 2016

Patients typically present with painful defecation, rectal bleeding, and itching [2]. Anal fissures that heal within 4–6 weeks with conservative treatment are considered acute, while chronic fissures persist for >6 weeks.

While the pathogenesis of anal fissures is unclear, the most common etiology is thought to be constipation and local anal trauma [1]. The fissure then initiates a cycle of pain, fear of defection, constipation, and sphincter spasm [3]. Increased resting internal sphincter tone paired with relative ischemia of the posterior anal canal has been implicated in chronic anal fissures [1].

Fissures are diagnosed by physical exam and can be associated with a sentinel skin tag and hypertrophied anal papilla. The majority (90 %) of fissures are located in the posterior midline (Fig. 28.1). Atypical fissures, those off the midline, are associated with other underlying diagnoses including Crohn's disease, sexually transmitted diseases (HIV, syphilis, herpes), anal cancer, and tuberculosis [4].

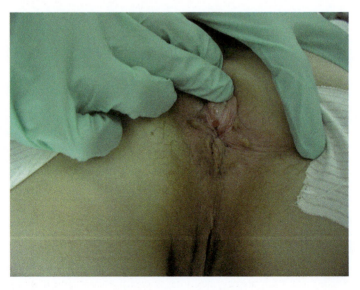

FIGURE 28.1 Anal fissure in posterior midline

Preoperative Care

Approximately half of all fissures resolve with conservative management, which consists of increased fiber and water intake and warm sitz baths. These measures have been found to heal nearly all fissures [1, 4, 5]. Various medical treatments may also be considered, including topical calcium channel blockers and botulinum toxin injection [5]. Medical therapies have been found to promote healing by decreasing sphincter pressures, however success rates are variable [6, 7]. Patients with persistent fissures or those associated with severe pain are candidates for surgical intervention [1, 4].

Indications for Surgical Approach

Lateral internal sphincterotomy (LIS) is the gold standard of treatment for chronic anal fissures with cure rates >90 % [1, 8]. Improvement in quality of life has also been described following LIS [9]. Overall, post-operative complications after this procedure are quite rare. While there is a potential risk of post-operative incontinence, incontinence rates after LIS have been found to be lower than reported in patients treated with medical therapies, such as calcium channel blockers and botulinum toxin injections [9, 10].

Description of Procedure

Positioning and choice of anesthesia are determined at the discretion of the surgeon. Many surgeons prefer the prone-jackknife position or high lithotomy for this procedure. General anesthesia is typically preferred, although a direct anal block may also be used. No preoperative bowel preparation is required.

Either a closed or open sphincterotomy may be performed, as both procedures have been found to result in similar outcomes [11]. In a closed sphincterotomy, the internal sphincter muscle is divided without incising the overlying anoderm. First, the groove between the internal and external sphincter is palpated and the index finger of the nondominant hand is inserted into the anal canal. A generous amount of 1 % lidocaine is injected into the intersphincteric groove. Then a No. 11 scalpel is inserted with the blade parallel to the fibers of the internal sphincter (Fig. 28.2). The blade is advanced to the dentate line, approximately 1.5 cm, or to the level of the apex of the fissure, and the scalpel is rotated 90° toward the mucosa. The knife is then advanced toward the inserted index finger with a sawing motion until the internal sphincter is transected taking care to not penetrate the mucosal surface (Fig. 28.3). The scalpel is removed and any remaining fibers are transected. This may be repeated on the opposite side of the anal canal if a deficiency cannot be palpated. Pressure should be applied to any bleeding. A foam sponge is then inserted to prevent hematoma formation. The sponge will be expelled during the patient's next bowel movement. Dry gauze over the wound can be removed on postoperative day 1.

An open sphincterotomy is performed by incising the anal mucosa to expose the internal sphincter muscle for division. A radial incision is made extending from the intersphincteric groove to a point just distal to the dentate line (Fig. 28.4). The

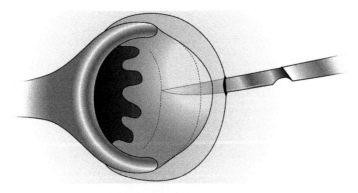

FIGURE 28.2 Lateral internal sphincterotomy incision

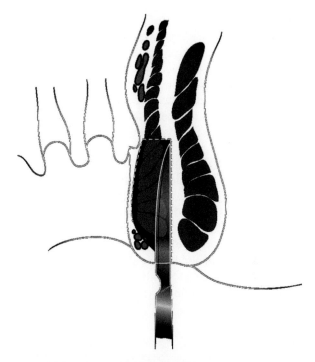

FIGURE 28.3 Division of the internal sphincter

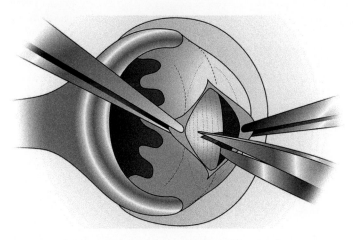

FIGURE 28.4 Open sphincterotomy technique

intersphincteric groove is identified and a small curved Kelly clamp is used to elevate the internal sphincter muscle. The fibers of the internal sphincter are divided to the level of the dentate line. Hemostasis is achieved with electrocautery. The wound is generally closed in a running fashion using a fine chromic suture. Care must be taken to ensure no sphincter muscle is caught in the closure. Alternatively, the wound may be allowed to heal by secondary intention.

Postoperative Considerations

Patients may be discharged home on the day of the procedure. All patients should be provided with medications for pain control. Patients should be instructed to take a fiber supplement, which will add bulk to the stool. Any wounds left open should be kept clean and dry. Warm sitz baths can be used for comfort and perianal hygiene.

References

1. Zaghiyan KN, Fleshner P. Anal fissure. Clin Colon Rectal Surg. 2011;24:22–30.
2. Sinha R, Kaiser AM. Efficacy of management algorithm for reducing need for sphincterotomy in chronic anal fissures. Colorectal Dis. 2011;14:760–4.
3. Farouk R, Duthie GS, MacGregor AB, Bartolo DC. Sustained internal sphincter hypertonia in patients with chronic anal fissure. Dis Colon Rectum. 1994;37:424–9.
4. American Gastroenterological Association. American Gastroenterological Association medical position statement: diagnosis and care of patients with anal fissure. Gastroenterology. 2003;124:233–4.
5. Jensen SL. Treatment of first episodes of acute anal fissure: prospective randomised study of lignocaine ointment versus hydrocortisone ointment or warm sitz baths plus bran. Br Med J (Clin Res Ed). 1986;292:1167–9.

6. Bhardwaj R, Vaizey CJ, Boulos PB, Hoyle CH. Neuromyogenic properties of the internal anal sphincter: therapeutic rationale for anal fissures. Gut. 2000;46:861–8.
7. Chrysos E, Xynos E, Tzovaras G, et al. Effect of nifedipine on rectoanal motility. Dis Colon Rectum. 1996;39:212–6.
8. Nicholls J. Anal fissure; surgery is the most effective treatment. Colorectal Dis. 2008;10:529–30.
9. Mentes BB, Tezcaner T, Yilmaz U, et al. Results of lateral internal sphincterotomy for chronic anal fissure with particular reference to quality of life. Dis Colon Rectum. 2006;49:1045–51.
10. Nelson R. Non surgical therapy for anal fissure. Cochrane Database Syst Rev. 2006;18:CD003431.
11. Nelson RL. Operative procedures for fissure in ano. Cochrane Database Syst Rev. 2011:CD002199.

Chapter 29
Hemorrhoids

Terrah J. Paul Olson and Gregory D. Kennedy

Abstract   Hemorrhoids, the mucosal vascular cushions in the anal canal, can lead to pain and bleeding when they become enlarged, prolapsed, or thrombosed. The locations of hemorrhoids are discussed, along with pertinent elements of the history and physical. Differences between the four degrees of hemorrhoids are also described. Preoperative preparation and positioning is outlined, including preoperative bowel preparation. The various methods for hemorrhoidectomy are described. Non-surgical procedures include injection of sclerosing agents, photocoagulation, and rubber-band ligation. Currently rubber-band ligation is the preferred non-excisional procedure. Various excisional techniques for hemorrhoidectomy exist, including open Milligan-Morgan procedure, closed Ferguson hemorrhoidectomy, excision with tissue sealing devices (Ligasure or Harmonic Scalpel), stapled hemorrhoidopexy, and transanal hemorrhoidal dearterialization. Additional study of long-term results of vessel

T.J. Paul Olson, MD (✉)
Department of General Surgery, University of Wisconsin Hospital and Clinics, 1629 Kings Mill Way, #310, 53718 Madison, WI, USA
e-mail: tpaulolson@uwhealth.org

G.D. Kennedy, MD, PhD
Department of Surgery, University of Alabama at Birmingham, Birmingham, AL, USA

H. Chen (ed.), *Illustrative Handbook of General Surgery*,   505
DOI 10.1007/978-3-319-24557-7_29,
© Springer International Publishing Switzerland 2016

sealing device hemorrhoidectomy, stapled hemorrhoidopexy and transanal hemorrhoidal dearterialization are needed to definitively say whether these are improvements on the traditional open or closed hemorrhoidectomies. Postoperative management including pain control, wound care, and bowel regimen is discussed.

Keywords Hemorrhoidectomy • Degrees of hemorrhoids • Non-surgical management of hemorrhoids • Outcomes of excisional hemorrhoidectomy • Stapled hemorrhoidopexy • Transanal hemorrhoidal dearterialization

Indications

Hemorrhoids are mucosal vascular cushions in the anal canal which are present in all individuals. They aid in closure of the anal canal at rest and help prevent incontinence to stool and flatus. They are classically located in the left, right posterior, and right anterior positions (from the patient perspective). Only when these cushions of tissue become symptomatic do they become what the general public refers to as "hemorrhoids." Hemorrhoidal disease is common with 75 % of people over the age of 45 experiencing hemorrhoids at some point in their lives. These cases account for 1.1 million ambulatory visits and 266,000 hospitalizations a year [1].

Prolapse, bleeding, thrombosis, pain, pruritis, and difficulty with hygiene are all chief complaints of symptomatic hemorrhoids [2]. Of these, painless bleeding is the most common complaint [3]. Many anorectal complaints are labeled "hemorrhoids", and therefore a careful history and physical exam are important prior to proceeding with treatment. Anal fissures, fistulae-in-ano, or rectal masses can all be mislabeled as hemorrhoids, and are managed differently than hemorrhoids. Additionally if these disorders are also present, this will affect the treatment of hemorrhoids [2, 4]. Hemorrhoids typically do not produce severe pain unless acutely throm-bosed. The degree of bleeding associated with hemorrhoids may be alarming to patients, but rarely is enough to produce significant anemia. Therefore severe pain and anemia should prompt further evaluation of other disorders. Physical exami-nation should include inspection while straining, digital rectal exam, and anoscopy to characterize the location and degree of hemorrhoids as well as to rule out other anorectal pathol-ogy [4].

Hemorrhoids may be external or internal to the dentate line. Internal hemorrhoids are classified by degree of pro-lapse. First degree hemorrhoids are characterized by lack of prolapse while fourth degree hemorrhoids are unable to be reduced and may become strangulated (Table 29.1). Figure 29.1 shows an example of third degree hemorrhoids.

The treatment of hemorrhoids is centered on relief of symptoms. Operations to improve appearance of the anus may lead to complications that are worse than the initial pre-sentation such as incontinence, fistula formation, or anal ste-nosis. Many symptomatic hemorrhoids are managed successfully by medical therapy. This includes dietary fiber supplements, stool softeners, increased fluid intake, and avoidance of straining. A Cochrane review demonstrated that fiber supplementation reduces overall symptoms from hem-orrhoids by 53 % in patients with grades 1–3 hemorrhoids. The authors also demonstrated that this effect is durable over time, making medical management of mildly symptomatic hemorrhoids a viable treatment strategy [5].

Hemorrhoids may occasionally present in an emergent situation. Acutely thrombosed external hemorrhoids are exquisitely painful and present as a hard prolapsed hemor-rhoid with surrounding erythema. Simple evacuation results in a high rate of future symptoms; therefore, these patients are best treated by excision of the thrombosed hemorrhoid. Thrombosis of internal hemorrhoids is less common and may not require surgical intervention, but excisional hemor-rhoidectomy is called for if surgical treatment is necessary [3]. Additionally, strangulated hemorrhoids are not only

TABLE 29.1 Classification of hemorrhoids and their typical symptoms

	First degree	Second degree	Third degree	Fourth degree
Findings	Bulge into the lumen of the anal canal ± painless bleeding	Protrude at the time of a bowel movement and reduce spontaneously	Protrude spontaneously or with bowel movement, require manual reduction	Permanently prolapsed and irreducible
Symptoms	Painless bleeding	Painless bleeding Anal mass with defecation Anal burning or pruritus	Painless bleeding Anal mass with defecation Feeling of incomplete evacuation Mucous leakage Fecal leakage Perianal burning or pruritus ani Difficulty with perianal hygiene	Painless or painful bleeding Irreducible anal mass Feeling of incomplete evacuation Mucous leakage Fecal leakage Perianal burning or pruritus ani Difficulty with perianal hygiene
Signs	Bright red bleeding Bleeding at the end of defecation Blood drips or squirts into toilet Bleeding may be occult	Bright red bleeding Prolapse with defecation	Bright red bleeding Blood drips or squirts into toilet Prolapsed hemorrhoids reduce manually Perianal stool or mucous Anemia extremely rare	Bright red bleeding Blood drips or squirts into toilet Prolapsed hemorrhoids always out Perianal stool or mucous Anemia extremely rare

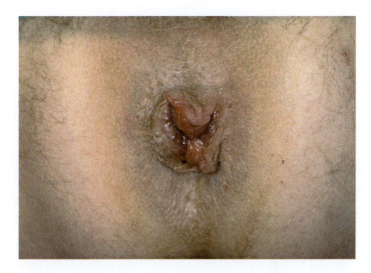

FIGURE 29.1 Third degree hemorrhoids. This patient has been placed in high lithotomy position for examination and treatment

thrombosed, but infarcted and can be infected. Closed hemorrhoidectomy may cause sepsis in these patients and open hemorrhoidectomy should be pursued [6].

Perioperative Care

Preoperative Preparation

Patients may undergo hemorrhoidal operations in the outpatient clinic, day surgery suite, or inpatient operating room. The preoperative care will vary slightly, but will generally have the same components. Full medical evaluation should be performed to ensure safety of anesthesia. A preoperative bowel prep is usually prescribed and may range from an enema or suppository to evacuate the rectum to a more complete prep with one or two doses of magnesium citrate followed by enemas the evening prior to and morning of the operation. All patients undergoing procedures in the operating room should not eat of drink anything after midnight. Antibiotics are administered prior to incision and should generally be targeted toward the normal colonic flora.

Positioning and Anesthesia

The patient may be placed in the lateral decubitus, jackknife, or high lithotomy position. Office procedures under local anesthetics are best served by the decubitus or jackknife approach, while either jackknife or high lithotomy may be used in the operating room. In the jackknife position, care needs to be taken to avoid pressure on facial structures. In high lithotomy, the patient's heels are placed in soft stirrups. Care should be taken to avoid pressure on the heels and calves. Choice of anesthesia involves extent of the planned procedure, patient anxiety and pain, likelihood of additional pathology, anesthetic risk, and patient preference. Local anesthesia alone may be used for simple procedures, but conscious sedation, spinal anesthesia, or general anesthesia with laryngeal mask or endotracheal tube may be needed for more complicated hemorrhoid treatment. In general, deep anesthesia is preferred when performing operations in the anal canal. This prevents the patient from straining against the anal speculum and traumatizing the sphincter mechanism. Preparation of the anus and perianal region should be performed with a full betadine scrub.

Description of the Procedure

Sclerosis

Injection of a sclerosing agent may be used to treat first, second and third degree hemorrhoids. One to five ml of sclerosing agent (5 % phenol in oil, ethanolamine, quinine urea, hypertonic saline, or aluminum potassium sulfate with tannic acid [ALTA]) is injected into the submucosa of each hemorrhoid [7]. The resultant ulceration and scarring prevent prolapse. Care should be taken in the anterior direction to inject superficially. The prostate or periprostatic venous plexus may be injured with deep injection [2, 6].

Infrared or Laser Photocoagulation

Either through an endoscope or using an anoscope, the tip of a fiberoptic probe is placed at the tip of the hemorrhoidal pedicle and infrared radiation is used to coagulate the underlying vascular plexus. This treatment is only suited for first and minor second degree hemorrhoids [2, 6, 7].

Doppler-guided laser photocoagulation (Hemorrhoid Laser Procedure, or HeLP) is a newer system of more targeted photocoagulation. Doppler ultrasound is used to identify the branches of the superior hemorrhoidal artery feeding into the hemorrhoidal plexuses about 3 cm above the dentate line, and a laser system is then used to coagulate the vascular supply. A small randomized controlled trial between HeLP and rubber band ligation demonstrated better postoperative pain control and more frequent resolution of symptoms at 6 months with HeLP as well as improved patient satisfaction [8]. Long-term follow up of this method is still needed [7].

Rubber-Band Ligation

Rubber-band ligation is best suited for first, second, and few third degree hemorrhoids. A Cochrane review comparing rubber band ligation to excisional hemorrhoidectomy concluded that this should be the initial treatment of choice for symptomatic grade 2 hemorrhoids, although higher-grade hemorrhoids respond better to surgical excision [9]. Rubber-band ligation involves the application of a rubber band to the mucosa above the hemorrhoidal tissue and 1–2 cm above the dentate line to include the feeding vessel of the hemorrhoid within the band. This causes necrosis of the captured tissue, ulceration and scarring, which prevents prolapse or bleeding. A slotted anoscope or anal speculum is inserted the hemorrhoidal tissue is allowed to protrude into the slot. Rubber-bands may be applied by a suction or non-suction device. The mucosa just above the hemorrhoidal cushion is either grasped with a clamp or suctioned into the tip of the banding device. The pre-loaded band is then deployed by squeezing the trigger on the device. The band must be employed above the dentate line to ensure that no sensate mucosa is included. Immediate and postoperative pain are indications of inclusion of this mucosa and removal of the bands may be necessary [2, 6].

Outcomes of the three office based procedures (sclerosis, infrared photocoagulation, and rubber band ligation) are similar. However, potential complications and longevity of the procedures are somewhat varied. If applied correctly, rubber band ligation has a lower complication rate, is better tolerated, and has a higher chance of long term success [10]. For that reason, we generally feel that rubber band ligation should be used preferentially over the alternative non-excisional therapies.

Hemorrhoidectomy

Open Hemorrhoidectomy

Open hemorrhoidectomy is also known as the Milligan-Morgan hemorrhoidectomy. The hemorrhoidal tissue is visualized with a slotted anoscope or speculum (See Fig. 29.2). Injection of a local anesthetic with epinephrine will aid in immediate post operative pain as well as operative bleeding. An elliptical incision is started proximal to the anal verge and carried across the dentate line to the anorectal ring. The vital step is to separate the fibers of the internal sphincter from the hemorrhoidal tissue. Metzenbaum scissors may be used to spread parallel and superficial to the fibers to separate them from the mucosal tissue, dissecting in a distal to proximal fashion (See Fig. 29.3). At the proximal corner, the pedicle of the hemorrhoid is suture ligated with non absorbable suture.

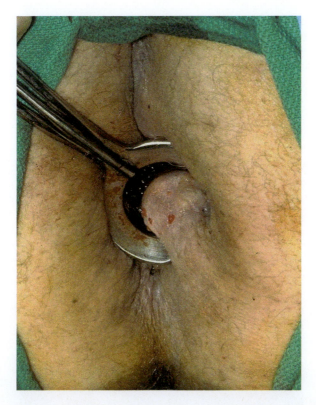

FIGURE 29.2 Combined internal-external hemorrhoid. A slotted anoscope is positioned to allow excision of the hemorrhoid

Electrocautery is used to achieve hemostasis along the bed. The pedicle is the transected, and the hemorrhoidal tissue removed. A gauze dressing is applied and the wound is left open to heal by secondary intent [2, 6].

Closed Hemorrhoidectomy

The Parks or Ferguson hemorrhoidectomy involves the same initial steps as the open operation except the wound is closed with suturing. The hemorrhoid is dissected out the same way,

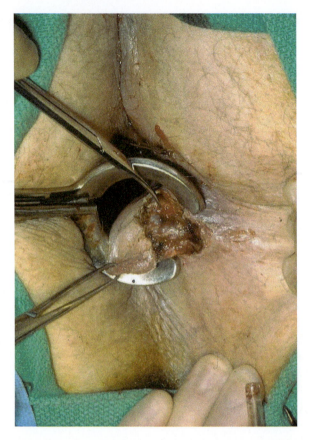

FIGURE 29.3 Hemorrhoidectomy. Dissection is carried proximally under the hemorrhoidal tissue taking care to separate the fibers of the internal sphincter with metzenbaum scissors

again with care to identify and separate the fibers of the internal sphincter. The pedicle is suture ligated, or encompassed in the anchoring stitch of the closing suture. The mucosa is then closed using a locking stitch to the dentate line and then a running stitch. A gauze dressing is then applied. We use an absorbable hemostatic dressing (Instat, Ethicon Inc.), rolled and inserted into the anus with Russian forceps [2, 6].

Ligasure and Harmonic Scalpel Hemorrhoidectomy

The bipolar electrothermic sealing device, or Ligasure, has been used for hemorrhoidectomy. A Cochrane review comparing outcomes of Ligasure and excisional hemorrhoidectomy revealed decreased operative time and lower blood loss with use of the Ligasure, as well as decreased immediate postoperative pain and a quicker return to work in patients who underwent hemorrhoidectomy with the Ligasure. Long-term results were not reported [11]. A randomized trial of closed hemorrhoidectomy versus Harmonic Scalpel ultrasonic vessel sealing device showed no difference in outcomes [12]. Another randomized trial compared Harmonic Scalpel hemorrhoidectomy, bipolar scissors hemorrhoidectomy, and sharp excision and found decreased bleeding with both Harmonic Scalpel and bipolar scissors. Additionally, pain was less with the Harmonic Scalpel [13]. A meta-analysis comparing outcomes between hemorrhoidectomy with the Ligasure and stapled hemorrhoidopexy revealed shorted operative time and lower rates of recurrence with the Ligasure, although other outcomes were equivalent [14]. While evidence appears to be mounting in favor of the Ligasure and the Harmonic Scalpel at least in the short term, long-term analysis of outcomes is still needed.

Stapled Hemorrhoidopexy/PPH

This technique involves removing a circumferential portion of rectal mucosa proximal to the dentate line. The goal is to ligate venules feeding the hemorrhoidal plexus and reduce redundant mucosa. This technique is based on the Whitehead's hemorrhoidectomy, which involved excision of this ring of tissue and manual approximation of the anal mucosa to the dentate line. Whitehead's procedure carries a risk of ectropion, or prolapsing rectal mucosa, known as Whitehead's deformity [2]. The stapled procedure involves placing an operating anoscope for visualization. A purse string suture is then placed around the rectal mucosa 4–5 cm proximal to the dentate line. The stapler is inserted in the anus with the anvil extended. The purse string allows the surgeon to draw the mucosa into the device as the stapler is fired. This excises the ring of tissue and approximates the remaining edges with staples. A Cochrane review comparing stapled hemorrhoidopexy with excisional hemorrhoidectomy revealed increased rates of recurrence, symptoms of prolapse, and need for additional operations both in the short term as well as at follow-up of greater than 1 year. Additionally, no statistically significant improvement in postoperative pain with stapled hemorrhoidopexy was demonstrated, which is often cited as the primary benefit of the stapled procedure [15]. Stapled hemorrhoidopexy was also initially associated with serious complications, such as severe pelvic sepsis, rectal perforation, and rectal occlusion, although rates of these complications appear to have decreased as surgeons have become more comfortable with the technique.

The role of stapled hemorrhoidopexy remains unclear and its use seems to be decreasing. If one plans to include the stapled hemorrhoidopexy in the treatment algorithm, a thorough discussion of uncertainties with the procedure should occur. Patients should clearly understand the goal of the operation as being to excise the redundant internal tissue that allows the internal hemorrhoids to prolapse. They should be advised of and willing to accept higher rates of long-term recurrence and potential need for reoperation. Additionally, patients with a large external component to their hemorrhoidal disease may not be good candidates as the stapled hemorrhoidopexy will not address this problem.

Transanal Hemorrhoidal Dearterialization (THD)

Transanal hemorrhoidal dearterialization (THD) with mucopexy uses a specially designed anoscope fitted with a Doppler ultrasound probe to identify the terminal branches of the hemorrhoidal arteries and then selectively ligate the six to eight branches feeding the hemorrhoidal submucosal plexuses. This decreases the inflow to the hemorrhoidal cushions, thereby reducing swelling. If there is an element of mucosal redundancy, sutured mucopexy can also be performed to reduce hemorrhoidal tissue back into the anal canal [16]. A recent systematic review of studies examining THD suggested that this non-excisional procedure can provide symptomatic relief with acceptable postoperative pain. However, especially with higher grade hemorrhoids, rates of recurrence can be as high as 50–60 %. Long-term follow up results are lacking [17]. Two prospective randomized controlled trials comparing THD and excisional hemorrhoidectomy suggested comparable outcomes, with no statistically significant differences in postoperative pain scores between procedures [18, 19]. De Nardi et al. also noted that THD is more expensive, although a formal cost analysis was not performed [18]. Another trial comparing THD and Ligasure suggested resolution of pain in the early postoperative period was better after THD, but by 1 year, there was no difference between groups in terms of pain, quality of life, and bowel function [20]. As with the other newer techniques discussed above, further study of long-term results and cost analysis is needed.

Special Postoperative Considerations

Postoperative pain is common following any excisional operation for hemorrhoids. Narcotic pain relievers are usually needed for adequate pain control. Sitz baths, muscle relaxers, NSAIDs, and topical analgesics may also help. Stool softeners and laxatives are needed to reduce pain with defecation and lower the risk of fecal impaction. Complications also include urinary retention, post-operative hemorrhage, anal fissure or fistula, anal stenosis, incontinence for flatus or stool, perirectal abscess, necrotizing soft tissue infection, and anorectal sepsis. Secondary hemorrhage following rubber-band ligation approximately 7–10 days is common and usually self-limited [2, 6].

References

1. Digestive Diseases Statistics. NDDIC. NIDDK. NIH Publication No. 13–3873. Sept 2013. http://digestive.niddk.nih.gov/statistics/statistics.aspx. Accessed 20 May 2014.
2. Brunicardi FC, et al., editors. Schwartz's principles of surgery. 9th ed. Columbus: The McGraw-Hill Companies, Inc; 2010.
3. Kaidar-Person O, Person B, Wexner SD. Hemorrhoidal disease: a comprehensive review. J Am Coll Surg. 2007;204(1):102–17.
4. Townsend CM, et al., editors. Sabiston textbook of surgery: the biological basis of modern surgical practice. 19th ed. Philadelphia: Elsevier Saunders; 2012.
5. Alonso-Coello P, Guyatt GH, Heels-Ansdell D, et al. Laxatives for the treatment of hemorrhoids. Cochrane Database Syst Rev. 2005;(4):CD004649. doi:10.1002/14651858.CD004649.pub2. Edited, no change to conclusions, published Issue 4, 2008.
6. Fischer JE, et al., editors. Fischer's mastery of surgery. 6th ed. Philadelphia: Wolters Kluwer Health/Lippincott Williams & Wilkins; 2011. p. 1616–20.
7. ASGE Technology Committee. Devices for the endoscopic treatment of hemorrhoids. Gastrointest Endosc. 2014;79(1):8–14.
8. Giamundo P, Salfi R, Geraci M, et al. The hemorrhoid laser procedure technique vs rubber band ligation: a randomized trial comparing two mini-invasive treatments for second- and third-degree hemorrhoids. Dis Colon Rectum. 2011;54(6):693–8.
9. Shanmugam V, Hakeem A, Campbell KL, et al. Rubber band ligation versus excisional haemorrhoidectomy for haemorrhoids. Cochrane Database Syst Rev. 2005;(1):CD005034. doi:10.1002/14651858.CD005034.pub2. Edited, no change to conclusions, published Issue 3, 2011.
10. Johanson JF, Rimm A. Optimal nonsurgical treatment of hemorrhoids: a comparative analysis of infrared coagulation, rubber band ligation, and injection sclerotherapy. Am J Gastroenterol. 1992;87:1600–6.
11. Nienhuijs SW, de Hingh IHJT. Conventional versus LigaSure hemorrhoidectomy for patients with symptomatic hemorrhoids. Cochrane Database Syst Rev. 2009;(1):CD006761. doi:10.1002/14651858.CD006761.pub2. Edited, no change to conclusions, published Issue 7, 2011.

12. Khan S, Pawlak SE, Eggenberger JC, et al. Surgical treatment of hemorrhoids: prospective, randomized trial comparing closed excisional hemorrhoidectomy and the Harmonic Scalpel technique of excisional hemorrhoidectomy. Dis Colon Rectum. 2001;44(6):845–9.

13. Chung CC, HA JP, Tai YP, et al. Double-blind, randomized trial comparing Harmonic Scalpel hemorrhoidectomy, bipolar scissors hemorrhoidectomy, and scissors excision: ligation technique. Dis Colon Rectum. 2002;45:789–94.

14. Chen H-L, Woo X-B, Cui J, et al. Ligasure versus stapled hemorrhoidectomy in the treatment of hemorrhoids: a meta-analysis of randomized control trials. Surg Laparosc Endosc Percutan Tech. 2014;24(4):285–9.

15. Lumb KJ, Colquhoun PH, Malthaner R, Jayaraman S. Stapled versus conventional surgery for hemorrhoids. Cochrane Database Syst Rev. 2006;(4):CD005393. doi:10.1002/14651858. CD005393.pub2. Edited, no change to conclusions, published Issue 9, 2010.

16. Ratto C. THD Doppler procedure for hemorrhoids: the surgical technique. Tech Coloproctol. 2014;18:291–8.

17. Giordano P, Overton J, Madeddu F, et al. Transanal hemorrhoidal dearterialization: a systematic review. Dis Colon Rectum. 2009;52(9):1665–71.

18. De Nardi P, Capretti G, Corsaro A, Staudacher C. A prospective, randomized trial comparing the short- and long-term results of Doppler-guided transanal hemorrhoid dearterialization with mucopexy versus excision hemorrhoidectomy for grade III hemorrhoids. Dis Colon Rectum. 2014;57:348–53.

19. Elmer SE, Nygren JO, Lenander CE. A randomized trial of transanal hemorrhoidal dearterialization with anopexy compared with open hemorrhoidectomy in the treatment of hemorrhoids. Dis Colon Rectum. 2013;56:484–90.

20. Zampieri Z, Castellani R, Andreoli R, Geccherle A. Long-term results and quality of life in patients treated with hemorrhoidectomy using two different techniques: Ligasure versus transanal hemorrhoidal dearterialization. Am J Surg. 2012;204:684–8.

Part VII
Hernia Surgery

Gregory D. Kennedy

Chapter 30
Lichtenstein Tension-Free Open Inguinal Hernia Repair

David M. Melnick

Abstract   Inguinal hernias represent a large burden of surgical disease and can be repaired by a variety of open and laparoscopic techniques. In the following chapter we will review our technique for the open repair of an inguinal hernia.

Keywords   Inguinal hernia • Open inguinal hernia repair • Lichtenstein • Tension-free herniorraphy • Groin hernia repair

Many techniques of open inguinal hernia repair exist [1, 2]. Historically, inguinal herniorraphies were performed utilizing tissue based repairs such as the Bassini repair, the McVay (Cooper's ligament) repair, or the Shouldice repair, among others. More recently, open tension-free repairs utilizing a variety of different mesh products have replaced these tissue-based repairs due to a significant decrease in hernia recurrence [3]. Newer techniques utilizing glue or self-adhering

D.M. Melnick, MD, MPH, FACS
Department of Surgery, University of Wisconsin School of Medicine and Public Health,
1 S. Park Street, Madison, WI 53715, USA
e-mail: melnick@surgery.wisc.edu

H. Chen (ed.), *Illustrative Handbook of General Surgery*,   523
DOI 10.1007/978-3-319-24557-7_30,
© Springer International Publishing Switzerland 2016

mesh instead of sutures are being developed with possible advantages of decreasing postoperative pain and operative time without increasing recurrence [4]. This section will describe the classic sutured Lichtenstein repair.

Positioning and Anesthesia

Have patients void preoperatively to decompress the bladder and avoid the need for foley catheter placement. Either monitored anesthesia combined with local anesthesia, spinal anesthesia, or general anesthesia may be used with good results. Use clippers (not a razor) for hair removal if needed. Prepare the skin with chlorhexadine or povidone-iodine and drape appropriately. Preoperative antibiotics are not mandatory but may be used in higher risk patients [5].

Obtaining Exposure

After prepping and draping the patient, identify the course of the inguinal ligament, extending from the anterior superior iliac spine to the pubic tubercle. Mark out the line of the incision 1–2 cm superior to the inguinal ligament, starting just lateral to the pubic tubercle and extending laterally approximately 5–6 cm. Use generous amounts of local anesthetic then incise the skin with a knife. Using electrocautery, dissect through the subcutaneous fat, then through the fatty layer of Scarpa's fascia. You will come to the areolar layer just superficial to the external oblique aponeurosis. Dissect this tissue off of the aponeurosis to completely expose the aponeurosis, including the inferior edge of the aponeurosis. Follow the inferior edge medially to identify and palpate the pubic tubercle. Identify and palpate the external ring of the external oblique aponeurosis, just superior and lateral to the tubercle. You can find the ilioinguinal nerve exiting the ring. Infiltrate the tissues just deep to the external oblique aponeurosis with local anesthetic. Incise the external oblique aponeurosis with a scalpel and then use a scissors to open up this layer in the direction of its fibers, medially to open up the external ring, then laterally to a position lateral to the deep ring to ensure adequate mesh overlap. Take care to identify and avoid injuring the ilioinguinal nerve which lies just beneath this aponeurosis (Fig. 30.1). Using a hemostat, grasp the inferior edge of the external oblique aponeurosis and lift it up. Use a "peanut" or "Kittner" to sweep the cord adhesions off the undersurface of the aponeurosis to expose the shelving edge of the inguinal ligament. You may also start dissecting behind the cord at this time. You can find the spermatic vessels and the genital branch of the genital femoral nerve during this dissection. Use a second hemostat to grasp the superior edge of the external oblique aponeurosis, lifting it up. In a similar manner, sweep the cord structures off of this structure to expose the conjoint tendon (also known as the *falx inguinalis*) lying deep to the aponeu-

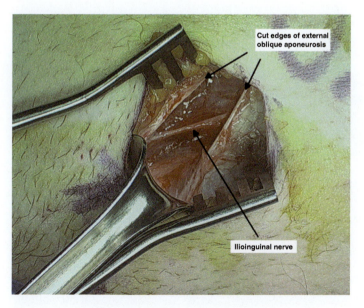

FIGURE 30.1 Exposure for open repair of left inguinal hernia

rosis. The conjoint tendon appears as the fibrous, white aponeurotic layer of the internal oblique aponeurosis (Fig. 30.2). You should mobilize the ilioinguinal nerve and retract it out of harm's way, behind the cut edge of the external oblique aponeurosis. For the repair, you will suture mesh to the conjoint tendon and to the shelving edge of the inguinal ligament.

Dissect around the spermatic cord, and secure the cord with a penrose drain. Palpate the vas deferens within the cord. The vas feels like a piece of *al dente* spaghetti. This ensures that you have correctly isolated the spermatic cord. Incise the cremasteric muscle fibers longitudinally to expose the spermatic cord. If the patient has an indirect inguinal hernia, you will find it on the anteromedial surface of the cord. You may find a lipoma, a piece of preperitoneal fat protruding through the internal ring. If you find a lipoma, either reduce it through the ring or ligate and excise it. If you

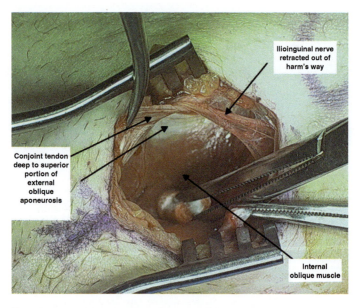

FIGURE 30.2 Exposure of conjoint tendon

find an indirect hernia, dissect the sac off the cord structures all the way back to the internal ring (Fig. 30.3). You may incise (with care to avoid bowel injury, especially in the case of a sliding hernia) and explore the peritoneal sac. If you open the sac, place your index finger in the hole, palpate for the iliac artery, then palpate medially to search for a femoral hernia. If you find a femoral hernia you will have to modify your technique to repair it (briefly discussed later.) You can then perform a high ligation of the sac by clamping it off around the level of the internal ring (with care to ensure no bowel is present in the sac,) tying it off, and reducing the stump through the internal ring. Alternatively, you may reduce the sac without opening it. You would note a direct hernia as an attenuation and bulging of the transversalis fascia in the medial aspect of the inguinal area, in Hesselbach's triangle, bordered inferiorly by the inguinal ligament, medially by the rectus muscle, and laterally by the inferior epigastric vessels.

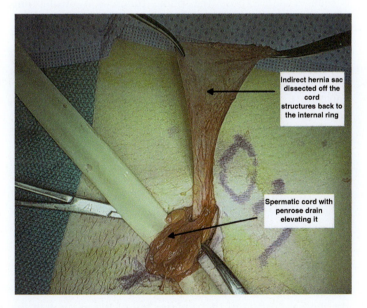

Indirect hernia sac dissected off the cord structures back to the internal ring

Spermatic cord with penrose drain elevating it

FIGURE 30.3 Dissection of hernia sac off of spermatic cord

Repair the Hernia Defect

The surgeon performs a Bassini type primary repair by approximating the conjoint tendon with the inguinal ligament using interrupted permanent sutures, such as 2-0 polyester sutures. The Lichtenstein repair performs the same basic anatomic repair but uses mesh to bridge the gap to prevent the tension seen in the primary Bassini repair. Importantly, neither a Bassini nor a Lichtenstein operation will repair a femoral hernia defect, since the Bassini and Lichtenstein repairs cover the space anterior to the inguinal ligament, while a femoral hernia occurs deep to the inguinal ligament, anterior to Cooper's ligament. To repair a femoral hernia defect, options include a McVay (Cooper's ligament) repair (approximating the conjoint tendon to Cooper's ligament), a primary or mesh plug closure of the femoral defect via an infrainguinal approach, or a laparoscopic repair.

For the Lichtenstein repair, fashion a piece of 3–4 inch by 6 inch mesh. Expose the pubic tubercle by using one Richardson retractor to retract the spermatic chord superiorly and another to retract the inferior edge of the external oblique aponeurosis inferiorly and medially. Palpate the pubic tubercle. Approximate the mesh to the aponeurotic tissues just medial to the pubic tubercle using 2-0 polypropylene suture. Then, using that stitch as a continuous suture, approximate the inferior edge of the mesh to the shelving edge of the inguinal ligament to a point lateral to the internal ring, then tie the stitch. Cut a longitudinal slit laterally in the mesh from the lateral edge of the mesh to a point around the internal ring. Pass the superior tail of the mesh underneath the cord and tuck both tails laterally under the external oblique aponeurosis. You may cut the tails shorter to allow for appropriate positioning under the external oblique aponeurosis. Reposition the retractors to retract the spermatic cord inferiorly and the superior edge of the external oblique aponeurosis superiorly to expose the conjoint tendon. Using a simple interrupted 2-0 polypropylene suture, approximate the medial portion of the superior tail of the mesh with the tissue around the pubic tubercle, close to the original stitch, to prevent a medial hernia recurrence. Using interrupted sutures and moving from medial to lateral, approximate the superior tail of the mesh with the conjoint tendon, stopping lateral to the internal ring. When completed, the mesh should appear flat, without excessive wrinkling.

The original description of the operation has the surgeon form the new internal ring by approximating the two tails of the mesh with the inguinal ligament, lateral to the cord [1]. Alternatively, many surgeons approximate the two tails with each other but not with the inguinal ligament, The new internal ring should be just large enough to admit the tip of a finger: tight enough to prevent an indirect hernia but loose enough to prevent cord ischemia. Adjust the size accordingly by either using a scissor to cut the mesh forming the hole to make the hole larger or by placing another stitch to make the hole smaller. Examine the quality of the repair (Fig. 30.4).

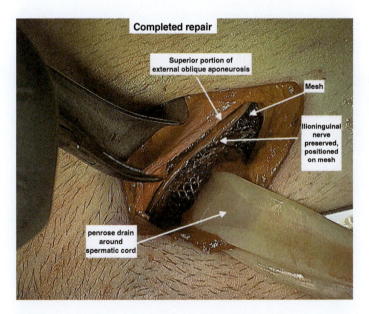

FIGURE 30.4 Appearance of mesh and ilioinguinal nerve after repair

Irrigate the wound if appropriate and ensure hemostasis. Replace the nerves in the correct anatomic position overlying the mesh, and ensure that no nerve injury or entrapment has occurred. If an injury or entrapment may have occurred, then divide the nerve laterally, excise the exposed portion to prevent pain relating to a nerve injury, and place the cut end of the nerve into muscle. Re-approximate the external oblique aponeurosis using a continuous absorbable suture. Finally, re-approximate Scarpa's fascia using a few interrupted absorbable sutures and close the skin with a subcutaneous absorbable suture and dressing.

References

1. Lichtenstein IL, Shulman AG, Amid PK, Montllor MM. The tension-free hernioplasty. Am J Surg. 1989;157(2):188–93.
2. Amid PK. Lichtenstein open tension-free hernioplasty; ACS collection, vol. 1. Hernia DVD. Cine-Med; 2001.
3. Scott N, Go PM, Graham P, McCormack K, Ross SJ, Grant AM. Open Mesh versus non-Mesh for groin hernia repair. Cochrane Database of Systematic Reviews 2001, Issue 3. Art. No.: CD002197. DOI: 10.1002/14651858.CD002197.
4. de Goede B. Meta-analysis of glue versus sutured mesh fixation for Lichtenstein inguinal hernia repair. Br J Surg. 2013;100(6):735–42 [0007–1323].
5. Sanchez-Manuel FJ, Lozano-García J, Seco-Gil JL. Antibiotic prophylaxis for hernia repai. Cochrane Database Syst Rev. 2012;2:CD003769.

Chapter 31
Laparoscopic Inguinal Hernia Repair: Transabdominal Preperitoneal (TAPP) Approach

Patrick J. Shabino and Jacob A. Greenberg

Abstract Inguinal hernias are one of the most common problems seen in surgical clinics across the world. While hernias may be repaired by a variety of open and laparoscopic techniques, this chapter we will review our technique for the laparoscopic transabdominal preperitoneal repair of an inguinal hernia.

P.J. Shabino, MD (✉)
Department of Surgery, University of Wisconsin,
600 Highland Ave, 53792 Madison, WI, USA
e-mail: pshabino@uwhealth.org

J.A. Greenberg, MD, EdM
Department of Surgery, University of Wisconsin,
K4/748 CSC, 600 Highland Avenue,
53792 Madison, WI, USA
e-mail: greenbergj@surgery.wisc.edu

H. Chen (ed.), *Illustrative Handbook of General Surgery*,
DOI 10.1007/978-3-319-24557-7_31,
© Springer International Publishing Switzerland 2016

532   P.J. Shabino and J.A. Greenberg

Keywords Inguinal hernia • Groin hernia • Laparoscopic • Transabdominal preperitoneal • TAPP • Laparoscopic inguinal hernia repair

The patient should be positioned with arms tucked at their sides allowing the surgeon and assistant to position themselves optimally for operating in the inferior abdomen and pelvis. The room and equipment should be organized to allow clear line of sight to a single monitor which is placed at the patients feet. The patient should void immediately prior to entry into the operating room. If they fail to void preoperatively, a foley catheter should be placed for bladder decompression.

Abdominal entry is performed at the inferior umbilical margin through a curvilinear incision. We utilize a Hasson technique and a 12 mm Hasson port is placed after the fascia is opened under direct visualization. Two additional 5 mm ports are then placed at the right and left midclavicular lines at the level of the umbilicus. The patient is then placed in trendelenburg position and both groins are inspected. Looking in the inferior abdomen and anteriorly, the hernia is identified sac extending through the defect in the abdominal wall in the indirect or direct space as well the epigastric vessels behind their covering of parietal peritoneum (Fig. 31.1). The peritoneum is then incised from the median umbilical fold laterally. The incision should be created cephalad to the groin defect and care should be taken not to injure the epigastric vessels which lie just anterior to the peritoneum at this location. At the lateral extent of this incision, the incision is curved inferiorly to just below the level of the defect (Fig. 31.2).

We begin our dissection in the indirect space where the testicular vessels and vas deferens are identified and bluntly dissected off the underlying peritoneum (Fig. 31.3a, b). In the female patient, the round ligament is generally quite adherent to the peritoneum and in order to avoid peritoneal

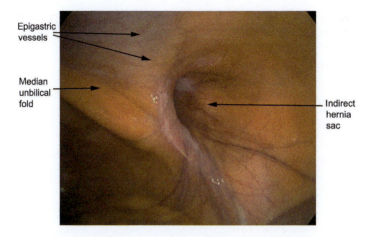

FIGURE 31.1 Right indirect inguinal hernia

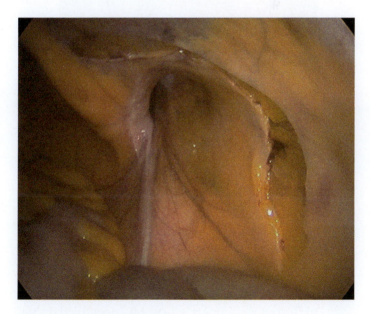

FIGURE 31.2 Peritoneal incision

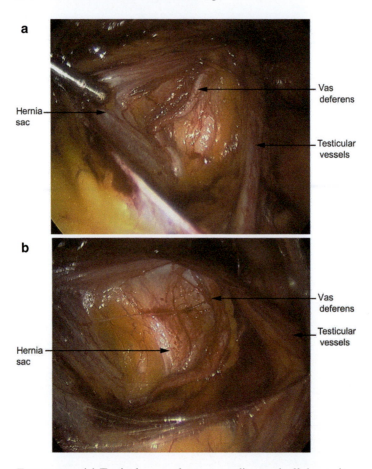

FIGURE 31.3 (**a**) Testicular vessels are seen dissected off the peritoneum while vas deferens are still attached. (**b**) Both testicular vessels and vas deferens are mobilized off the peritoneum

tears, the round ligament is clipped and divided. The preperitoneal space is then bluntly dissected along the medial
portion of our incision. The bladder is mobilized in the
space of Retzius and Cooper's ligament is identified on both
the right and left sides (Fig. 31.4). Direct defects will be
found in this location and can be reduced by pulling the

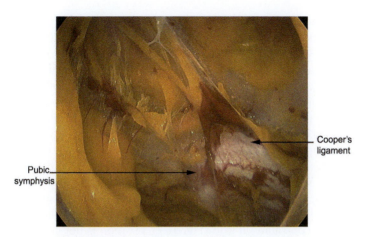

FIGURE 31.4 Bladder mobilization to expose the pubic symphysis and Cooper's ligaments

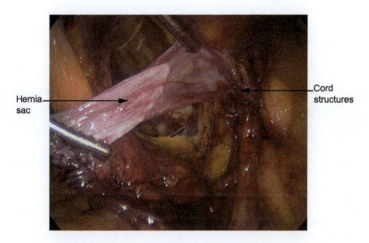

FIGURE 31.5 Reduction of an indirect hernia sac

perperitoneal fat off of the overlying transversalis fascia. Indirect defects should then be reduced by pulling the peritoneal hernia sac medially and bluntly pushing the vas deferens and testicular vessels laterally (Fig. 31.5).

Once the hernia sac has been completely reduced, adequate space must be created in order to accommodate our mesh. Careful dissection along the iliac vessels is performed in an avascular plane in order to expose the femoral space and create adequate room for mesh reinforcement. Take care to avoid vessels in this area such as the obturator vein and corona mortis as it traverses coopers ligament. The completed dissection is seen in Fig. 31.6.

Proper mesh placement should focus on covering the entire myopectineal orifice with wide overlap in all directions. We use an anatomically shaped polypropylene mesh which is inserted through the 12 mm trocar and extends medially to at least the pubic symphysis and most commonly to the contralateral side (Fig. 31.7). Fixation is not generally required but can be performed with permanent or absorbable tacks or fibrin glue. If tack fixation is desired, tacks should be placed medially into Cooper's ligament or the rectus muscles and laterally above the level of the iliopubic tract. Great care must be taken not to place tacks below Cooper's ligament medially or the iliopubic tract laterally as vascular or nerve injuries could occur.

The peritoneal defect needs to be closed over the mesh to prevent bowel exposure to the mesh and minimize adhesions. This may be completed with a variety of methods. We prefer

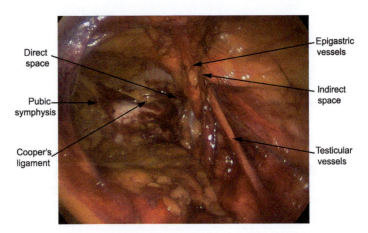

FIGURE 31.6 Completed dissection

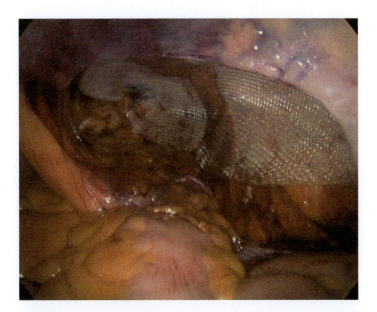

FIGURE 31.7 Mesh placement

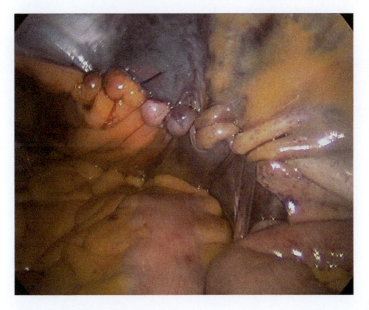

FIGURE 31.8 Peritoneal closure

to suture the defect with a continuous running barbed slowly absorbable suture (Fig. 31.8). Alternatively, tacks or staples may be used for peritoneal closure. With the peritoneal defect closed, the trocars are removed, the abdomen is desufflated and the fascial defect at the 12 mm port site is closed with interrupted absorbable suture. Skin sites are closed and covered with a protective dressing. The scrotum is inspected following the procedure to ensure both testicles are present.

Chapter 32
Laparoscopic Inguinal Hernia Repair Total Extraperitoneal (TEP) Approach

Michael J. Garren

Abstract Inguinal hernias are extremely common and can be repaired through a variety of open and laparoscopic techniques. The following chapter reviews our approach to the laparoscopic Totally Extraperitoneal Inguinal Hernia Repair.

Keywords Inguinal hernia • Groin hernia • Extraperitoneal • TEP • Laparoscopic inguinal hernia repair

A variety of approaches to inguinal hernia repair are available to surgeons. Both open traditional repair and laparoscopic repair provide excellent results with low recurrence rates. The laparoscopic totally extraperitoneal (TEP) approach allows for mesh placement within the preperitoneal space without entering the abdominal cavity, thereby avoiding the incision and closure of the peritoneum required of the transabdominal preperitoneal approach (TAPP). In this chapter, I will describe the technique of laparoscopic TEP inguinal hernia repair.

M.J. Garren, MD
Department of Surgery, University of Wisconsin,
K4/752 CSC, 600 Highland Avenue, 53792 Madison, WI, USA
e-mail: garren@surgery.wisc.edu

H. Chen (ed.), *Illustrative Handbook of General Surgery*, 539
DOI 10.1007/978-3-319-24557-7_32,
© Springer International Publishing Switzerland 2016

The procedure is overwhelmingly performed utilizing general anesthesia, although regional anesthesia (spinal, epidural) approaches have been described. The patient is instructed to void on call to the operating room and if successful, intraoperative bladder decompression is not routinely performed. The patient is positioned supine with the arms tucked to the side. Preoperative antibiotics are administered within 30 min of incision and lower extremity pneumatic compression stockings are utilized for DVT prophylaxis. The abdomen and groin areas are prepped and draped.

Initial incision is made in the infraumbilical position. Dissection is carried to the anterior rectus fascia, just lateral to the midline. The anterior fascia is incised longitudinally and the rectus muscle retracted laterally to expose the posterior fascia. I routinely make the incision to the right of midline, although either side is acceptable. The dissection tends to be better on the side of the fascial incision. Dissection is initiated between the rectus muscle and posterior fascia with a finger or blunt dissecting instrument. The dissecting balloon is inserted into the space between the rectus muscle and posterior fascia and directed to the symphysis pubis. Avoid over-aggressive insertion posterior to the symphysis due to the risk of bladder injury. The dissecting balloon is inflated while the space is viewed with the laparoscope. The pubis and Cooper's ligaments should be seen bilaterally, the rectus fibers and inferior epigastric vessels anteriorly and the urinary bladder posteriorly (Figs. 32.1 and 32.2). The balloon is deflated, removed and replaced with a Hassan-type trocar. Carbon dioxide flow is maintained at 12 mmHg and the patient is placed in moderate Trendelenburg position. Two 5 mm trocars are placed; one approximately one finger breadth above the symphysis, the other halfway between the two previously placed trocars.

Direct inguinal hernias are typically seen and oftentimes reduced as the balloon dissector inflates. The same is true of femoral and obturator hernias. Unreduced direct hernias should be carefully reduced, clearing Cooper's ligament and allowing for visualization of lateral structures (Figs. 32.3 and 32.4). Prior to lateral dissection, the position of the inferior

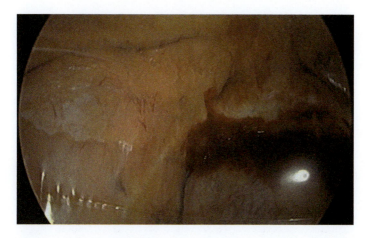

FIGURE 32.1 View through dissecting balloon. Note pubis and Cooper's ligament bilaterally

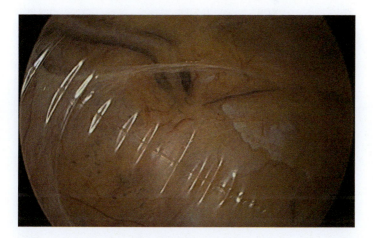

FIGURE 32.2 View through dissecting balloon showing left inferior epigastric vessels and direct hernia

epigastric vessels should be identified as occasionally, these vessels will be pushed posteriorly by the dissecting balloon. It is important that lateral peritoneal dissection occur posterior to the plane of the epigastric vessels. In rare circumstances,

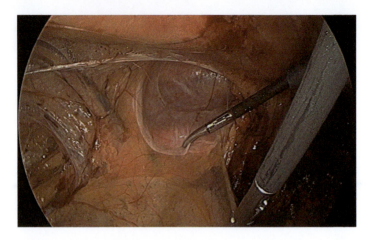

FIGURE 32.3 Attenuated transversalis fascia of left direct hernia, medial to inferior epigastric vessels

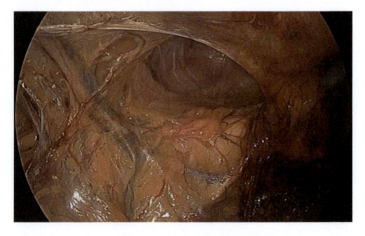

FIGURE 32.4 Left direct inguinal hernia fully reduced

the epigastric vessels may be clipped and divided should they dissect free from the rectus bed.

Lateral peritoneal blunt dissection will expose the arcuate line anteriorly and the psoas muscle posteriorly. The three cutaneous nerves, ilioinguinal, genitofemoral and lateral

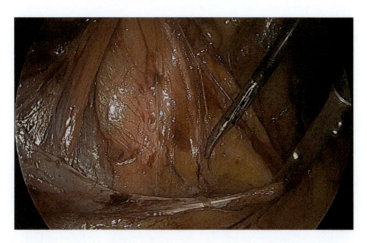

FIGURE 32.5 Left side view of spermatic cord vessels lateral and vas deferens medial. Peritoneum dissected in cephalad direction to a point where the vas deferens courses inferomedially toward bladder

femoral cutaneous, lay on the psoas muscle and should be avoided during dissection and mesh fixation. Lateral dissection will expose the lateral aspect of an indirect hernia sac. This sac should be reduced from the internal ring with bimanual traction and careful dissection. Spermatic cord structures are dissected off of the lateral aspect of the indirect sac and carefully preserved. The indirect sac should be dissected in a cephalad direction to the point at which the vas deferens turns inferiorly toward the bladder (Fig. 32.5). The internal ring should be examined for evidence of a lipoma, which, if noted, should be dissected from the ring.

There are a variety of mesh products that may be used for the repair. Polyester or lightweight polypropylene, 4×6 inch, or precontoured mesh products are commonly employed. Mesh is inserted through the Hassan port and positioned in only fashion over the inguinal floor, covering direct, indirect, femoral and obturator spaces (Fig. 32.6). It is essential that the mesh cover these spaces widely, while avoiding peritoneal migration beneath the posterior aspect of the mesh. Mesh fixation may be utilized routinely or selectively (direct hernias,

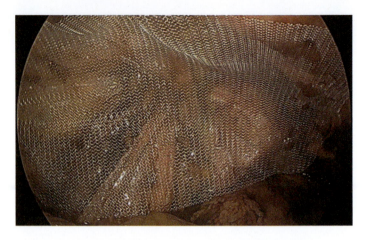

FIGURE 32.6 Mesh fixation to pubis with absorbable straps

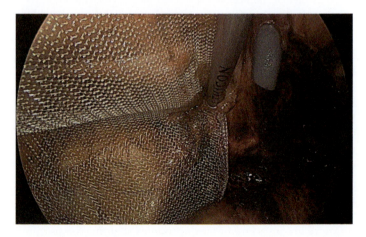

FIGURE 32.7 Absorbable straps being deployed anterior to symphysis pubis

large indirect hernias). The author's preference is to routinely fix mesh with absorbable tacks. Fixation should occur in three areas: Cooper's ligament, anteromedial and anterolateral (Fig. 32.7). Posterolateral fixation is to be avoided due to risk to the cutaneous nerves.

For bilateral hernias, the two pieces of mesh should overlap at the midline. For all repairs, 10 mL of 0.25 % bupivacaine with epinephrine is sprayed over the psoas muscle(s) as a field block for postoperative analgesia. Special attention is paid to the inferolateral corner of the mesh as the CO_2 is evacuated to assure the mesh remain entirely extraperitoneal. Failure to do so will result in an early recurrence of the hernia. Ports are removed as the space is de-sufflated and all gas is evacuated. The anterior rectus sheath is closed with absorbable suture as are skin incisions. Sterile band-aids or dermabond are applied to the skin.

Chapter 33
Open Umbilical Hernia Repair

Rebecca Gunter and Jacob A. Greenberg

Abstract Umbilical hernias are common primary ventral hernias and many become symptomatic over time. In the following chapter, we will review the open repair of umbilical hernias with and without mesh reinforcement.

Keywords Umbilical Hernia • Ventral Hernia • Mesh • Open Umbilical Henria Repair • Mesh Herniorraphy

The procedure can be performed under general anesthesia with an endotracheal tube or a laryngeal mask airway, or utilizing local anesthetics and sedation. The surgeon should

R. Gunter, MD
Department of General Surgery, University of Wisconsin Hospital and Clinics, 600 Highland Ave, H4/785A Clinical Science Center, Madison, WI 53792, USA
e-mail: rgunter@uwhealth.org

J.A. Greenberg, MD, EdM (✉)
Department of Surgery, University of Wisconsin Hospital and Clinics, K4/748 CSC, 600 Highland Avenue, Madison, WI 53792, USA
e-mail: greenbergj@surgery.wisc.edu

H. Chen (ed.), *Illustrative Handbook of General Surgery*,   547
DOI 10.1007/978-3-319-24557-7_33,
© Springer International Publishing Switzerland 2016

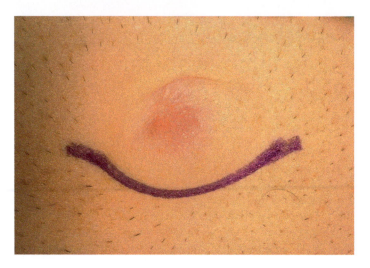

FIGURE 33.1 An infraumbilical, semicircular incision is made

appropriately anesthetize the periumbilical area prior to incision. A semicircular infraumbilical incision is made (Fig. 33.1),
and the subcutaneous tissue is dissected down to the underlying fascia. The umbilical stalk is isolated, encircled, and
divided (Fig. 33.2). Care must be taken to avoid injuring the
umbilical skin during this portion of the procedure. The hernia sac and its contents are dissected from the fascia and the
hernia defect, and then reduced into the abdominal cavity
(Fig. 33.3). Hernia defects less than 2 cm are then closed primarily, while larger defects are repaired with mesh in order to
decrease recurrence rates [1, 2].

Primary Repair

For a primary repair, the fascial edges are dissected out and
reapproximated with interrupted braided polyester sutures
(Ethibond, Johnson & Johnson) (Fig. 33.4). This can be done
with interrupted or figure of 8 type sutures or utilizing a vest
over pants technique. The base of the umbilicus is resecured

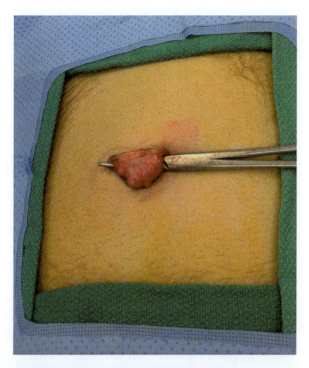

FIGURE 33.2 A clamp around the isolated umbilical stalk. Division of the stalk allows access to the hernia defect below

to the underlying fascia with a single simple absorbable suture, and the overlying skin is then closed. In order to prevent seroma formation we place a cotton ball in the umbilicus, cover it with an occlusive dressing, and aspirate the air with a needle to create a pressure dressing (Fig. 33.5).

Preperitoneal Mesh Repair

Once the hernia has been reduced, the preperitoneal space is cleared to make space for the mesh to extend 3–5 cm beyond the edges of the defect. Blunt dissection with the surgeon's finger or a surgical sponge through the hernia defect can

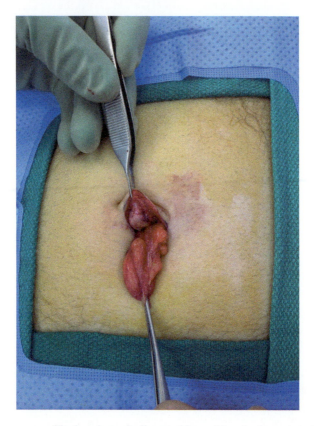

FIGURE 33.3 The hernia sac is dissected free of its attachments to the fascia and replaced within the abdomen

create the preperitoneal pocket for mesh placement. The PROCEED Ventral Patch (PVP, Ethicon, Johnson & Johnson) is a composite, polypropylene based circular mesh used for small umbilical and ventral hernias. It is available in two sizes, 4.3 and 6.4 cm, and has two anchoring straps on the external surface. For use, the PVP is moistened with saline, folded into a semicircle, and placed in the hernia defect, taking care to secure the anchoring straps prior to insertion

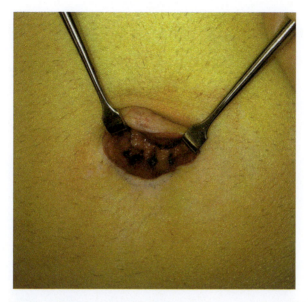

FIGURE 33.4 Simple interrupted sutures close the hernia defect in this primary repair

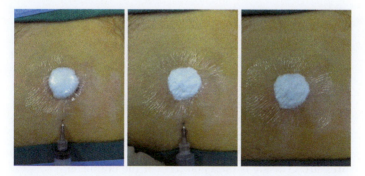

FIGURE 33.5 A cotton ball pressure dressing is created by covering the umbilicus with a cotton ball and occlusive dressing, and aspirating the excess air with an empty syringe

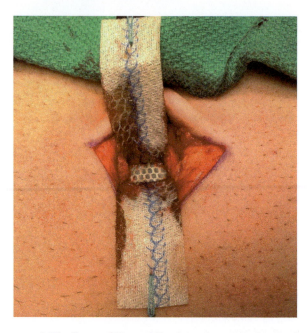

FIGURE 33.6 The Proceed Ventral Patch in place, covering the fascial defect. The anchoring straps are sutured to the edges of the fascial defect and the excess strap is trimmed

(Fig. 33.6). The mesh is self-expanding, though this may be aided either by manipulating the straps or using the back of a forceps. Once the mesh is in position, the fascia is closed laterally to the anchoring straps with interrupted polyester sutures. The medial closure incorporates the anchoring straps in the fascial closure to hold the mesh in place (Fig. 33.7). The excess strap is then trimmed. The base of the umbilicus is secured to the underlying fascia with a single simple absorbable suture, and the overlying skin closed. The cotton ball pressure dressing is then placed over the umbilicus.

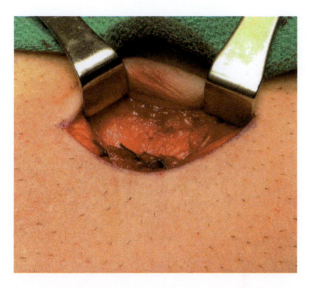

FIGURE 33.7   Fascial closure incorporating the Proceed Ventral Patch

References

1. Nguyen MT et al. Comparison of outcomes of synthetic mesh vs suture repair of elective primary ventral herniorrhaphy: a systematic review and meta-analysis. JAMA Surg. 2014;149(5):415–21.
2. Tollens T et al. A prospective study of one-year clinical outcomes utilizing a composite three-dimensional device with a tissue-separating layer for repair of primary ventral and small incisional hernia. Surg Technol Int. 2014;24:195–202.

Chapter 34
Laparoscopic Ventral Hernia Repair

Luke M. Funk

Abstract   Ventral and Incisional hernias are a common problem encountered by general surgeons. While there are open and laparoscopic approaches for the repair of these hernias, this chapter will focus on the laparoscopic repair of ventral hernias.

Keywords   Ventral Hernia • Incisional Hernia • Laparoscopy • Laparoscopic Ventral Hernia Repair • Mesh

Positioning and Anesthesia

The patient is placed in the supine position for most hernias of the upper abdomen. If the fascial defect is in the lower abdomen, the arms are tucked to enable the surgeon and assistant to stand closer to the patient's head to facilitate dissection in the lower abdomen. Care is taken to pad potential

L.M. Funk, MD, MPH
Department of Surgery, University of Wisconsin School of
Medicine and Public Health, University of Wisconsin,
600 Highland Ave., CSC H4/728, Madison, WI 53792, USA
e-mail: funk@surgery.wisc.edu

H. Chen (ed.), *Illustrative Handbook of General Surgery*,   555
DOI 10.1007/978-3-319-24557-7_34,
© Springer International Publishing Switzerland 2016

pressure points along the arms to prevent peripheral neu-ropathies which may develop after prolonged compression of the upper or lower extremities. Extra padding is also placed between IV lines and the skin to prevent skin breakdown after the case. General anesthesia is administered given that pneumoperitoneum is an essential part of the operation. Muscle paralysis is also critical to ensure adequate visualiza-tion of the peritoneal cavity during the operation.

Patient Preparation

Following induction with general anesthesia and placement of the endotracheal tube, an orogastric tube is placed into the stomach and connected to suction for gastric decompression. This is important given that the first port will be placed into the left upper quadrant. If the case is expected to take longer than 2 hours, a foley catheter is typically placed. For lower abdominal hernias, a three-way foley catheter may be placed to facilitate injection of methylene blue through the one of the catheter ports to ensure that the bladder has not been injured. The abdomen is prepped and draped and an antimi-crobial drape (e.g., Ioban™) is placed onto the abdomen to secure the drapes along the lateral edges and minimize mesh contact with the skin (a potential source for infection).

Description of Procedure

Abdominal Access and Port Placement

Access may be obtained through a variety of approaches including the, Hasson technique or use of a Veress needle. We prefer the latter technique. A Veress needle is introduced into the left upper quadrant immediately inferior to the costal margin at the mid-clavicular line (Fig. 34.1). Following a negative saline drop test, the abdomen is inflated to a pres-sure of 15 mmHg. The Veress needle is then withdrawn and a

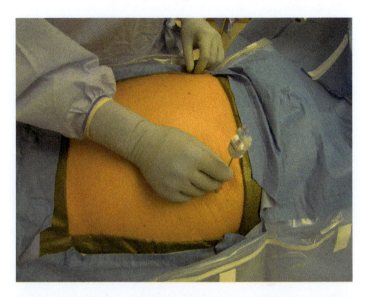

FIGURE 34.1 Veress needle placement. A Veress needle is placed into the left upper quadrant. After a negative saline drop test, the abdomen is insufflated to a pressure of 15 mmHg

5 or 12 mm port is introduced into the abdomen either blindly or under direct visualization with an optical trocar. Depending on the size and location of the hernia defect, two to four additional ports are placed along the right and left lateral margins of the abdomen (Fig. 34.2). It is critical that these ports are placed away from the fascial defect. If they are placed too close to the fascial defect, they will become non-functional when the mesh is placed because the mesh will overlap with the port locations.

At least one of the ports is typically a 12 mm port to allow passage of the mesh. If a small piece of mesh is used (e.g., a 9 cm round), an 8 mm port may be used or one of the 5 mm ports may be removed so the mesh can be placed through the port site incision. For most medium sized hernia defects, three ports are placed on the patient's left so the surgeon can have two working ports on the same side of the abdomen that

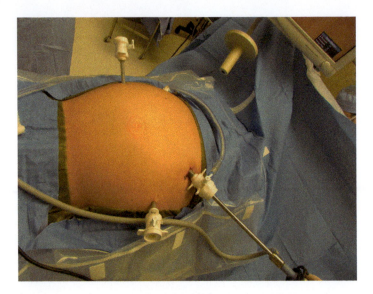

FIGURE 34.2 Abdominal port positioning. This patient has a 2 cm umbilical hernia. Only 3 ports are needed given that we typically use a small mesh (9 cm round) for this type of hernia. The ports are placed quite lateral both on the right and left side to ensure an adequate working space once the mesh is placed into the abdomen

the camera is located. A single right-sided port is usually necessary for fixation of the mesh along the left margin of the mesh. If this is too difficult with the camera on the left side, an additional 5 mm port can be placed on the patient's right such that the surgeon is not working opposite the camera.

Dissection and Characterization of Hernia Defect

A combination of blunt and sharp dissection with scissors is used to reduce herniated abdominal contents from the abdominal wall. The most commonly herniated contents are omentum and small bowel although the transverse colon and other organs such as the liver or stomach can be present within the hernia (Fig. 34.3). Tedious dissection is critical

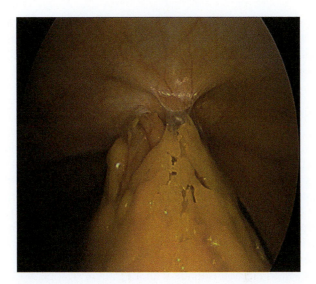

FIGURE 34.3 Herniated omentum. Herniated omentum can be seen exiting through the umbilical defect while an adhesion can be seen in the foreground. This herniated tissue was easily reduced with blunt dissection using atraumatic graspers. Care was taken to avoid ripping the omentum as this frequently causes bleeding

during this phase of the operation to avoid the dreaded complication of a missed enteric injury. Our preference is to avoid usage of cautery or bipolar energy devices if possible given the possibility of enteric injury. Often, a combination of gentle pushing and pulling using atraumatic graspers will result in separation of the omentum from the hernia sac. If the omentum is densely adherent to the abdominal wall and cannot be easily reduced, judicious use of cautery or bipolar energy devices is reasonable if we are able to ensure that no bowel is in close proximity. If the anatomy is unclear or we are unable to reduce the herniated contents laparoscopically, we do not hesitate to convert to an open approach to finish the hernia reduction.

A plastic ruler is then introduced into the abdomen to measure the length and width of the fascial defect. Two atraumatic graspers are used to stretch the ruler in both the cranial-caudal and lateral directions to abdomen these measurements. We prefer at least 3 cm of overlap between the mesh and fascial edges on each side to minimize the likelihood of hernia recurrence.

Closure of the Hernia Defect

Given that laparoscopic ventral hernia repairs are typically performed for small to medium sized hernia defects, it is usually possible to close these hernia defects primarily before placing the intra-abdominal mesh. While there is no consensus on whether this maneuver decreases hernia recurrence, it helps decrease the dead space superficial to the intraperitoneal mesh and closes the hernia defect. To perform this closure, the center of the fascial defect is marked with a pen and a stab incision is made with a 15 blade scalpel. A #1 or 0 suture is then passed transfascially with a suture passer (e.g., Endo Close™ or Carter-Thomason device) (Fig. 34.4). Multiple sutures can be placed along the fascia from the same skin incision site. This minimizes the number of stab incisions that are needed. For most defects, 2–3 stab incisions are used to pass 5–10 transfascial sutures. Alternatively, the fascia can be sutured closed intracorporeally using a slowly absorbable barbed suture.

Mesh Selection and Orientation

A round mesh is typically selected for small to medium size umbilical hernia defects while a rectangular mesh is used for "swiss cheese" type defects which may occur after laparotomies. We prefer to use a composite mesh with an anterior later that promotes ingrowth into the abdominal wall and a posterior layer that is designed to minimize visceral attachments to the mesh. Once the mesh is selected, the mesh is folded in half and a pen is used to bisect the mesh. The mesh is then placed onto the abdomen and centered along the

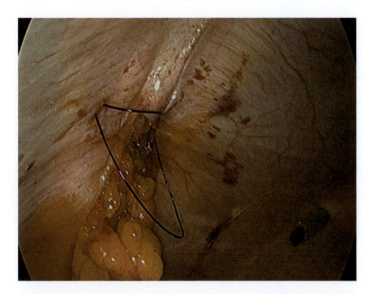

FIGURE 34.4 Primary fascial closure. The first transfascial suture is being placed with the aid of a transfascial suture passer (not pictured). Three transfascial sutures were used in this case to close the fascial defect

hernia defect using the previous placed pen mark in the center of the hernia defect (Fig. 34.5). The mesh is then outlined on the abdominal wall and an "x" is placed 1 cm peripheral to where each line on the mesh intersected with the outline of the mesh on the abdominal wall (Fig. 34.6). These "X's" mark the spot where the transfascial sutures in the mesh will be pulled up through the abdominal wall. These X's are placed 1 cm peripheral to the mesh outline because the abdominal wall has a round shape and since the suture passer is advanced perpendicular to the abdominal wall, it will typically pierce the peritoneal lining in a location that allows the mesh to be pulled up taught to the abdominal wall. The insufflation pressure may also be decreased so that the abdominal wall takes on its more routine shape.

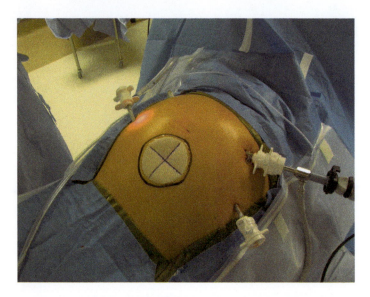

FIGURE 34.5 Mesh positioning. A 9 cm round mesh has been bisected with two perpendicular lines drawn on the abdominal wall side of the mesh. The mesh has been outlined on the abdominal wall for subsequent marking which will be used for transfascial suture placement

Depending on the size of the mesh, two to eight sutures are placed through the outer layer of the mesh near the edge. If a small piece of mesh is used (e.g., 9 cm round), two sutures placed across from each other are adequate to fixate the mesh to the abdominal wall and facilitate tacking. For larger, rectangular pieces of mesh, numerous sutures may be needed to facilitate fixation and tacking. Alternatively, there are now several commercially available mesh deployment devices which may aid in mesh positioning. Once the sutures have been placed into the mesh and the needles have been removed, the mesh is briefly placed in saline and subsequently rolled up and placed into the abdomen through the 12 mm port (Fig. 34.7).

Orientation is checked to ensure that the non-adherent side faces the viscera. This is verified by noting the location of the suture knots which are on the abdominal wall side of the mesh. If a non-circular piece of mesh is used, proper

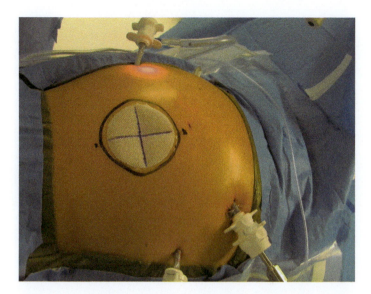

FIGURE 34.6 Mesh positioning (cont). Given that a small round mesh was used in this case, only two transfascial sutures were placed. X's mark the spot approximately 1 cm peripheral to where the vertical line in the mesh intersects with the outline of the mesh. In this case, the two X's are made in the midline, rather than the laterally to minimize the likelihood of inferior epigastric vascular injury during passage of the transfascial suture device

cranial-caudal mesh orientation is verified. We prefer to draw on the abdominal wall side of the mesh prior to mesh insertion so that orientation is obvious once in the abdomen (e.g., a stick figure; the head of the figure corresponds with the cranial positioning of the mesh).

Securing the Mesh

An empty suture passer is placed through the previously placed stab incisions where the "X's" were previously marked 1 cm peripheral to the outline of the mesh. The assistant uses a bullet-nosed grasper or Maryland device (not an atraumatic grasper which holds suture poorly) to grasp and deliver the

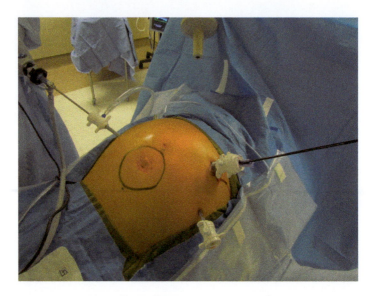

FIGURE 34.7 Mesh placement into the abdomen. The mesh has been rolled up and is being passed with an atraumatic grasper through the 12 mm port. The non-adhesive barrier side is protected by rolling up the mesh so that the abdominal wall side faces outward. Suture tails from the two sutures placed into the mesh can be seen exiting the 12 mm port

suture to the transfascial suturing device. The surgeon then pulls the device out of the abdomen and snaps the suture near the tail. The surgeon then advances the passer through the same skin incision and alters the location where the tip pierces the peritoneum by approximately 1 cm. The passer is removed and both tails are snapped at their ends. Once all suture tails have been pulled through the fascia, they are pulled up in unison and tied sequentially. The mesh is then tacked into place using a double-crown technique and absorbable tacks (Fig. 34.8). Placement of the tacks for each of the two rows is approximately one centimeter away from the next tack near the margins of the mesh. This is very important because it helps prevent herniation of intra-abdominal contents above the mesh which can result in bowel incarceration and ischemia.

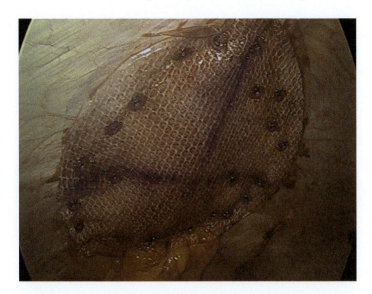

FIGURE 34.8 Securing the mesh. The transfascial sutures have been secured at the upper and lower margins of the mesh and the first row of absorbable sutures has been placed at approximately 1 cm intervals along the outer circumference of the mesh. A second row of tacks will be placed approximately 1 cm inward from the initial outer row creating a 'double crown' row of tacks. The pre-peritoneal fat seen along the inferior portion of the mesh occasionally needs to be mobilized away from the hernia defect to ensure that intra-abdominal contents will not herniate above the inferior margin of the mesh

Identification and Avoidance of Epigastric Vessels

It is critical to identify and avoid the inferior epigastric vessels during passage of the transfascial suture passer and tacking. If they are inadvertently injured, two sutures should be placed using the transfascial suture passer: one above the bleeding point and encompassing the bleeding vessel and one below. These may be simple sutures or figure of eight's. A large abdominal wall hematoma or intra-abdominal hemorrhage may ensue if this injury is not addressed appropriately.

Wound Closure

Following mesh fixation, the abdominal cavity is explored to ensure that there is no ongoing bleeding. Specifically, the abdominal wall and omentum are examined. Actively bleeding areas can either be cauterized or clipped. Once hemostasis is achieved, we typically close the 12 mm port site with a #1 suture on a suture passer. Fascial defects at the 5 mm port sites are not closed. The ports are then removed under direct visualization and the abdomen is desufflated. Absorbable sutures and topical glue are used to close the skin incision. Topical glue alone is used to close the stab incisions for the transfascial suture device. An abdominal binder may be applied if the hernia defect was moderate or large in size.

Postoperative Care

Unless there was significant manipulation of the bowel or concern for delayed return of bowel function (e.g., the patient was obstructed at the time of an urgent hernia operation), the orogastric tube and foley are typically removed at the end of the case and the patient is given a liquid diet. Advancement is dictated by the patient's condition. IV and oral narcotics are provided on an as needed basis. Most patients are able to go home within 1–2 days after surgery. Excellent pain control and adequate mobility are essential prior to discharge.

Chapter 35
Open Retromuscular Ventral Hernia Repair

Jacob A. Greenberg

Abstract   Large ventral and incisional hernias are challenging procedures often associated with significant morbidity and high risks of recurrence. While there are a variety of options available for the repair of these hernias, this chapter will focus on the open retromuscular technique for Ventral Hernia repairs.

Keywords   Open Ventral Hernia Repair • Retromuscular • Rives-Stoppa • Incisional Hernia • Ventral Hernia • Mesh

The use of mesh in the repair of ventral and incisional hernias has led to a significant decrease in the rate of recurrence compared to primary repair [1]. During ventral hernia repair, mesh can be placed in the onlay, inlay, sublay, or underlay position, which describes where the mesh lies with respect to

J.A. Greenberg, MD, EdM
Department of Surgery, University of Wisconsin Hospital
and Clinics, Madison, WI, USA
e-mail: greenbergj@surgery.wisc.edu

H. Chen (ed.), *Illustrative Handbook of General Surgery*,   567
DOI 10.1007/978-3-319-24557-7_35,
© Springer International Publishing Switzerland 2016

the fascia. In this chapter we will describe the technique of sublay mesh placement in the retrorectus position as it was popularized by Rives and Stoppa [2, 3].

We routinely use epidural analgesia for these operations as they are associated with significant pain during the early postoperative period. The patient is laid supine on the table with the arms out. The abdomen is widely prepped and draped making sure to extend the prep wider than the original incision as the mesh will extend beyond the incision in all directions. We routinely give preoperative antibiotics for skin flora and utilize both pneumatic boots and subcutaneous heparin administration for DVT prophylaxis. The old scar is excised and the abdomen is opened widely over the entire length of the previous incision. The fascia is opened cephalad or caudad to the defect in virgin territory in order to decrease the risk of bowel injury on entry. The incision is then opened widely and adhesiolysis is performed to a point lateral to the linea semilunaris so that the posterior rectus sheath can be opened widely and safely. If the hernia is located in the sub-xiphoid or suprapubic location, these areas are also freed of adhesions.

Once the adhesiolysis is complete we turn our attention to dissection of the posterior rectus sheath. Kocher clamps are placed on the medial edge of the fascia and the fascia is elevated anteriorly. Aliss clamps are used to grasp the posterior sheath 1 cm lateral to the linea alba and the posterior sheath is opened with electrocautery (Fig. 35.1). The rectus abdominis muscle should be identified to ensure that you are in the correct plane and not simply preperitoneal. Using a peanut or the surgeons finger the rectus muscle can bluntly be dissected off of the underlying posterior sheath. The sheath is then opened both cephalad and caudad over the entire length of the fascial defect and extending several centimeters both above and below the defect (Fig. 35.2). Using Richardson retractors, the rectus muscle is retracted laterally while constant medial tension is kept on the posterior sheath in order to dissect the retrorectus space to its lateral extent at the

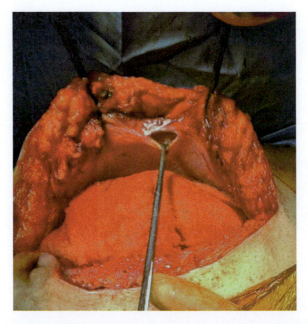

FIGURE 35.1 Beginning dissection of the posterior sheath. The posterior sheath is incised 1 cm lateral to the linea alba and grasped with an Aliss clamp to aid in retraction

linea semilunaris. Perforating neurovascular bundles and the inferior epigastric vessels can be seen laterally and should be preserved (Fig. 35.3). Once the linea semilunaris is reached the dissection is completed in a similar fashion on the contralateral side.

After the posterior sheath dissection is complete, the posterior sheath is closed using a running 2-0 Polydiaxanone (PDS) suture (Ethicon, Cincinnati, OH) (Fig. 35.4). Sponge and needle counts should be completed at this time as the abdomen will be essentially closed at this point. The retrorectus space is then measured and an appropriately sized piece of mesh is selected. There are a wide variety of mesh products that can be utilized in this space. For all clean cases,

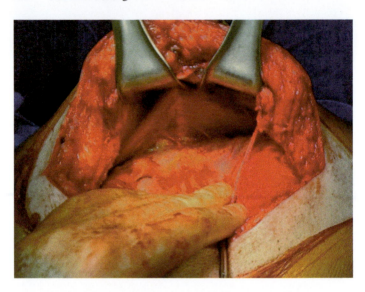

FIGURE 35.2 Complete posterior sheath dissection. Retractors are on the rectus abdominis muscle

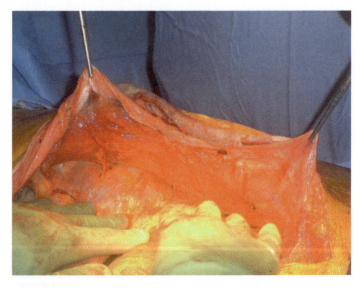

FIGURE 35.3 Perforating neurovascular bundles can be seen laterally at the linea semilunaris

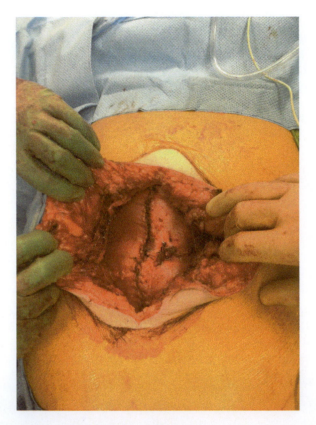

FIGURE 35.4 Posterior sheath closure

we prefer a midweight macroporous synthetic mesh. This mesh is cut to fit the retrorectus space and 0 PDS sutures are preplaced on the mesh at the top, bottom, and along both sides at regular intervals. As there is limited room for the mesh to migrate 6-8 sutures are generally all that is needed for adequate fixation. The mesh is then placed in the retrorectus space and the sutures are passed transfascially through separate stab incisions using the Reverdin suture passer (Figs. 35.5 and 35.6). Once all of the sutures have been passed, they are tied down and a 15 Fr closed suction drain is placed on top of the mesh in order to prevent seroma formation. The anterior sheath is then closed with a running 0 PDS suture

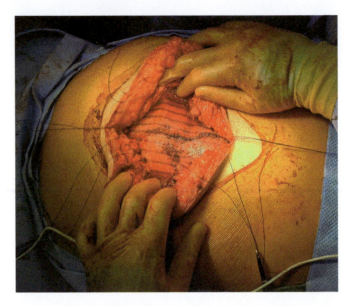

FIGURE 35.5 Mesh Placement in the retromuscular position. Snaps are on the preplaced sutures

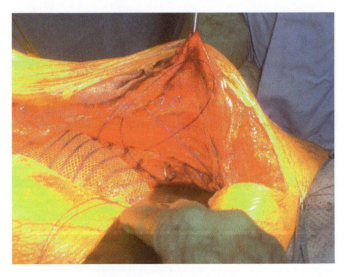

FIGURE 35.6 The Reverdin Suture Passer is seen passing through the rectus muscle above the malleable retractor

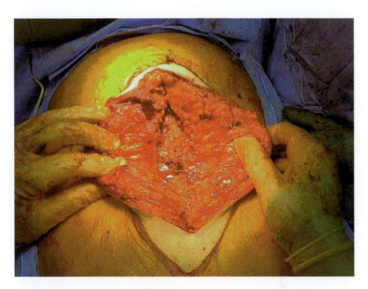

FIGURE 35.7 Anterior sheath closure

using small, frequent bites (Fig. 35.7). The incision is then closed with staples on interrupted nylon sutures and a dry sterile dressing is placed over the wound.

References

1. Luijendijk RW, et al. A comparison of suture repair with mesh repair for incisional hernia. N Engl J Med. 2000;343(6):392–8.
2. Rives J, et al. Treatment of large eventrations. New therapeutic indications apropos of 322 cases. Chirurgie. 1985;111(3):215–25.
3. Stoppa RE. The treatment of complicated groin and incisional hernias. World J Surg. 1989;13(5):545–54.

Part VIII
Hepatobiliary Surgery

Clifford S. Cho

Chapter 36
Open Hepatic and Biliary Procedures

Andrew J. Russ and Clifford S. Cho

Abstract In this chapter, the operative conduct of common hepatobiliary procedures will be described. It is important to recognize that the surgical management of many hepatobiliary disorders will require a combination of procedures; for example, surgical extirpation of hilar cholangiocarcinoma with predominant left-sided involvement will require cholecystectomy, extrahepatic bile duct resection, portal lymphadenectomy, left hemihepatectomy, and biliary-enteric reconstruction. Operations of the liver and bile ducts demand solid familiarity with hepatobiliary anatomy, which can vary greatly from patient to patient. Therefore, careful preoperative study of individual patient imaging studies is of critical importance.

A.J. Russ, MD
Department of Surgery, University of Tennessee Graduate School of Medicine, University of Tennessee Medical Center,
1924 Alcoa Highway, Box U-94, Knoxville, TN 37920, USA

C.S. Cho, MD (✉)
Department of Surgery, University of Wisconsin School of Medicine and Public Health, J4/703 Clinical Sciences Center,
600 Highland Avenue, Madison, WI 53792, USA
e-mail: cho@surgery.wisc.edu

H. Chen (ed.), *Illustrative Handbook of General Surgery*,   577
DOI 10.1007/978-3-319-24557-7_36,
© Springer International Publishing Switzerland 2016

Keywords   Liver resection • Hepatectomy • Cholecystectomy • Hilar dissection • Portal vein • Hepatic artery • Hepatic vein • Portal lymphadenectomy • Hepaticojejunostomy

Hepatobiliary

Hepatic Procedures

Incision

A generous right subcostal incision (dotted line) or vertical upper midline incision with right lateral extension (solid line) permits adequate exposure of the entire liver. Left lateral sectionectomy can be performed through a vertical upper midline incision without lateral extension (Fig. 36.1).

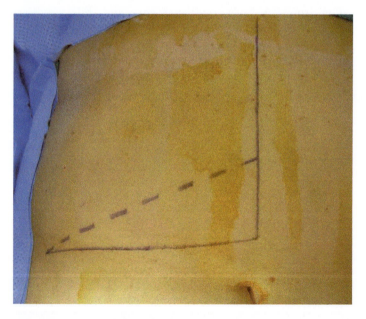

FIGURE 36.1 Subcostal incision (*dotted line*) and vertical upper midline incision (*solid line*)

For oncological resections, careful inspection and palpation of the liver and peritoneal surfaces is performed to identify occult metastases that may potentially alter operative conduct. In selected cases, diagnostic laparoscopy may be useful in this regard (Fig. 36.2).

Exposure

The ligamentum teres is ligated and divided, and its proximal aspect can be used as a handle with which to elevate the left hemiliver (Fig. 36.3).

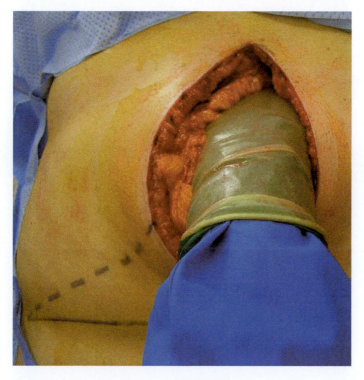

FIGURE 36.2 The abdomen is carefully explored

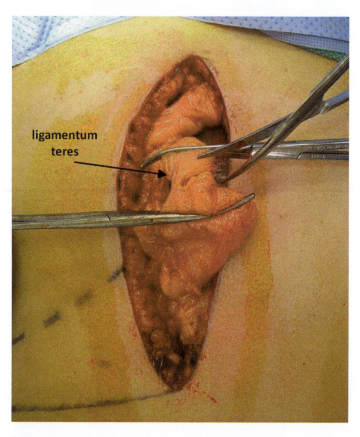

ligamentum
teres

FIGURE 36.3 The ligamentum teres is ligated and divided

The falciform ligament is divided close to the liver from the ligamentum teres toward the confluence of the hepatic veins, and retractors are positioned to provide exposure of the liver (Fig. 36.4).

Intraoperative hepatic ultrasonography is performed for evaluation of hepatic anatomy, tumor localization, and to exclude previously unidentified pathology (Fig. 36.5).

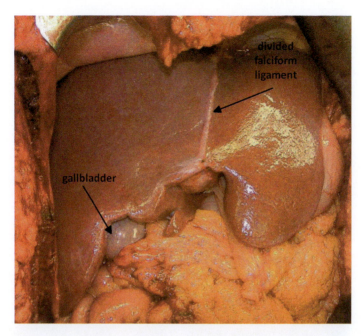

FIGURE 36.4 The falciform ligament is divided close to the liver from the ligamentum teres toward the confluence of the hepatic veins

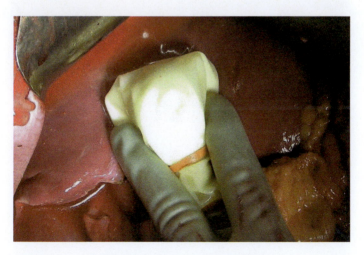

FIGURE 36.5 Intraoperative hepatic ultrasonogrphy

Right Hemihepatectomy (Segmentectomy V-VIII)

Exposure

The retroperitoneal attachments of the right hemiliver are incised, permitting elevation and medial rotation of the right hemiliver off the inferior vena cava and right adrenal gland. Here, the right triangular ligament is being incised (Fig. 36.6).

Cholecystectomy

A cholecystectomy is performed (see section "Open cholecystectomy").

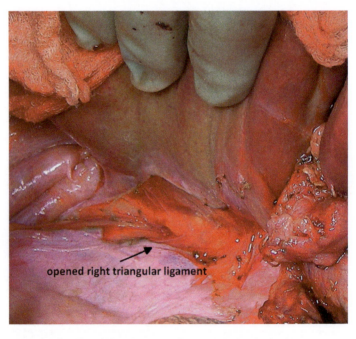

FIGURE 36.6 The right triangular ligament being incised

Inflow Control

The peritoneum overlying the porta hepatis is incised (Fig. 36.7).

The right hepatic artery is identified, ligated, and divided (Figs. 36.8 and 36.9).

Division of the right hepatic artery facilitates exposure of the right portal vein, which is ligated and divided (Figs. 36.10 and 36.11).

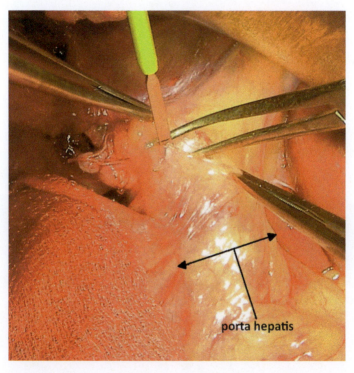

FIGURE 36.7 The peritoneum overlying the porta hepatis being incised

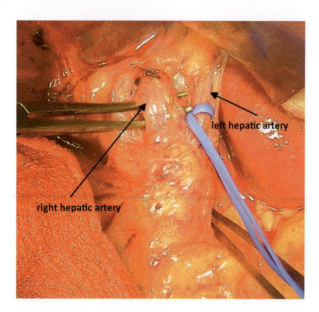

FIGURE 36.8 The right hepatic artery is identified, ligated, and divided (view 1)

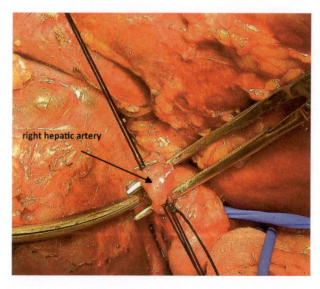

FIGURE 36.9 The right hepatic artery is identified, ligated, and divided (view 2)

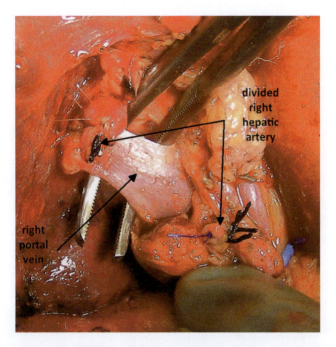

FIGURE 36.10 Division of the right hepatic artery

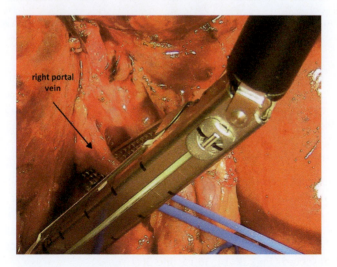

FIGURE 36.11 The right portal vein is ligated and divided

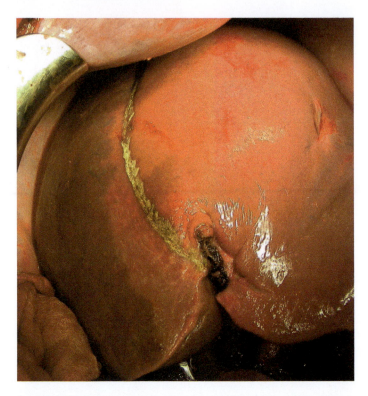

FIGURE 36.12 The line of planned parenchymal transection is marked with electrocautery

Division of the right hepatic inflow results in ischemic demarcation of the right hemiliver. The line of planned parenchymal transection is marked with electrocautery (Fig. 36.12).

Outflow Control

Multiple draining veins between the right hemiliver and inferior vena cava are individually ligated and divided (Fig. 36.13).

Dissection along the confluence of the hepatic veins permits identification of the junction between the right and middle hepatic veins. The right hepatic vein is encircled and transected (Figs. 36.14, 36.15, and 36.16).

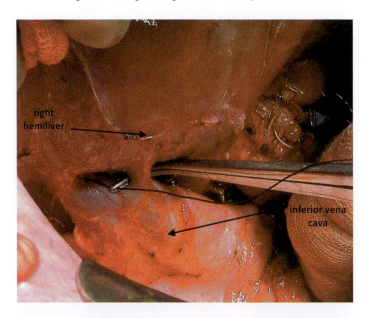

FIGURE 36.13 Multiple draining veins between the right hemiliver and inferior vena cava are individually ligated and divided

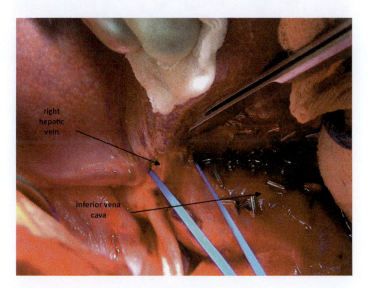

FIGURE 36.14 The right hepatic vein is encircled

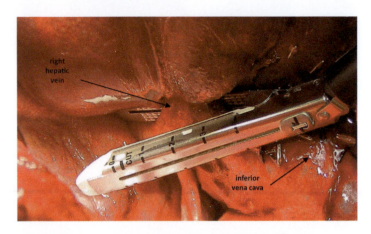

FIGURE 36.15 The right hepatic vein is transected

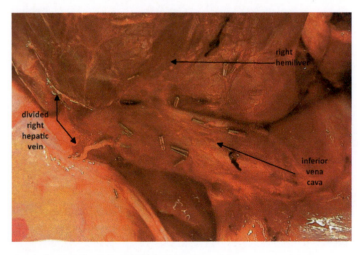

FIGURE 36.16 The retrohepatic inferior vena cava is exposed

Parenchymal Transection

A Pringle maneuver may be performed by intermittently occluding the porta hepatis (Fig. 36.17).

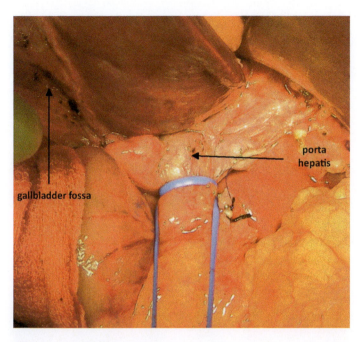

FIGURE 36.17 Pringle maneuver

Stay sutures placed along either side of the planned parenchymal transaction plane permit elevation and separation of the right and left hemilivers, facilitating exposure (Fig. 36.18).

Glisson's capsule can be divided sharply; alternatively, parenchymal transaction can also be initiated using the harmonic scalpel (Figs. 36.19, 36.20, and 36.21).

Crushing the hepatic parenchyma with a clamp permits visualization of biliary and vascular structures, which are individually ligated and divided (Figs. 36.22, 36.23, and 36.24).

Larger structures such as the middle hepatic vein may be divided with a stapler (Figs. 36.25 and 36.26).

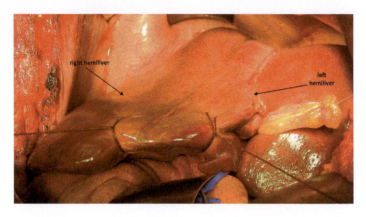

FIGURE 36.18 Stay sutures facilitate exposure of right and left hemilivers

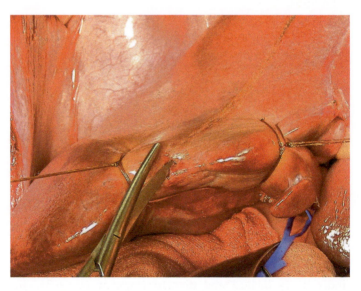

FIGURE 36.19 Glisson's capsule being divided sharply

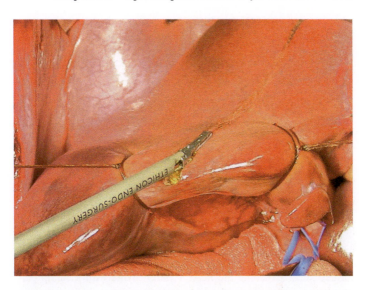

FIGURE 36.20 Parenchymal transaction initiated using the harmonic scalpel (view 1)

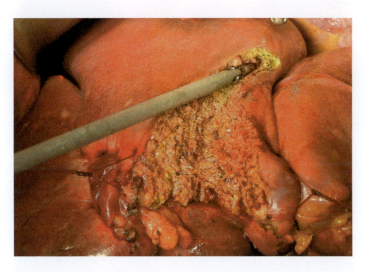

FIGURE 36.21 Parenchymal transaction initiated using the harmonic scalpel (view 2)

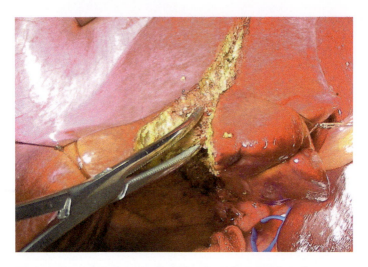

FIGURE 36.22 Crushing the hepatic parenchyma with a clamp permits visualization of biliary and vascular structures

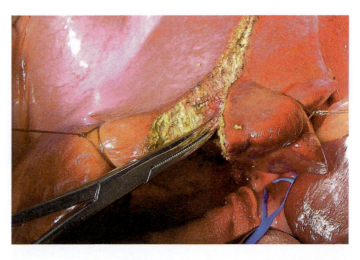

FIGURE 36.23 Biliary and vascular structures are individually ligated and divided (view 1)

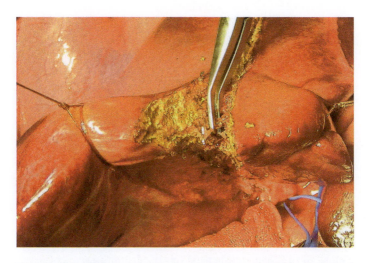

FIGURE 36.24 Biliary and vascular structures are individually ligated and divided (view 2)

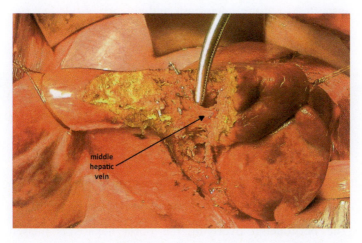

FIGURE 36.25 The middle hepatic vein divided with a stapler (view 1)

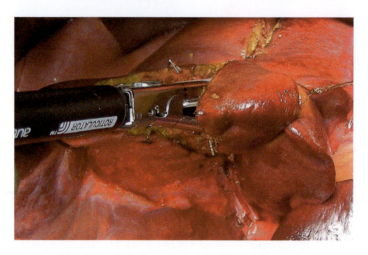

FIGURE 36.26 The middle hepatic vein divided with a stapler (view 2)

The specimen is removed, the cut surface of the liver is inspected to insure hemostasis and absence of bile leakage, and the abdomen is closed.

Left Hemihepatectomy (Segmentectomy II, III, IV)

Exposure

The diaphragmatic attachments of the left hemiliver (the left triangular ligament) are divided, permitting medial rotation of the left lateral section of the liver (Fig. 36.27).

Cholecystectomy (see section "Open cholecystectomy")

Inflow Control

The peritoneum overlying the porta hepatis is incised (Fig. 36.28).

The left hepatic artery is identified, ligated, and divided (Figs. 36.29 and 36.30).

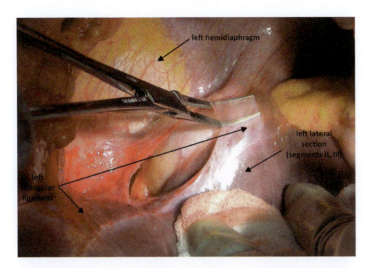

FIGURE 36.27 The diaphragmatic attachments of the left hemiliver are divided

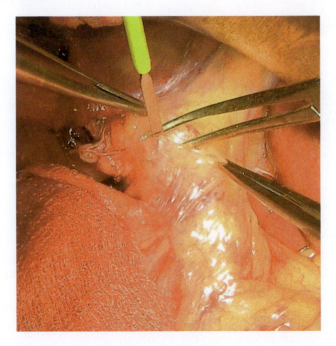

FIGURE 36.28 The peritoneum overlying the porta hepatis is incised

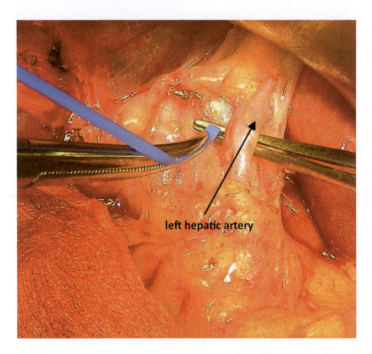

FIGURE 36.29 The left hepatic artery is identified, ligated, and divided (view 1)

Division of the left hepatic artery facilitates exposure of the left portal vein, which is ligated and divided. If the caudate lobe (segment I) is to be preserved, care is taken to divided the left portal vein distal to the segment I branch (Figs. 36.31, 36.32, 36.33, and 36.34).

Division of the left hepatic inflow results in ischemic demarcation of the left hemiliver (Fig. 36.35).

Outflow Control

Dissection along the confluence of the hepatic veins permits identification of the junction between the left and middle hepatic veins (Figs. 36.36 and 36.37).

Division of the ligamentum venosum along the undersurface of the left lateral section of the liver facilitates exposure of the left hepatic vein (Fig. 36.38).

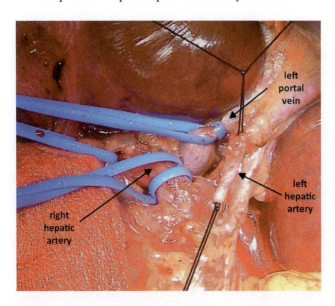

FIGURE 36.30 The left hepatic artery is identified, ligated, and divided (view 2)

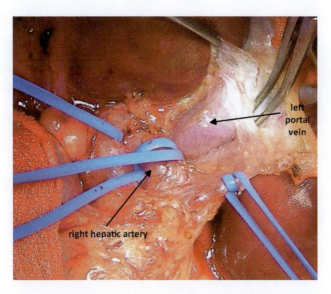

FIGURE 36.31 Division of the left hepatic artery facilitates exposure of the left portal vein

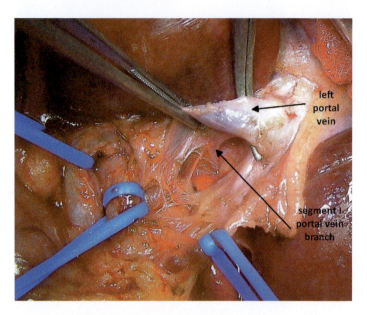

FIGURE 36.32 The left portal vein is ligated and divided

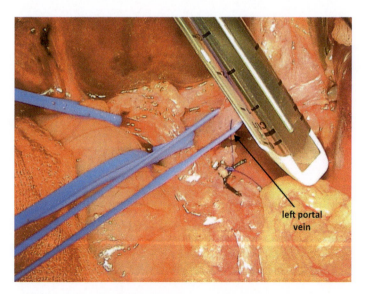

FIGURE 36.33 To preserve the caudate lobe (segment I), the left portal vein is divided distal to the segment I branch

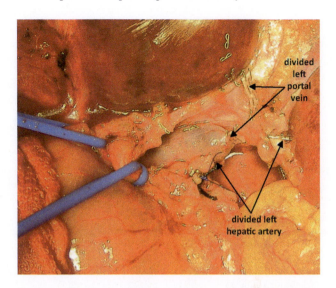

FIGURE 36.34 Divided left hepatic artery and left portal vein

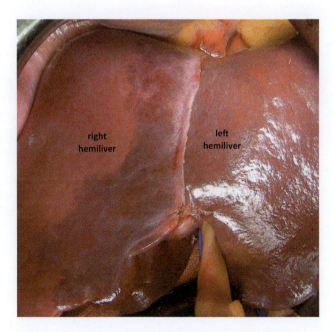

FIGURE 36.35 Ischemic demarcation of the left hemiliver

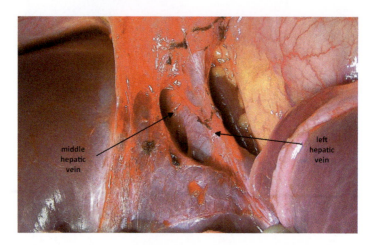

FIGURE 36.36 Dissection along the confluence of the hepatic veins permits identification of the junction between the left and middle hepatic veins (view 1)

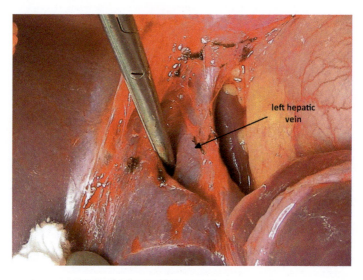

FIGURE 36.37 Dissection along the confluence of the hepatic veins permits identification of the junction between the left and middle hepatic veins (view 2)

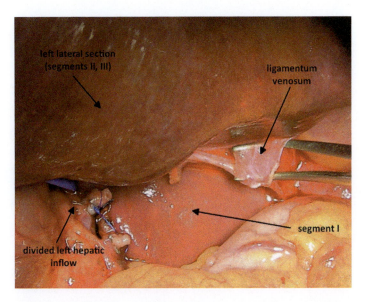

FIGURE 36.38 Division of the ligamentum venosum along the under-surface of the left lateral section of the liver

The left hepatic vein is encircled and divided (Figs. 36.39, 36.40, and 36.41).

Parenchymal Transection

A Pringle maneuver may be performed by intermittently occluding the porta hepatis (Fig. 36.42).

Stay sutures placed along either side of the planned parenchymal transection plane permit elevation and separation of the right and left hemilivers, facilitating exposure (Fig. 36.43).

Glisson's capsule can be divided sharply; alternatively, parenchymal transection can also be initiated using the harmonic scalpel (Figs. 36.44, 36.45, and 36.46).

Crushing the hepatic parenchyma with a clamp permits visualization of biliary and vascular structures, which are individually ligated and divided (Figs. 36.47, 36.48, and 36.49).

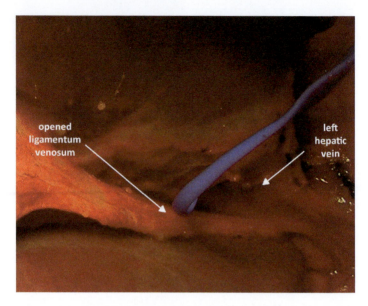

FIGURE 36.39 The left hepatic vein is encircled and divided (view 1)

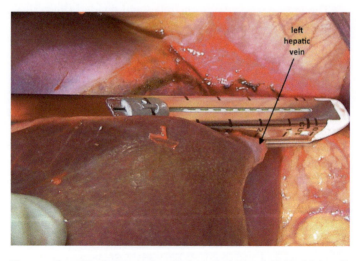

FIGURE 36.40 The left hepatic vein is encircled and divided (view 2)

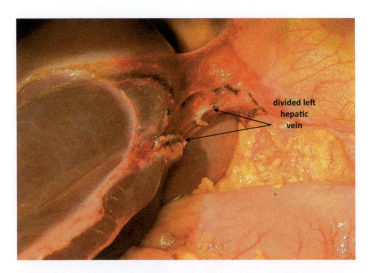

FIGURE 36.41 The left hepatic vein is encircled and divided (view 2)

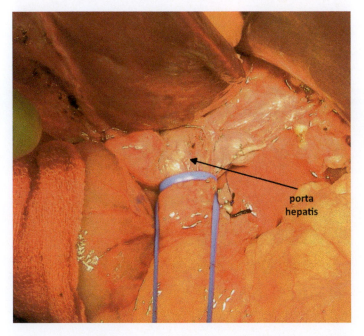

FIGURE 36.42 Pringle maneuver performed by intermittently occluding the porta hepatis

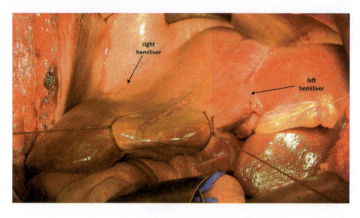

FIGURE 36.43 Stay sutures facilitate elevation, separation, and exposure of the right and left hemilivers

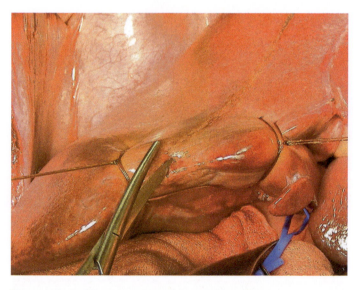

FIGURE 36.44 Glisson's capsule being divided sharply

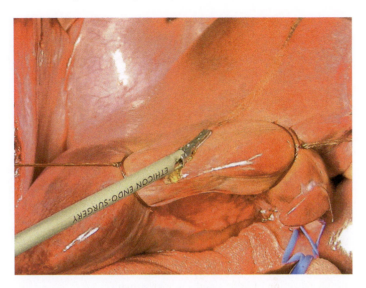

FIGURE 36.45 Parenchymal transaction of the Glisson's capsule initiated using the harmonic scalpel (view 1)

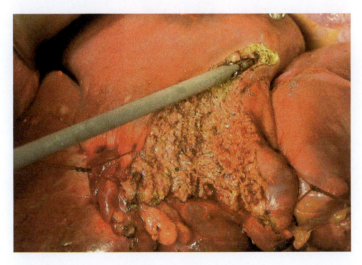

FIGURE 36.46 Parenchymal transaction of the Glisson's capsule initiated using the harmonic scalpel (view 2)

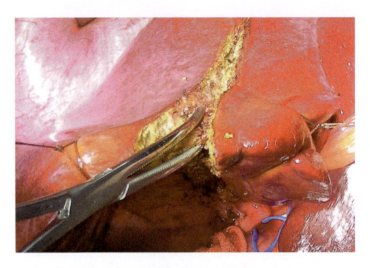

FIGURE 36.47 Crushing the hepatic parenchyma with clamp to permit visualization of biliary and vascular structures

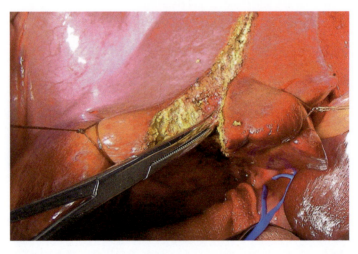

FIGURE 36.48 Biliary and vascular structures are individually ligated and divided (view 1)

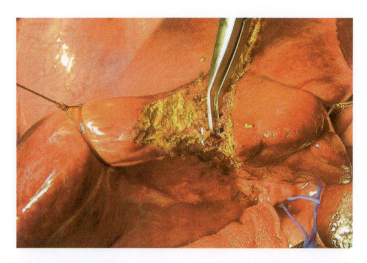

FIGURE 36.49 Biliary and vascular structures are individually ligated and divided (view 2)

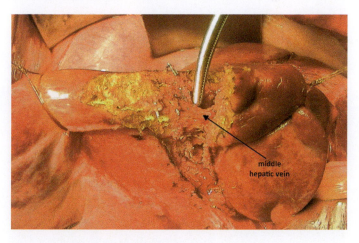

FIGURE 36.50 The middle hepatic vein

Larger structures such as the middle hepatic vein may be divided with a stapler (Figs. 36.50 and 36.51).

The specimen is removed, the cut surface of the liver is inspected to insure hemostasis and absence of bile leakage, and the abdomen is closed (Fig. 36.52).

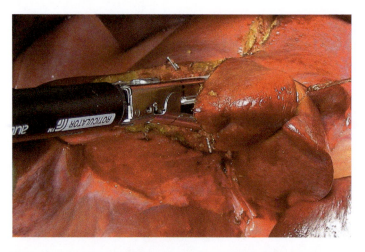

FIGURE 36.51 The middle hepatic vein is divided with a stapler

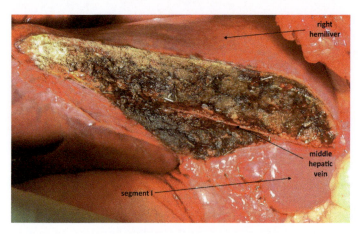

FIGURE 36.52 The cut surface of the liver is inspected

Left Lateral Sectionectomy (Segmentectomy II, III)

Exposure

The diaphgramatic attachments of the left hemiliver (the left triangular ligament) are divided, permitting medial rotation of the left lateral section of the liver (Fig. 36.53).

Inflow Control

The ligamentum teres is elevated, and any hepatic parenchyma overlying the umbilical fissure is divided (Fig. 36.54).

The inflow vessels into segments II and III are ligated (Fig. 36.55).

Division of the segment II/III inflow results in demarcation of the left lateral section (Fig. 36.56).

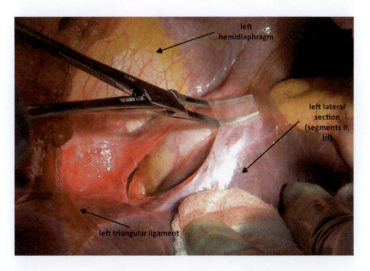

FIGURE 36.53 Diaphgramatic attachments of the left hemiliver

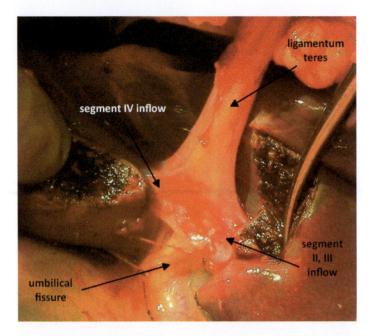

FIGURE 36.54 The ligamentum teres is elevated

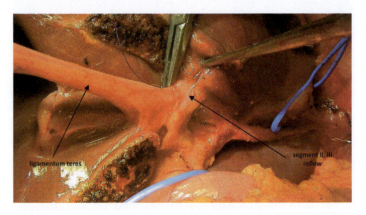

FIGURE 36.55 Inflow vessels into segments II and III are ligated

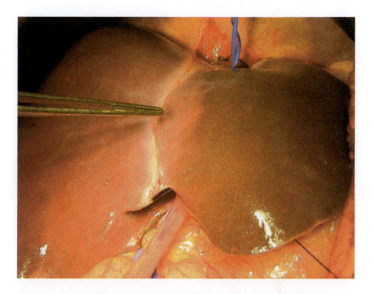

FIGURE 36.56 Ischemic demarcation of segments II and III

Parenchymal Transection

A Pringle maneuver may be performed by intermittently occluding the porta hepatis (Fig. 36.57).

Stay sutures placed along either side of the planned parenchymal transection plane permit separation and elevation of the left lateral section of the liver, facilitating exposure. Glisson's capsule can be divided sharply; alternatively, parenchymal transaction can also be initiated using the harmonic scalpel (Fig. 36.58).

Crushing the hepatic parenchyma permits visualization of biliary and vascular structures, which are ligated and divided. Larger structures including the left hepatic vein may be divided with a stapler (see sections "Parenchymal transection", "Right hemihepatectomy (segmentectomy V-VIII)" or "Left hemihepatectomy (segmentectomy II, III, IV)").

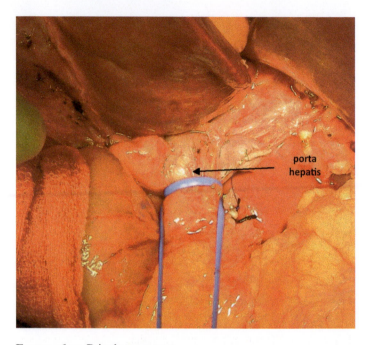

FIGURE 36.57 Pringle maneuver

The specimen is removed, and the cut surface of the liver is inspected to insure hemostasis and absence of bile leakage (Fig. 36.59).

Biliary Procedures

Incision

A right subcostal incision (dotted line) permits adequate exposure of the liver hilus (Fig. 36.60).

Open Cholecystectomy

The peritoneum overlying the fundus of the gallbladder is incised (Fig. 36.61).

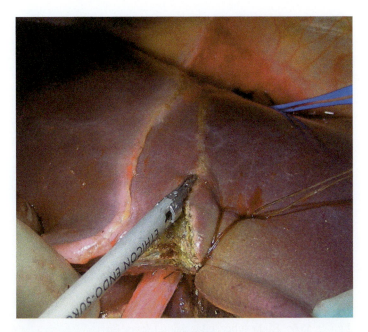

FIGURE 36.58 Stay sutures permit separation of the left lateral section of the liver

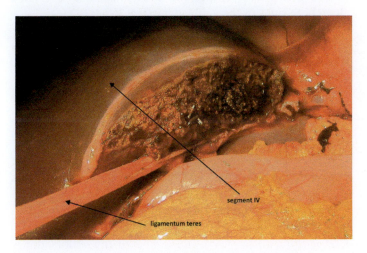

FIGURE 36.59 After removal of specimen, liver is inspected

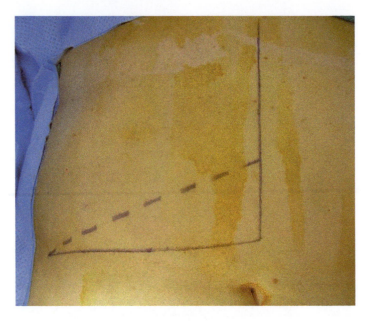

FIGURE 36.60 Right subcostal incision (*dotted line*)

The peritoneum enveloping the gallbladder is incised along both sides of the gallbladder (Fig. 36.62).

The course of the cystic artery is shown here (Fig. 36.63).

The gallbladder is dissected out of the gallbladder fossa (Figs. 36.64 and 36.65).

The cystic artery is ligated and divided (Fig. 36.66).

The cystic duct is ligated and divided (Figs. 36.67 and 36.68).

Common Bile Duct Exploration

The common bile duct is exposed in the porta hepatis (Fig. 36.69).

Stay sutures are placed on either side of the planned choledochotomy, and the common bile duct is opened (Fig. 36.70).

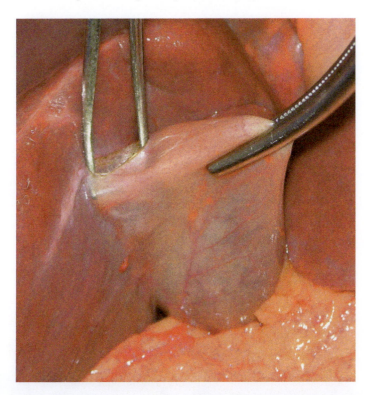

FIGURE 36.61 Peritoneum overlying the fundus of the gallbladder is incised

The common bile duct is explored, then closed over a T-tube (Fig. 36.71).

Extrahepatic Bile Duct Resection

The peritoneum is incised to permit identification of the common bile duct (Fig. 36.72).

The common bile duct is transected at the base of the porta hepatis (Figs. 36.73 and 36.74).

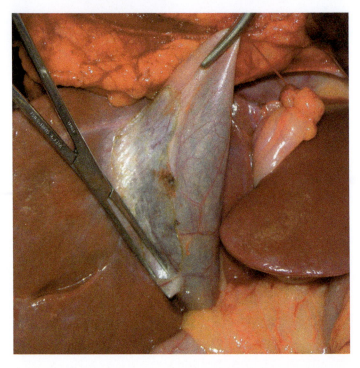

FIGURE 36.62 Peritoneum enveloping the gallbladder is incised

The transected bile duct is elevated in a cephalad direction and portal lymphadenectomy is performed by sweeping all nodal tissues off the hepatic artery and portal vein toward the hepatic hilus (Fig. 36.75) (see section "Portal lymphadenectomy").

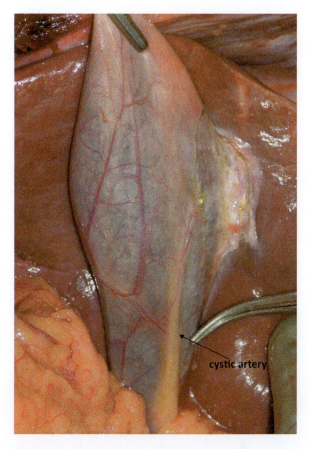

FIGURE 36.63 The course of the cystic artery

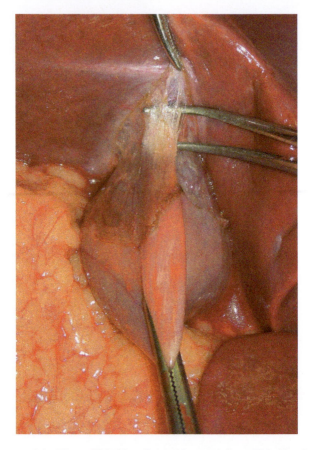

FIGURE 36.64 The gallbladder dissected out of the gallbladder fossa (view 1)

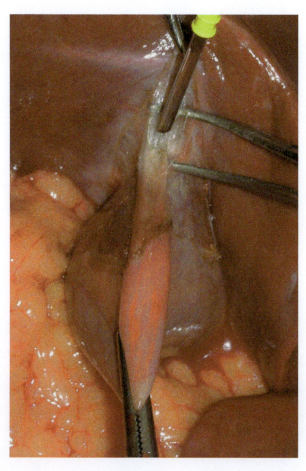

FIGURE 36.65 The gallbladder dissected out of the gallbladder fossa (view 2)

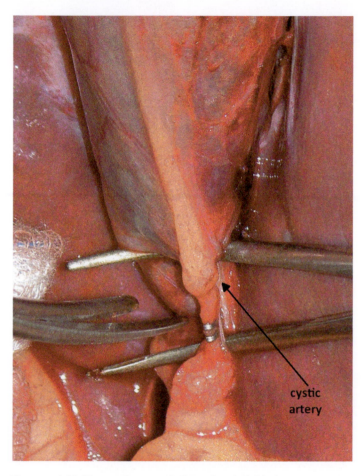

FIGURE 36.66 The cystic artery is ligated and divided

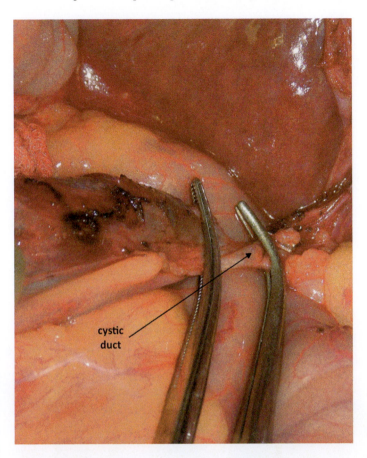

FIGURE 36.67 The cystic duct is ligated and divided (view 1)

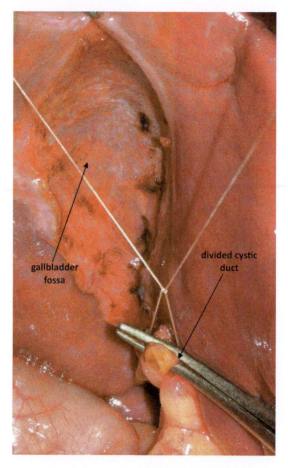

FIGURE 36.68 The cystic duct is ligated and divided (view 2)

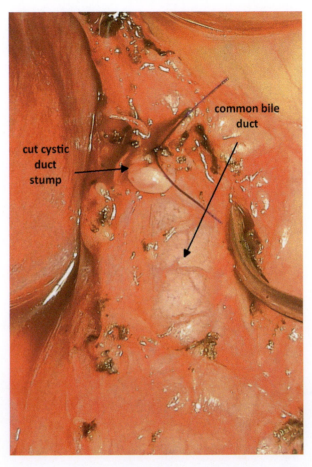

FIGURE 36.69 The common bile duct is exposed in the porta hepatis

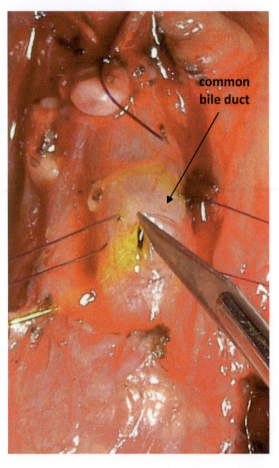

FIGURE 36.70 Stay sutures are placed on either side of the planned choledochotomy

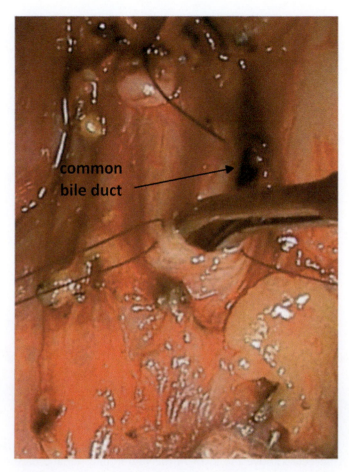

FIGURE 36.71 The common bile duct is explored

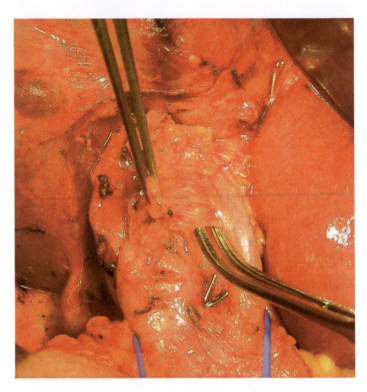

FIGURE 36.72 The peritoneum is incised to permit identification of the common bile duct

The hepatic duct draining the planned liver remnant is transected above the level of the tumor, and hepatic parenchymal transection is performed (see sections "Right hemihepatectomy (segmentectomy V-VIII)" or "Left hemihepatectomy (segmentectomy II, III, IV)").

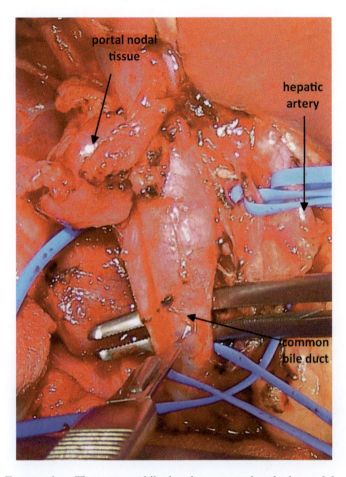

FIGURE 36.73 The common bile duct is transected at the base of the porta hepatis (view 1)

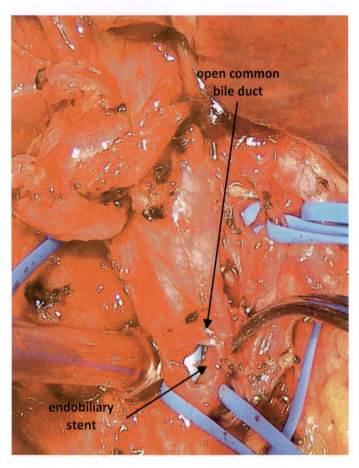

FIGURE 36.74 The common bile duct is transected at the base of the porta hepatis (view 2)

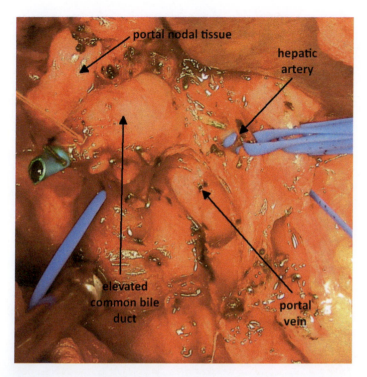

FIGURE 36.75 The transected bile duct is elevated in a cephalad direction

Portal Lymphadenectomy

The peritoneum is incised to permit identification of the common bile duct (Fig. 36.76).

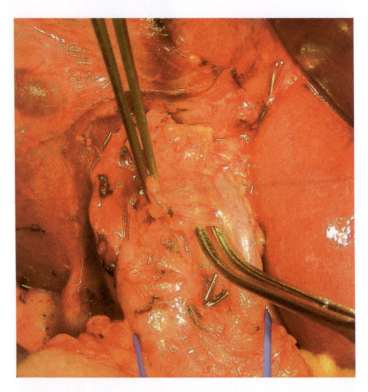

FIGURE 36.76 The peritoneum is incised to permit identification of the common bile duct

Nodal tissue is swept off of the underlying porta hepatis structures from the duodenum to the hepatic hilus, with care taken to ligate all lymphovascular structures (Fig. 36.77).

Biliary-Enteric Reconstruction

The cut hepatic duct is anastomosed to a small jejunotomy fashioned in a Roux limb, which is delivered toward the liver through the transverse colonic mesentery (Fig. 36.78).

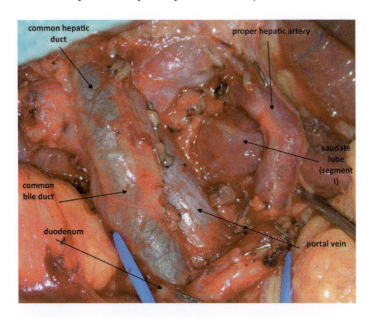

FIGURE 36.77 Nodal tissue is swept off the underlying porta hepatis structures from the duodenum to the hepatic hilus

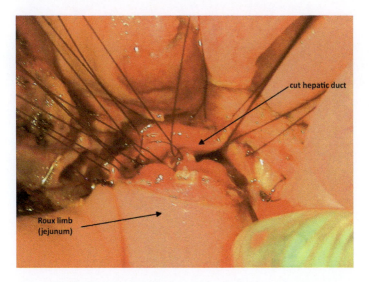

FIGURE 36.78 The cut hepatic duct anastomosed to a small jejunotomy fashioned in a Roux limb

Chapter 37
Minimally Invasive Liver and Biliary Procedures

M. Shirin Sabbaghian and Allan Tsung

Abstract Minimally invasive techniques have been applied to hepatobiliary surgery more frequently as comfort with and understanding of hepatobiliary surgery has grown. The goal is to technically perform the case as if it is an open procedure while taking advantage of the benefits minimally invasive surgery can bring, including decreased post-operative pain, time of ileus, and length of stay, as well as improved cosmesis. Techniques for minimally invasive hepatobiliary surgery include pure laparoscopic, hand-assisted laparoscopic, the hybrid approach (operation is started laparoscopically for

M.S. Sabbaghian, MD
Riverside Surgical Group, Department of Surgery,
Lexington Medical Center,
146 North Hospital Drive, Suite 430, West Columbia,
SC 29169, USA

Surgical Oncology and General Surgery, Private Practice,
Louisiana State University Health Sciences Center,
1307 Crowley Rayne Highway, Suite D Crowley,
LA 70526, USA
e-mail: shirin.sabbaghian@gmail.com

A. Tsung, MD (✉)
Division of Hepatobiliary and Pancreatic Surgery,
University of Pittsburgh Medical Center, UPMC Liver
Cancer Center, Montefiore Hospital, Pittsburgh, PA 15213, USA
e-mail: tsunga@upmc.edu

H. Chen (ed.), *Illustrative Handbook of General Surgery*,   633
DOI 10.1007/978-3-319-24557-7_37,
© Springer International Publishing Switzerland 2016

mobilization of the liver and early dissection and followed by a small laparotomy for completion of the hepatic parenchymal transection], and more recently robotic-assisted. The following chapter describes minimally invasive techniques used for common hepatobiliary procedures. The illustrations and pictures that follow are adapted from a combination of laparoscopic, hand-assisted, and robotic-assisted cases, but note that regardless of the minimally invasive technology used, the approach and technique remain essentially the same.

Keywords   Liver resection • Minimally invasive hepatobiliary surgery • Robotic liver resection • Laparoscopic liver resection • Hybrid approach liver resection • Hand-assisted

Minimally Invasive Hepatobiliary Surgery

Minimally invasive techniques have been applied to hepatobiliary surgery more frequently as comfort with and understanding of hepatobiliary surgery has grown. The goal is to technically perform the case as if it is an open procedure while taking advantage of the benefits minimally invasive surgery can bring, including decreased post-operative pain, time of ileus, and length of stay, as well as improved cosmesis [1–3]. Techniques for minimally invasive hepatobiliary surgery include pure *laparoscopic*, *hand-assisted laparoscopic*, the *hybrid approach* (operation is started laparoscopically for mobilization of the liver and early dissection and followed by a small laparotomy for completion of the hepatic parenchymal transection], and more recently *robotic-assisted* [4–6]. The following chapter describes minimally invasive techniques used for common hepatobiliary procedures. The illustrations and pictures that follow are adapted from a combination of laparoscopic, hand-assisted, and robotic-assisted cases, but note that regardless of the minimally invasive technology used, the approach and technique remain essentially the same.

Cholecystectomy

Carl Langenbuch was the first to describe open cholecystectomy in 1882 [7]; approximately 100 years later in 1985, Eric Muhe performed the first laparoscopic cholecystectomy [7]. Many benefits to the laparoscopic approach were recognized with time – these included decreased postoperative pain as well as quicker recovery time and thus shorter hospital stays [8–10]. As a result, cholecystectomy has become one of the most commonly performed operations in the United States. As robotic-assisted surgery has emerged, surgeons interested in the technology are beginning to perform robotic-assisted cholecystectomy. Robotic-assisted cholecystectomy has served as a prototype procedure for surgeons who are first using robotic technology.

Step 1

Ports are placed.

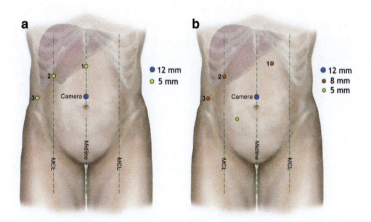

FIGURE 37.1 (a) Port placement for laparoscopic cholecystectomy. (b) Port placement for multiport, robotic-assisted cholecystectomy. An optional 5 mm assist port is used in the right lower quadrant if needed

Step 2

Positioning and exposure. With the patient positioned in reverse Trendelenberg and with the right side up, the fundus of the gallbladder is grasped and retracted superolaterally. The infundibulum of the gallbladder is retracted inferolaterally. It is good practice at this point to identify the porta hepatis in proper position and without adjacent severe inflammation to ensure a safe gallbladder dissection. If severe inflammation is identified, alternate methods for cholecystectomy (including open cholecystectomy) should be considered.

Step 3

Exposure of the critical view and ligation of cystic structures. Peritoneum overlying the gallbladder is dissected on the medial and lateral surfaces of the gallbladder to eventually expose the cystic structures. The cystic duct and artery are identified, and the tissue between the two is dissected to expose the base of the liver. The critical view – view of the cystic duct and cystic artery directly entering the gallbladder with the base of liver seen in between – is identified. Cholangiogram can be performed at this point either as a routine procedure or selectively based on surgeon preference. Cystic duct and artery are then clipped and divided with scissors.

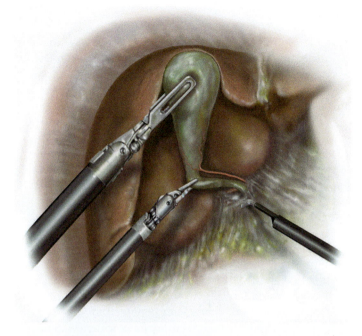

FIGURE 37.2 Illustration of laparoscopic cholecystectomy demonstrating exposure of the critical view

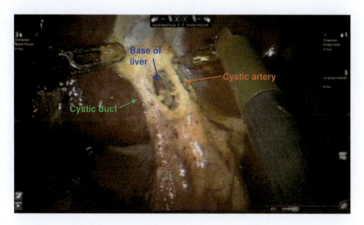

FIGURE 37.3 Picture of multiport robotic cholecystectomy demonstrating exposure of the critical view

Step 4

Completion of cholecystectomy. The gallbladder is dissected off of the gallbladder fossa using cautery. Hemostasis of the dissection bed is ensured, and clips are evaluated to make sure they have remained in place. The gallbladder is removed through a specimen bag. Fascia is closed.

Hepatic Resection

Langenbuch later described elective hepatectomy in 1888 [11]; liver surgery has since evolved very significantly with experience as well as with the evolution of technology. Improved knowledge of liver anatomy [12–15], advances in both surgical technique and anesthesia care [16–21], use of intraoperative ultrasound [22,23], better preoperative imaging quality, and the use of vascular stapling devices [24] as well as energy-induced hemostasis [25–27] have all contributed to improved outcomes after hepatectomy [28–30]. As a result, indications for hepatectomy have widened to include patients with certain benign diseases as well as select patients with abnormal liver function. As laparoscopic experience and technology have improved, interest in using minimally invasive techniques for liver surgery has grown with the intent to take advantage of the potential benefits as noted with laparoscopic cholecystectomy. Many groups have suggested less post-operative pain, earlier return of bowel function, decreased hospital length of stay, fewer post-operative complications, and improved cosmesis [1–3] with minimally invasive hepatectomy. Most recently, robotic technology has been used for liver resection with the first robot-assisted hepatectomy reported from Japan in 2004 [31]. Multiple centers across the world have since started to apply robotic technology to the practice of minimally invasive hepatectomy. Successful procedures have been reported, and outcomes have been comparable to the laparoscopic approach [32].

Right Hepatectomy

Step 1

The room is set up, ports are placed, the patient is positioned in reverse Trendelenberg position with the right side slightly up.

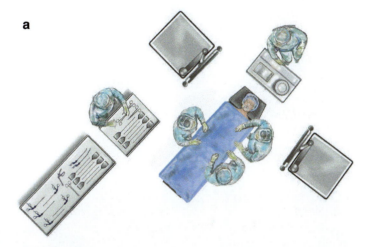

a

FIGURE 37.4 (**a**) Room setup for laparoscopic hepatectomy. Patient is positioned in the center of the room. Anesthesia sits at the patient's head. Surgeons and assistant stand at either side of the operating room (OR) table. The technician stands at the surgeon's preferred side of the table. (**b**) Room setup for robotic assisted hepatectomy. Patient is positioned in the center of the room in split-leg position. Anesthesia sits at the patient's left shoulder. One surgeon and assistant stand at either side of the operating room (OR) table or between the legs. The robotic surgeon sits at the robotic console. The technician stands at the surgeon's preferred side of the table. (**c**) Illustration of port placement for hand-assisted laparoscopic right hepatectomy. Note that for pure laparoscopic right hepatectomy, the hand-port can be switched for a 10–12 assist port. *MCL* mid clavicuar line. (**d**) Illustration of port placement for robotic-assisted right hepatectomy. Robotic ports for robotic instruments are represented by the 8 mm ports

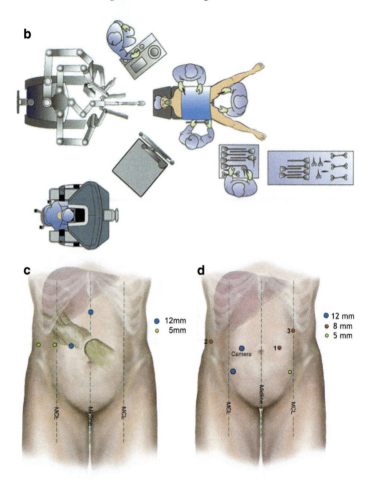

FIGURE 37.4 (continued)

Step 2

Laparoscopic dissection of ligamentous attachments of the liver.

First, the falciform ligament is dissected to the hepatic veins using cautery or a sealing device. Next, the right triangular and coronary ligaments are dissected to mobilize the right liver.

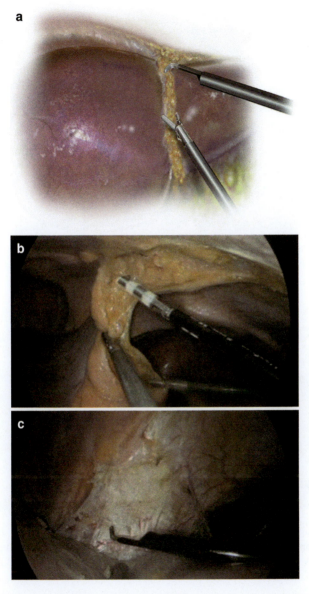

FIGURE 37.5 (**a**) Illustration of the falciform dissected. (**b**) The falciform is dissected. (**c**) Dissection is continued to the anterior surface of the hepatic veins

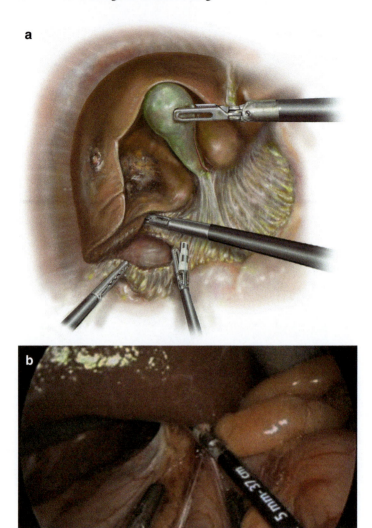

FIGURE 37.6 (**a**) Illustration of the triangular and coronary ligaments dissected. (**b**) The right lobe liver is lifted anteriorly and medially to dissect the triangular ligament

Step 3

Ultrasound the liver, map the lesion(s).

Intraoperative imaging should confirm location of the suspected lesion(s) to ensure no other unexpected lesions are present anywhere else in the liver, to ensure that the pathology suspected is resectable, and to confirm the appropriate resection plan as decided preoperatively (ie to confirm a right hepatectomy is appropriate instead of a wedge resection or trisegmentectomy).

Step 4

If robotic technology is to be used, the robot is docked now. Robotic instruments, including the robotic camera, are introduced.

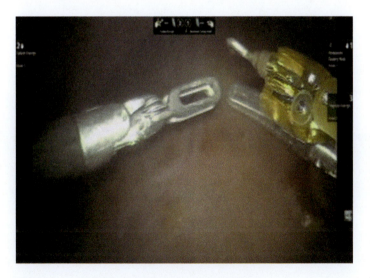

FIGURE 37.7 Robotic instruments are introduced

Step 5

Short hepatic veins are dissected and ligated. With the liver retracted anteriorly, short hepatic veins (SHV) that return blood directly from the liver to the IVC are dissected, ligated, and divided.

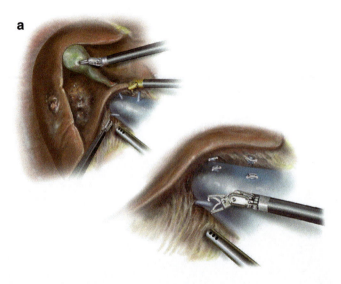

FIGURE 37.8 (**a**) Illustration of the liver retracted anteriorly, and short hepatic veins (SHV) are dissected and ligated. (**b**) The liver is retracted anteriorly, and short hepatic veins are dissected. (**c**) SHV ligated with clips. Shears are in the background to cut between clips

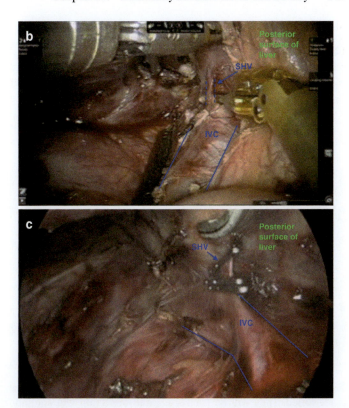

FIGURE 37.8 (continued)

Step 6. Inflow Dissection

(a) Lower the hilar plate.

To accomplish this, cholecystectomy is initiated. Please refer to cholecystectomy portion of this chapter for details. After transecting the cystic duct and artery, tissue overlying the porta hepatis is dissected at the base of the liver and toward the right, exposing the right portal structures.

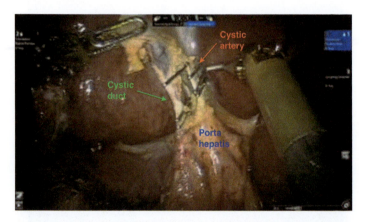

FIGURE 37.9 Cystic artery and duct are clipped after the critical view is identified. They will be transected, and dissection will continue along the porta

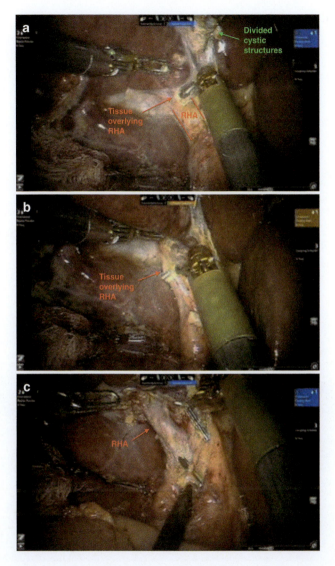

FIGURE 37.10 (**a–c**) Dissection of portal tissue at the base of the right liver leads to exposure of the right hepatic structures. The right hepatic artery is the first structure to be exposed as it is most antero-lateral

(b) Isolate, ligate, and divide the right hepatic artery

   After exposing the right hepatic artery, the tissue surrounding it is further dissected to completely isolate the vessel. This includes tissue posterior to it. It is then ligated with ties and divided. Alternatively, a stapling device can be used as space allows.

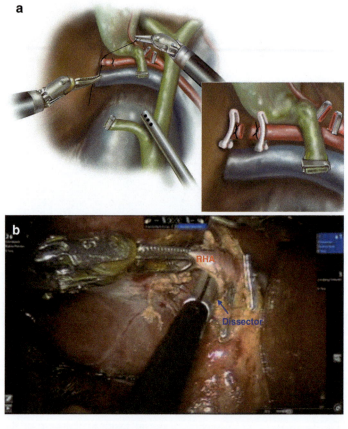

FIGURE 37.11 (a) Illustration demonstrating ligation and division of the right hepatic artery. (b) Tissue behind the artery is dissected with dissector. (c) Right hepatic artery is ligated with clips and ties and divided

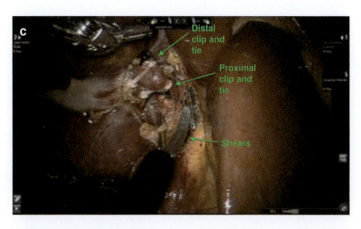

FIGURE 37.11 (continued)

(c) Isolate, ligate, and divide the right portal vein.

The right portal vein (RPV) rests posterior to the right hepatic artery. It is exposed after transection of the RHA. After exposing the right portal vein (RPV), the tissue surrounding it is further dissected to completely isolate the vessel. A branch to the caudate is typically seen running laterally, and this should be ligated and divided.

Once the right portal vein is completely isolated, a silk tie can be placed around it to retract and facilitate introduction of a laparoscopic, roticulating stapler across it. The vessel is ligated and divided using the stapler.

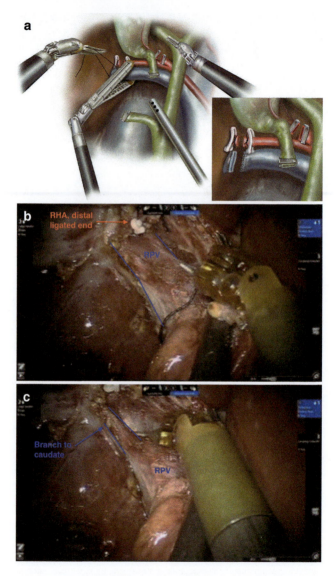

FIGURE 37.12 (a) Illustration of the right portal vein (RPV) isolated, ligated, and divided. (b) The RPV is identified posterior to the RHA after the RHA is transected. (c) Branch running laterally and to the caudate is identified, isolated, and eventually ligated and divided

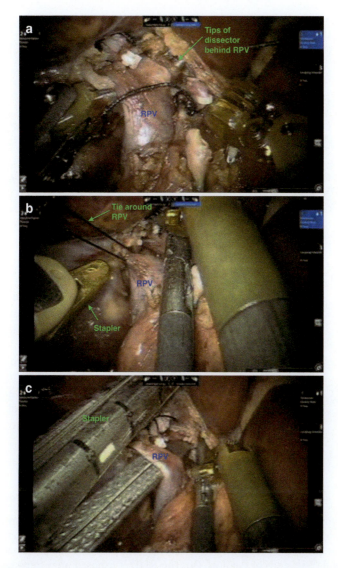

FIGURE 37.13 (a) RPV completely isolated with dissector across it posteriorly. (b) Tie around RPV helps retract and expose it optimally for introduction of stapler around it. (c) Stapler around RPV. (d) Stapled RPV

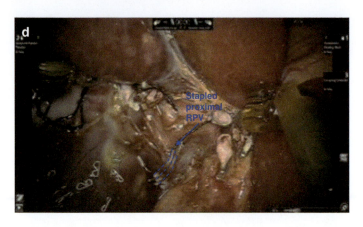

FIGURE 37.13 (continued)

(d) Isolate, ligate, and divide the right hepatic duct.

Note that the duct can also alternatively be ligated intrahepatically if able to help avoid injury to the left ductal system. The right hepatic duct is routinely found as the medial-most structure. It is best exposed after transection of the right hepatic artery and portal vein. After isolating the duct, it is tied distally, then cut proximally to allow visualization of bile draining from the proximal duct. This allows for definite identification of the duct. The duct is then fully transected, and additional clips are placed on the distal duct to ensure it is sealed.

⸻⸻⸻⸻⸻⸻⸻⸻⸻⸻⸻⸻⟶

FIGURE 37.14 (**a**) Illustration of the right hepatic duct (RHD) isolated. It is ligated distally and cut proximally to confirm bile from the proximal duct. Additional clips are then placed to the proximal and distal ends of the duct. (**b**). The RHD is exposed after transection of the right portal vein. (**c**) The RHD is fully dissected. (**d**). The RHD is ligated distally. (**e**) The proximal duct is cut to identify bile coming from it. (**f**) Additional clips are placed on the proximal and distal duct ends. (**g**) Cholecystectomy is completed. The gallbladder is dissected from the gallbladder fossa. It is placed in a laparoscopic bag and removed from the abdominal cavity

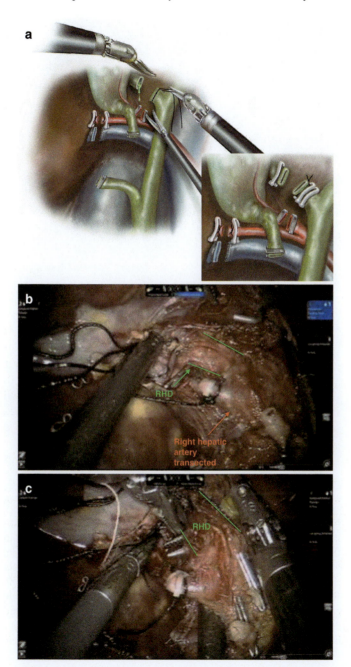

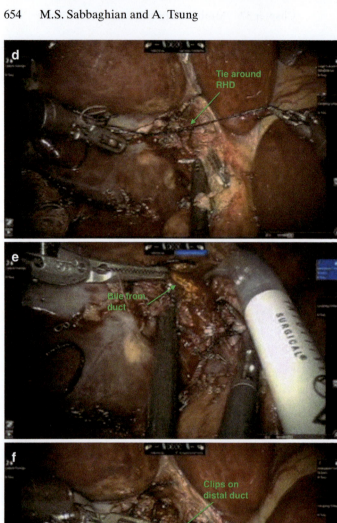
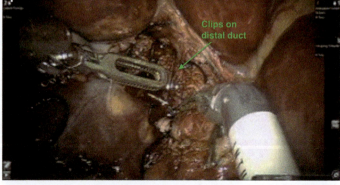

FIGURE 37.14 (continued)

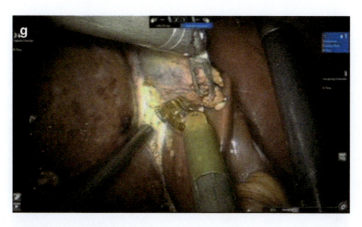

FIGURE 37.14 (continued)

Outflow Dissection

The right hepatic vein can be isolated in an extrahepatic manner, as depicted below, if the tumor rests near the inferior
vena cava. Alternatively, the right hepatic vein can be isolated
within the hepatic parenchyma during parenchymal dissection. For extrahepatic dissection:

(a) On the anterior surface of the liver, the right hepatic vein
    is dissected along its medial edge, creating a window to
    the undersurface of the liver.

(b) While lifting the liver anteriorly, the right hepatic vein is
    dissected from the undersurface of the liver.

(c) While along the undersurface of the liver, a bending
    grasper is placed anterior to the RHV and advanced
    through the window that has been created.

(d) The liver is allowed to fall back into place, and the bend-
    ing grasper is visualized from the anterior surface of the
    liver through the window created. A vessel loop is fed to
    the grasper, and the grasper gently pulls back through to
    the undersurface of the liver. The other end of the vessel
    loop is fed around the lateral border of the RHV from an
    anterior approach, as well. The lateral edge of the liver is

retracted anteriorly again, and both ends of the vessel loops should be around the RHV, thus having a defined isolation of this vein.

(e) The vessel loop can then retract the vein gently, acting as a guide while a stapler is introduced. The vessel is ligated and transected with a vascular loaded roticulating stapler.

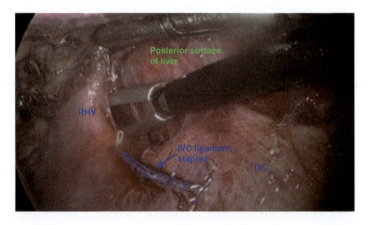

FIGURE 37.15 The right liver is lifted anteriorly, and the right hepatic vein is dissected from the liver's undersurface

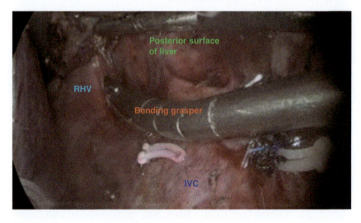

FIGURE 37.16 Along the undersurface of the liver, a bending grasper is placed anterior to the RHV. It is advanced through the window created

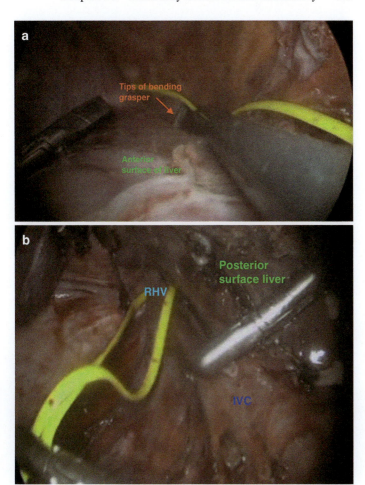

FIGURE 37.17 (**a**) The liver is allowed to fall back into place, and the tips of the bending grasper can be seen across the anterior surface of the liver. A vessel loop is fed to this grasper. (**b**) The vessel loop is fully around the RHV as seen here from the undersurface of the liver. The vessel loop helps to guide the stapler across the vein

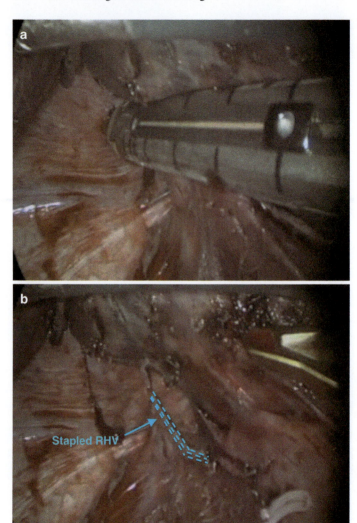

FIGURE 37.18 (**a**) The RHV is stapled from the undersurface of the liver. (**b**) The RHV stapled and transected. Highlighted is the distal end of the RHV on the IVC

Parenchymal Transection

Large caliber, figure of eight, stay stitches are placed on either side of the line of parenchymal transection, which should also be the "line of demarcation" that appears after inflow has been ligated. These stitches help retract the liver. The line of transection is defined using hook cautery. Ultrasound is repeated to ensure that the pathology is included within the resection specimen. The parenchyma is coagulated, and ducts/vessels are controlled with ties, clips, or staples, as appropriate. The specimen is placed in a specimen bag and removed from the abdominal cavity. Hemostasis is ensured at the resection bed, and the falciform ligament is tacked to the diaphragm.

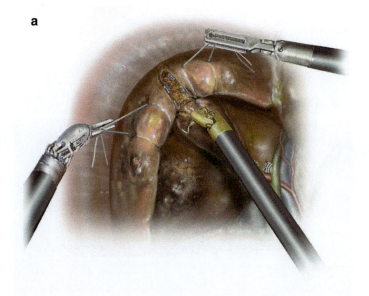

a

FIGURE 37.19 (a) Illustration of large, absorbable stitches placed on both sides of the transection line. (b) Large, absorbable stitches are placed on either side of the line of demarcation. (c) After complete parenchymal transection, specimen is placed in a specimen bag and retrieved from the abdominal cavity

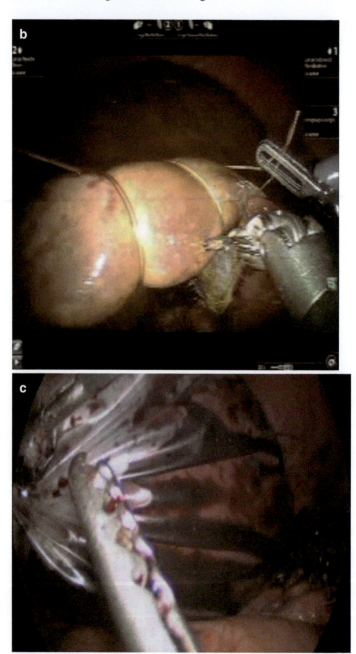

FIGURE 37.19 (continued)

Left Hepatectomy

Step 1

The room is set up similar to right hepatectomy, ports are placed, the patient is positioned in reverse Trendelenberg position with the left side slightly up.

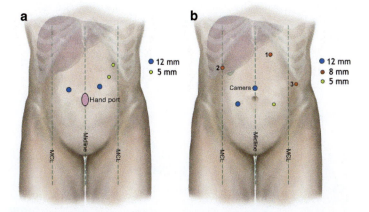

FIGURE 37.20 (**a**) Illustration of port placement for hand-assisted laparoscopic left hepatectomy. Note that for pure laparoscopic left hepatectomy, the hand-port can be switched for a 10–12 assist port. (**b**) Port placement for robotic assisted left hepatectomy

Step 2

Laparoscopic dissection of ligamentous attachments of the liver.

The round and falciform ligaments are divided to expose the anterior surface of the hepatic veins (Refer to pictures from Step 3 Right hepatectomy). The left triangular and coronary ligaments are dissected with a cautery or sealing device up to the left hepatic vein. The left hepatic vein can be identified by following the left phrenic vein along the diaphragm to its junction with the left hepatic vein. Note that the left and middle hepatic veins join a common trunk before entering the inferior vena cava 95 % of the time.

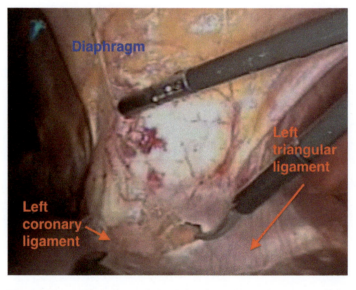

FIGURE 37.21 Dissection of the left triangular and coronary ligaments at the hepatic veins

Step 3

Ultrasound the liver, map the lesion(s).

Step 4

If using robotic technology, the robot is docked now. Robotic instruments, including the robotic camera, are introduced into the abdominal cavity.

Step 5

The left liver is retracted anteriorly with a closed grasper, and the undersurface of the left liver is exposed. The gastrohepatic ligament is divided close to the left lateral segments and caudate lobe using cautery while a grasper is used to retract. If a replaced left hepatic artery is present, it is isolated and divided.

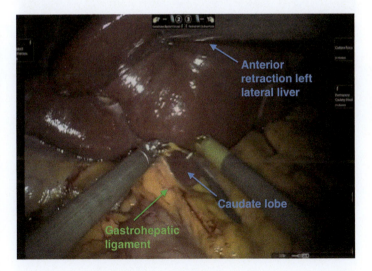

FIGURE 37.22 The left liver is retracted anteriorly, and the gastrohepatic ligament is dissected open with cautery

Step 6. Inflow Dissection

(a) Lower the hilar plate

The left liver at the base of the falciform is retracted anteriorly using a closed grasper. Cautery is used to dissect tissue overlying left portal structures at the base of the falciform. Assistance can be given via additional ports as necessary.

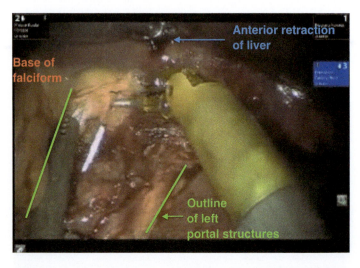

FIGURE 37.23 The hilar plate is lowered at the base of the falciform ligament, and the left portal structures are exposed

(b) Isolate, ligate, and divide the left hepatic artery.

  The left hepatic artery is identified and dissected to completely isolate the vessel. This includes tissue posterior to it. It is ligated and then transected. A stapling device can be used as space allows.

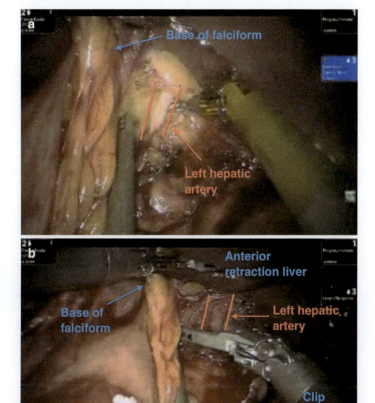

FIGURE 37.24 (**a**) Identification of the left hepatic artery (LHA). (**b**) Ligation of the LHA

(c) Isolate, ligate, and divide left portal vein (LPV).

The LPV sits deep to the left hepatic artery. It is exposed after transection of the LHA. A grasper grasps the ligamentum teres to retract the liver anteriorly, and another grasper is used to retract portal tissue. The vein is fully exposed by dissecting tissue around it with a cautery device. Once the left portal vein is further defined, a silk tie or vessel loop is placed around it for this to be used to retract and expose the full length of the vein. It can then be ligated and divided using a vascular load, roticulating stapler. Alternatively, the vein can be controlled using a tie and suture ligature of non-absorbable material on the proximal vein and a tie or clip on the distal vein – it is then divided.

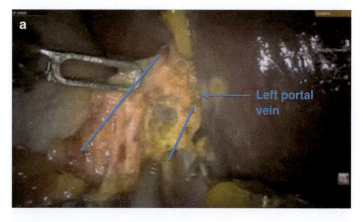

FIGURE 37.25 (**a**) Retraction of tissue overlying the LPV. (**b**) Tissue surrounding the LPV is dissected with a cautery device. (**c**) The LPV is fully exposed. A dissector is seen around the posterior surface of the vein. (**d**) A vessel loop is placed around the LPV

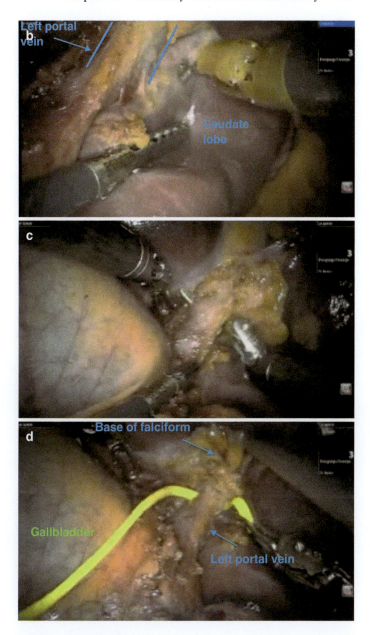

FIGURE 37.25 (continued)

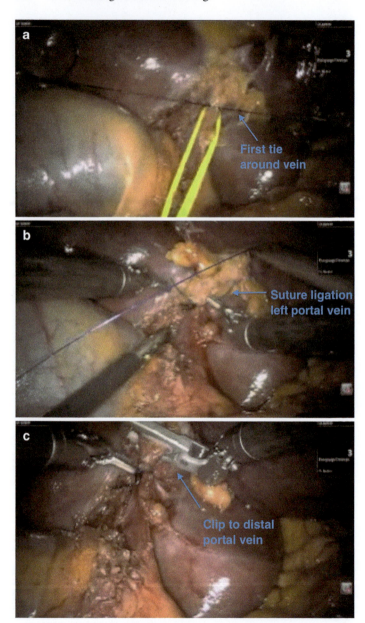

FIGURE 37.26 (**a**) Tie around the proximal LPV. (**b**) Suture ligation of the proximal LPV. (**c**) Clip to the distal LPV. (**d**) The LPV is divided with shears

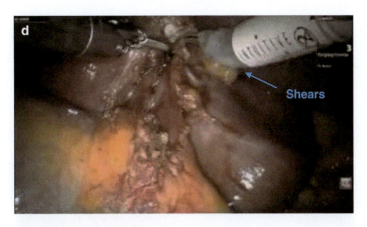

FIGURE 37.26 (continued)

(d) Isolate, ligate, and divide the left hepatic duct (LHD).

The LHD can be isolated and divided in an extra or intrahepatic manner depending on what is needed. After isolating the duct with dissection, the duct is tied and clipped distally and transected proximally, identifying bile from the proximal duct (as with right hepatectomy described previously in this chapter). The proximal end can be clipped to maintain a clean field during the remainder of the case.

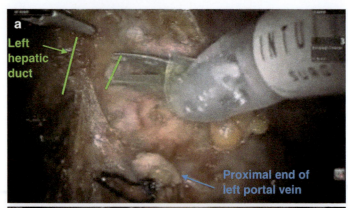

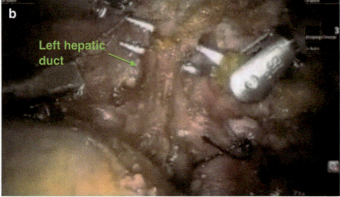

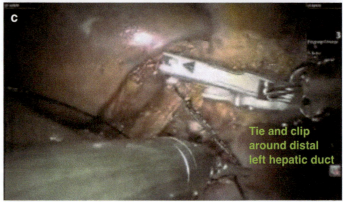

FIGURE 37.27 (**a**) The LHD is identified and dissected. (**b**) The LHD is further dissected. (**c**) A tie and clip are placed around the distal LHD. (**d**) The proximal duct is cut with shears

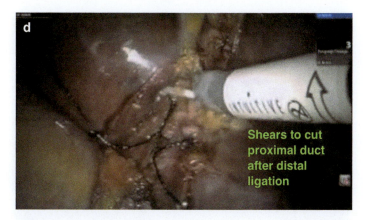

Figure 37.27 (continued)

Step 7. Outflow Dissection

If isolating the left hepatic vein in an extrahepatic manner, outflow dissection is performed now. The left and middle hepatic veins join at a common trunk in 95 % of patients. This trunk is first dissected from the anterior surface of the liver. The left liver is then retracted anteriorly, and the left/middle hepatic vein trunk is further dissected. A vessel loop is placed around this vein to help direct a vascular load, roticulating stapler across the vein. The vessel loop is removed, and the vein is then ligated and divided with the stapling device. Alternatively, the left hepatic vein is isolated and ligated within hepatic parenchyma during the last parts of the parenchymal dissection.

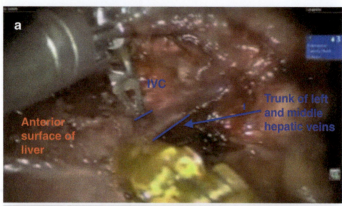

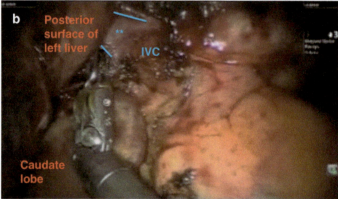

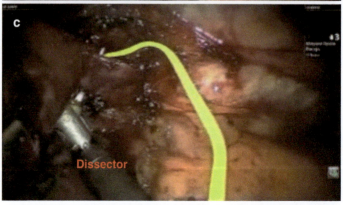

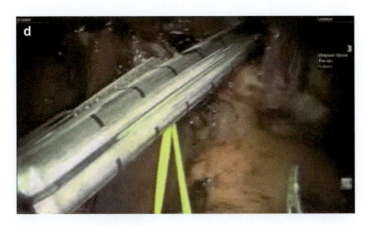

FIGURE 37.28 (continued)

FIGURE 37.28 (**a**) The trunk of the left and middle hepatic veins is visualized anteriorly. A dissector is used to dissect the space between this vein and the IVC. (**b**) The trunk of the left and middle hepatic veins is visualized along the posterior surface of the liver (indicated by **). The posterior surface of the liver is retracted anteriorly, and the plane around the LHV/MHV trunk is developed further. (**c**) A dissector is demonstrated around the left/middle hepatic vein trunk, and a vessel loop is fed. (**d**) The vessel loop helps direct a vascular load roticulating stapler across the vein trunk

Step 8. Parenchymal Transection

The line of transection is defined using hook cautery, following the line of demarcation on the liver's anterior surface. Ultrasound is repeated to ensure that the pathology is included within the resection specimen. Heavy figure of eight stitches are placed on either side of the line of transection, and these are retracted to either side (as in right hepatectomy). The parenchyma is then coagulated and divided using cautery and/or a sealing device and placing clips when needed. Note that if the caudate lobe is to be resected during left hepatectomy, additional dissection of portal and systemic venous tributaries should be performed. In this demonstration, the caudate lobe remains *in situ*. The specimen is collected in a bag, and hemostasis is ensured. The falciform ligament does not need to be tacked to the diaphragm.

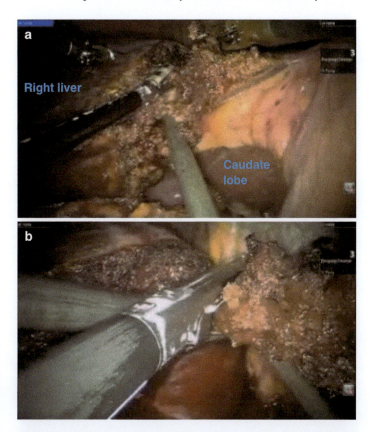

FIGURE 37.29 (**a**, **b**) If the left hepatic vein is isolated intrahepatically, a vascular load stapler that can crush tissue well is used to ligate and divide the LHV at the end of the parenchymal dissection

Left Lateral Segmentectomy

Patient positioning and port placement is the same as left hepatectomy. When ready for parenchymal transection, the line of transection is defined to the left of the falciform ligament to include only the pedicles of segments II and III (transecting to the right of the falciform disrupts the pedicles for segments IVa and IVb). Ultrasound is repeated. With appropriate retraction, the parenchyma is then coagulated and divided using a sealing device. The pedicles to segments III and II are ligated with the sealing device, ties, or a stapling device as appropriate. A roticulating, vascular load stapler is used via the 12 mm port to control the left hepatic vein as it is encountered intrahepatically. Specimen is removed from the abdominal cavity, hemostasis is ensured.

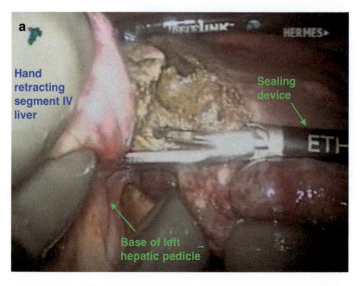

FIGURE 37.30 (**a**) Control of hepatic parenchyma and pedicles of segments III and II with sealing device. Hand is used to retract the liver laterally. (**b**) LHV is controlled intrahepatically with a stapling device

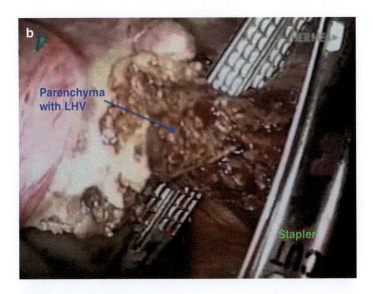

FIGURE 37.30 (continued)

Wedge Hepatectomy

Optimal port placement varies dependent on where the lesion is. Ligamentous attachments are taken down as necessary. Laparoscopic ultrasound is performed prior to resecting the lesion to ensure that the specimen can be removed in its entirety by wedge resection. If using a robotic system, the robot is docked, and instruments are placed in the abdominal cavity. The circumference of resection is defined with hook cautery according to what is appropriate by surgical or oncologic guidelines. Ultrasound can be used to guide this. A heavy, absorbable figure of eight stitch is placed along the line of transection, and this is retracted to allow for exposure. The parenchyma is coagulated and divided, placing clips when appropriate, delivering the lesion out of the liver bed. The specimen is placed in a laparoscopic specimen bag, hemostasis is ensured, and the specimen is removed. The robot is undocked. Laparoscopic equipment is used to close fascia and remove ports under direct visualization. Skin is closed.

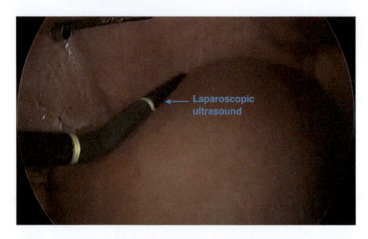

FIGURE 37.31 Laparoscopic ultrasound is performed

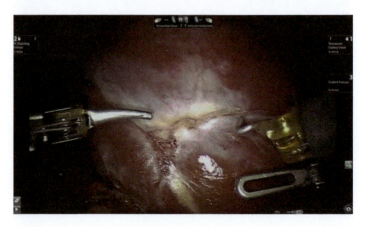

FIGURE 37.32 Robotic is docked, and robotic instruments are introduced

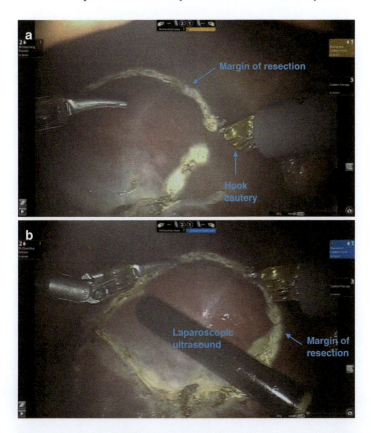

FIGURE 37.33 (**a**) Cautery is used to define the line of parenchymal dissection. (**b**) Ultrasound can be helpful to draw this line, ensuring that the whole of the lesion is included

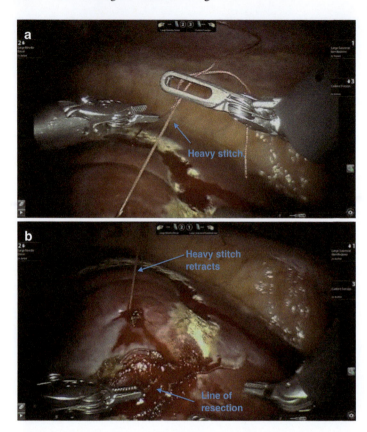

FIGURE 37.34 (**a**) Figure of eight stitch is placed along the line of transection. (**b**) Stitch placed is used to aide in retraction during dissection

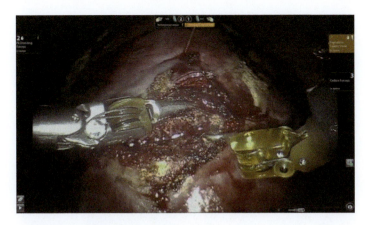

FIGURE 37.35 Parenchyma is dissected

Portal Lymphadenectomy

Portal lymphadenectomy is usually performed as part of treatment for gallbladder cancer or for cholangiocarcinoma.

Step 1.

Ports Are Placed

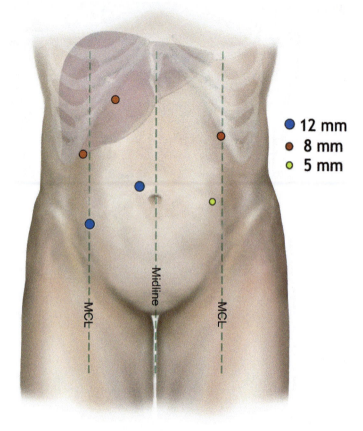

FIGURE 37.36 Port placement for robotic assisted portal lymphade-nectomy. For laparoscopic approach, please refer to port illustration for right hepatectomy

Step 2

Identification of porta hepatis, Kocher maneuver, exposure posterolateral porta hepatis.

The porta is identified after the gallbladder is grasped and retracted anterolaterally. Kocher maneuver is performed to expose the posterolateral portion of the porta hepatis. With the porta hepatis rotated/retracted anteromedially, the retro-portal space is exposed. Care should be taken to identify and prevent injury to the inferior vena cava, which runs just posterior to the porta.

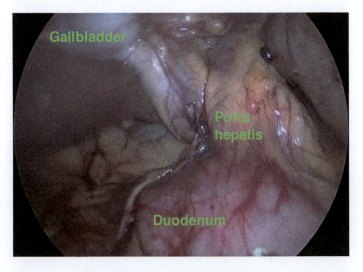

FIGURE 37.37 Identification of the porta hepatis

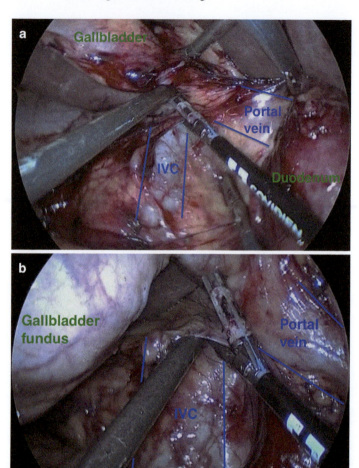

FIGURE 37.38 (**a**) Exposure of the posterolateral portion of the porta hepatis. The IVC rests behind the porta and injury should be avoided. (**b**) Tissue between the porta and IVC is further dissected

Step 3

Portal lymphatic tissue is dissected.

After releasing the porta to its natural position and starting at the anterior surface of the porta hepatis, the adventitial and nodal tissue is dissected using cautery or a sealing device. Tissue on the anterior, posterior (portocaval nodes), and lateral surfaces of the porta should be taken. The right gastric artery is ligated to aid in this dissection. Consideration of the portal anatomy is taken. Aberrant anatomy should be recognized preoperatively (such as a replaced or accessory right or left hepatic artery) based on imaging; however, a surgeon should be on the lookout for aberrant anatomy even if it is not suspected preoperatively.

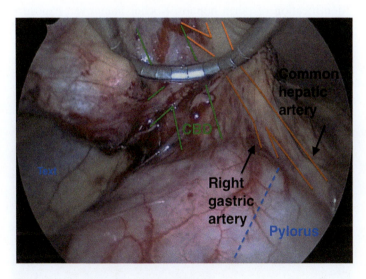

FIGURE 37.39 Anatomy of porta hepatis

Extrahepatic Bile Duct Resection

Cases of minimally invasive extrahepatic bile duct surgery have been reported – these cases have been reported as solely bile duct cases or in the setting of cases involving the liver, gallbladder, or pancreas [33–42].

Step 1

Positioning and port placement is similar to that for portal lymphadenectomy.

Step 2

Identification of porta hepatis, Kocher maneuver, exposure posterolateral porta hepatis. This is performed as with portal lymphadenectomy. Tissue overlying the porta hepatis is dissected using cautery or a sealing device. If the gallbladder remains in situ, the cystic duct can be dissected, ligated, and divided just at its entry to the common bile duct. Portal anatomy is exposed with dissection.

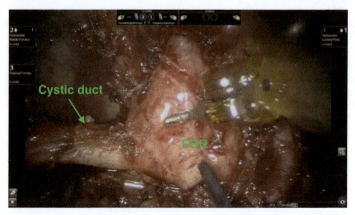

FIGURE 37.40 Cystic duct entering the lateral wall of the common bile duct

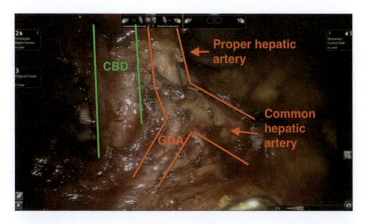

FIGURE 37.41 Exposure of distal portal anatomy. *GDA* gastroduodenal artery

Step 3

Dissection of the common bile duct.

The common bile duct is dissected up to its bifurcation at the base of the liver using cautery or a sealing device. Note that, as the most posterior structure of the porta hepatis, the portal vein can be seen behind the common bile duct as the common bile duct is dissected. A vessel loop can be placed around the fully dissected common bile duct for exposure before transection.

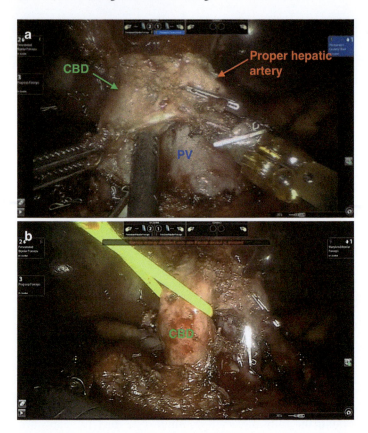

FIGURE 37.42 (a) Dissection of tissue between the common bile duct and proper hepatic artery exposes the portal vein posteriorly. (b) Vessel loop around the common bile duct

Step 4

Roux en Y hepaticojejunostomy.

Roux en Y hepaticojejunostomy with the common hepatic duct is created using either a running or interrupted absorbable stitch.

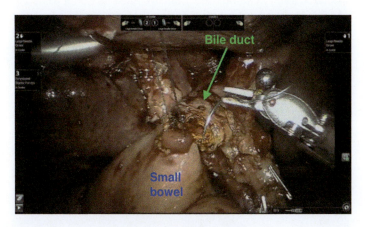

Figure 37.43 Creation of hepaticojejunostomy

Hepatic Cyst Unroofing

Ports are placed based on location of the cyst(s) to be treated. Adhesions to the cyst are dissected free, if present. The cyst is intentionally ruptured in a controlled manner with a suction catheter used to suction the fluid.

The cyst is then unroofed using either a sealing device or a stapler. Cautery can be used, but care must be taken to detect small bile ducts potentially tracking through a thin layer of liver that may overly the wall of the cyst. The excised cyst wall is sent for pathologic evaluation – a cystadenoma warrants complete cyst resection of the cyst and adjacent liver because of its malignant potential.

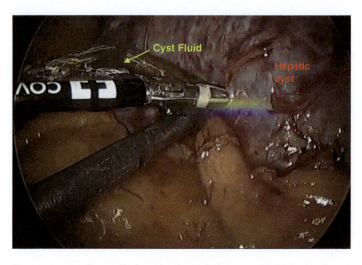

FIGURE 37.44 Controlled aspiration of the cyst. Fluid is suctioned after creation of a defect in the cyst wall

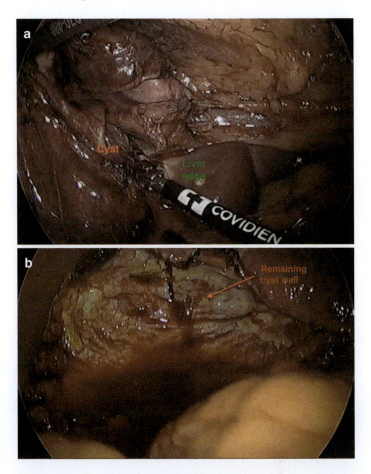

FIGURE 37.45 (**a**) Collapsed cyst wall is unroofed. (**b**) The inside of the remaining cyst wall is inspected for bleeding or bile leak

Acknowledgments Illustrations used with kind permission from Randal S. McKenzie/McKenzie Illustrations.

References

1. Cai XJ, Yang J, Yu H, Liang X, Wang YF, Zhu ZY, et al. Clinical study of laparoscopic versus open hepatectomy for malignant liver tumors. Surg Endosc. 2008;22(11):2350–6.
2. Koffron AJ, Auffenberg G, Kung R, Abecassis M. Evaluation of 300 minimally invasive liver resections at a single institution: less is more. Ann Surg. 2007;246(3):385–92. discussion 392–4.
3. Nguyen KT, Gamblin TC, Geller DA. World review of laparoscopic liver resection-2,804 patients. Ann Surg. 2009;250(5):831–41.
4. Koffron AJ, Kung RD, Auffenberg GB, Abecassis MM. Laparoscopic liver surgery for everyone: the hybrid method. Surgery. 2007;142(4):463–8; discussion 468.e1–2.
5. Nitta H, Sasaki A, Fujita T, Itabashi H, Hoshikawa K, Takahara T, et al. Laparoscopy-assisted major liver resections employing a hanging technique: the original procedure. Ann Surg. 2010;251(3):450–3.
6. Kitisin K, Packiam V, Bartlett DL, Tsung A. A current update on the evolution of robotic liver surgery. Minerva Chir. 2011;66(4):281–93.
7. Reynolds Jr W. The first laparoscopic cholecystectomy. JSLS J Soc Laparoendosc Surg. 2001;5(1):89–94.
8. Velanovich V. Laparoscopic vs open surgery: a preliminary comparison of quality-of-life outcomes. Surg Endosc. 2000;14(1):16–21.
9. McIntyre Jr RC, Zoeter MA, Weil KC, Cohen MM. A comparison of outcome and cost of open vs. laparoscopic cholecystectomy. J Laparoendosc Surg. 1992;2(3):143–8; discussion 149.
10. Barkun JS, Barkun AN, Sampalis JS, Fried G, Taylor B, Wexler MJ, et al. Randomised controlled trial of laparoscopic versus mini cholecystectomy. The McGill Gallstone Treatment Group. Lancet. 1992;340(8828):1116–9.
11. Langenbuch D. Ein fall von resektion eines linksseitigen schnurlappens der leber. Heilung Berl Klin Wochenschr. 1888;25:37–8.
12. Couinaud C, editor. Etudes anatomiques et chirurgales. Paris: Masson; 1957.

13. Cantlie J. On a new arrangement of the right and left lobes of the liver. J Anat Physiol. 1897;32:iv–x.
14. Hjortsjo CH. The topography of the intrahepatic duct systems. Acta Anat (Basel). 1951;11(4):599–615.
15. McIndoe AHCV. The bilaterality of the liver. Arch Surg. 1927;15:589–612.
16. Fortner JG, Shiu MH, Kinne DW, Kim DK, Castro EB, Watson RC, et al. Major hepatic resection using vascular isolation and hypothermic perfusion. Ann Surg. 1974;180(4):644–52.
17. Huguet C, Nordlinger B, Bloch P, Conard J. Tolerance of the human liver to prolonged normothermic ischemia. A biological study of 20 patients submitted to extensive hepatectomy. Arch Surg. 1978;113(12):1448–51.
18. Huguet C, Nordlinger B, Galopin JJ, Bloch P, Gallot D. Normothermic hepatic vascular exclusion for extensive hepatectomy. Surg Gynecol Obstet. 1978;147(5):689–93.
19. Kousnetzoff MPJ. Sur la resection partielle du foie. Rev Chir. 1896;16:954–92.
20. Melendez JA, Arslan V, Fischer ME, Wuest D, Jarnagin WR, Fong Y, et al. Perioperative outcomes of major hepatic resections under low central venous pressure anesthesia: blood loss, blood transfusion, and the risk of postoperative renal dysfunction. J Am Coll Surg. 1998;187(6):620–5.
21. Pringle JH. V. Notes on the arrest of hepatic hemorrhage due to trauma. Ann Surg. 1908;48(4):541–9.
22. Bismuth H, Castaing D, Garden OJ. The use of operative ultrasound in surgery of primary liver tumors. World J Surg. 1987;11(5):610–4.
23. Castaing D, Kunstlinger F, Habib N, Bismuth H. Intraoperative ultrasonographic study of the liver. Methods and anatomic results. Am J Surg. 1985;149(5):676–82.
24. Fong Y, Blumgart LH. Useful stapling techniques in liver surgery. J Am Coll Surg. 1997;185(1):93–100.
25. Geller DA, Tsung A, Maheshwari V, Rutstein LA, Fung JJ, Marsh JW. Hepatic resection in 170 patients using saline-cooled radiofrequency coagulation. HPB (Oxford). 2005;7(3):208–13.
26. Saiura A, Yamamoto J, Koga R, Sakamoto Y, Kokudo N, Seki M, et al. Usefulness of LigaSure for liver resection: analysis by randomized clinical trial. Am J Surg. 2006;192(1):41–5.
27. Weber JC, Navarra G, Jiao LR, Nicholls JP, Jensen SL, Habib NA. New technique for liver resection using heat coagulative necrosis. Ann Surg. 2002;236(5):560–3.

28. Belghiti J, Hiramatsu K, Benoist S, Massault P, Sauvanet A, Farges O. Seven hundred forty-seven hepatectomies in the 1990s: an update to evaluate the actual risk of liver resection. J Am Coll Surg. 2000;191(1):38–46.

29. Dimick JB, Pronovost PJ, Cowan Jr JA, Lipsett PA. Postoperative complication rates after hepatic resection in Maryland hospitals. Arch Surg. 2003;138(1):41–6.

30. Jarnagin WR, Gonen M, Fong Y, DeMatteo RP, Ben-Porat L, Little S, et al. Improvement in perioperative outcome after hepatic resection: analysis of 1,803 consecutive cases over the past decade. Ann Surg. 2002;236(4):397–406; discussion 406–7.

31. Wakabayashi G, Sasaki A, Nishizuka S, Furukawa T, Kitajima M. Our initial experience with robotic hepato-biliary-pancreatic surgery. J Hepatobiliary Pancreat Sci. 2011;18(4):481–7.

32. Tsung A, Geller DA, Sukato DC, Sabbaghian S, Tohme S, Steel J, et al. Robotic versus laparoscopic hepatectomy: a matched comparison. Ann Surg. 2014;259:549–55.

33. Alkhamesi NA, Davies WT, Pinto RF, Schlachta CM. Robot-assisted common bile duct exploration as an option for complex choledocholithiasis. Surg Endosc. 2013;27(1):263–6.

34. Giulianotti PC, Coratti A, Angelini M, Sbrana F, Cecconi S, Balestracci T, et al. Robotics in general surgery: personal experience in a large community hospital. Arch Surg. 2003;138(7):777–84.

35. Ji WB, Zhao ZM, Dong JH, Wang HG, Lu F, Lu HW. One-stage robotic-assisted laparoscopic cholecystectomy and common bile duct exploration with primary closure in 5 patients. Surg Laparosc Endosc Percutan Tech. 2011;21(2):123–6.

36. Tung KL, Tang CN, Lai EC, Yang GP, Chan OC, Li MK. Robot-assisted laparoscopic approach of management for Mirizzi syndrome. Surg Laparosc Endosc Percutan Tech. 2013;23(1):e17–21.

37. Wang Z, Liu Q, Chen J, Duan W, Zhou N. Da Vinci robot-assisted anatomic left hemihepatectomy and biliary reconstruction. Surg Laparosc Endosc Percutan Tech. 2013;23(3):e89.

38. Giulianotti PC, Sbrana F, Bianco FM, Addeo P. Robot-assisted laparoscopic extended right hepatectomy with biliary reconstruction. J Laparoendosc Adv Surg Tech A. 2010;20(2):159–63.

39. Zureikat AH, Moser AJ, Boone BA, Bartlett DL, Zenati M, Zeh 3rd HJ. 250 robotic pancreatic resections: safety and feasibility. Ann Surg. 2013;258(4):554–62.

40. Roeyen G, Chapelle T, Ysebaert D. Robot-assisted choledo-chotomy: feasibility. Surg Endosc. 2004;18(1):165–6.
41. Li S, Wang W, Yu Z, Xu W. Laparoscopically assisted extrahe-patic bile duct excision with ductoplasty and a widened hepati-cojejunostomy for complicated hepatobiliary dilatation. Pediatr Surg Int. 2014;30(6):593–8.
42. Tian Y, Wu SD, Zhu AD, Chen DX. Management of type I cho-ledochal cyst in adult: totally laparoscopic resection and Roux-en-Y hepaticoenterostomy. J Gastrointest Surg. 2010;14(9):1381–8.

Part IX
Pancreatic Surgery

Emily Winslow

Chapter 38
Pancreaticoduodenectomy (Whipple Procedure)

Scott N. Pinchot and Sharon M. Weber

Abstract Pancreaticoduodenectomy is the treatment of choice of pancreas head lesions, and can be performed as a pylorus-sparing or standard (pylorus resecting) operation. This complex operation is fraught with a high rate of complications, and mortality increases in lower-volume hospitals and is best performed by an experienced team.

Keywords Pancreas resection • Pancreas cancer

Indications

Carcinoma of the exocrine pancreas affects nearly 38,000 people in the United States each year and results in 35,000 deaths annually, making it the fifth leading cause of cancer-related death in this country each year [1]. Ductal adenocarcinoma and

S.N. Pinchot (✉)
Department of Surgery, Northwest Community Healthcare,
Arlington Heights, IL, USA
e-mail: S1pinchot@nchmedicalgroup.com

S.M. Weber
Department of Surgery, University of Wisconsin,
Madison, WI, USA

H. Chen (ed.), *Illustrative Handbook of General Surgery*,
DOI 10.1007/978-3-319-24557-7_38,
© Springer International Publishing Switzerland 2016

its variants account for 80–90 % of all pancreatic neoplasms and for an even greater fraction of malignant pancreatic lesions. The remaining 10–20 % of pancreatic neoplasms include other tumors of the exocrine pancreas (e.g., serous cystadenomas, mucinous cystadenomas), acinar cell cancers, and pancreatic neuroendocrine tumors (e.g., insulinomas, gastrinomas). As tumors of the head, neck, and uncinate process of the pancreas account for about 70 % of pancreatic tumors, pancreaticoduodenectomy (PD), with or without preservation of the pylorus and proximal duodenum, remains the recommended treatment for patients with periampullary adenocarcinomas arising in the head of the pancreas, the ampulla, the distal common bile duct, or the duodenum. Recently, indications for PD have been extended to include intraductal papillary mucinous neoplasms arising in the head of the pancreas [2, 3] and periampullary tumors invading the mesenteric-portal vein [4, 5]. Nevertheless, PD continues to be an extensive operation with a postoperative mortality rate of less than 5 % but a high morbidity rate of close to 40 %, even in recent series [6, 7].

Perioperative Care

Preoperative Preparation

Preoperative cardiac clearance should be performed in all patients with a history of uncontrolled hypertension, coronary artery disease, previous coronary artery bypass grafting, or an abnormal preoperative electrocardiogram. Every attempt at normalizing electrolyte levels and renal function, as shown by creatinine and blood urea nitrogen, in the preoperative setting should be made. A Foley urinary catheter and nasogastric tube should be inserted to closely monitor fluid status. Administration of preoperative antibiotic prophylaxis is appropriate, as icteric patients and those patients receiving preoperative biliary drainage procedures have been shown to have higher rates of bacterial contamination of the bile and a higher rate of postoperative infectious complications following PD [8].

Positioning and Anesthesia

The patient is placed supine on a standard operating table. General anesthesia with endotracheal intubation is utilized.

Description of the Procedure

Pancreaticoduodenectomy (Whipple Procedure)

PD with hemigastrectomy (standard PD) has long been the standard approach to malignant neoplasms arising in the periampullary region. The operative procedure may be performed through either a bilateral subcostal or an upper abdominal midline incision. While the upper midline incision extending inferiorly below the umbilicus is useful, more extensive and free visualization of the upper abdomen may be afforded by the oblique or curved incision paralleling the costal margins. Regardless of the incision used, care must be taken to maintain meticulous hemostasis by carefully clamping and tying all bleeding points, especially in the jaundiced patient. After making the skin incision, the rectus muscles are slowly transected with bipolar electrocautery Fig. 38.1. Once the abdomen is entered, curved clamps may be utilized to assist ligation and division of the round ligament. Division of the falciform ligament superior to the dome of the liver may assist with further hepatic mobility.

Before irreversible steps are taken, a thorough exploration of the abdomen must be carried out to determine the location and extent of the pathologic process and to detect any evidence of tumor spread outside the limits of resection. The liver and all serosal surfaces should be carefully examined for metastatic spread or peritoneal dissemination. In addition, metastatic spread to the periportal and celiac axis lymph nodes, the root of the transverse mesocolon, the region above the pancreas, and the hepatoduodenal ligament should be sought by careful examination. The discovery of involved peripancreatic lymph nodes, even along the cephalad border of the pancreas near the portal vein, does not preclude resec-

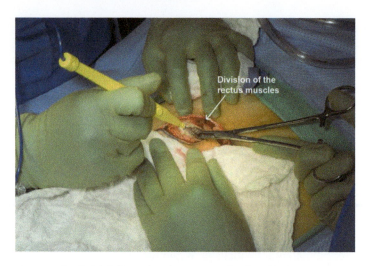

FIGURE 38.1 Initial dissection for pancreaticoduodenectomy. A curvilinear, subcostal incision is first carried out over the right upper quadrant and is subsequently extended across the midline as far as is necessary for adequate surgical exposure. Excessive care must be taken to maintain meticulous hemostasis, especially in the jaundiced patient. After making the skin incision, the rectus muscles are carefully transected with bipolar electrocautery (shown above)

tion, although it worsens prognosis [9]. Ultrasound may be helpful in ruling out metastatic spread to the liver.

Once disseminated disease has been ruled out, the surgeon proceeds with mobilization of the duodenum and head of the pancreas by the Kocher maneuver. Dissection of the lateral peritoneal attachments of the duodenum, which facilitates inspection of the duodenum, head of the pancreas, and periampullary tumor is usually bloodless; an avascular cleavage plane can be easily developed as the posterior wall of the pancreas is bluntly separated from the underlying vena cava and right kidney. Extensive kocherization should be performed to allow the surgeon to be comfortable that there is no extension of tumor beyond the uncinate process. Special care should be taken to identify and preserve the right

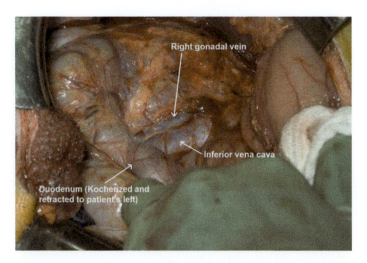

FIGURE 38.2 Relationship of retroperitoneal structures encountered in the early stages of pancreaticoduodenectomy (Picture taken from patients left side). Once disseminated disease has been ruled out, the surgeon may proceed with mobilization of the duodenum and head of the pancreas by the Kocher maneuver. With adequate duodenal mobilization, the surgeon should identify and preserve the right gonadal vein, which arises from and often runs parallel to the inferior vena cava at this point in the retroperitoneal dissection

gonadal vein, which often runs parallel to the inferior vena cava at this point in the retroperitoneal dissection Fig. 38.2. Further mobilization of the second and third portion of the duodenum is carried out to adequately determine resectability of the lesion.

Before concluding that the lesion is resectable, the lesser sac must be entered to facilitate visualization and mobilization of the pancreas. The greater omentum is retracted upward and the gastrocolic ligament is incised all the way to the splenic flexure, allowing entry into the lesser sac. The right gastroepiploic artery and vein are identified and a thorough evaluation of potential metastases above the pancreas and adjacent to the celiac axis lymph nodes should be performed. The middle colic vein with its origin at the supe-

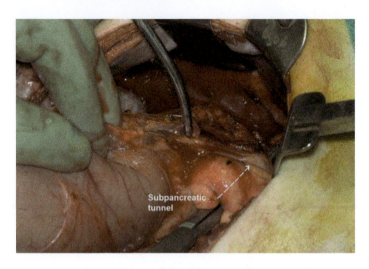

FIGURE 38.3 Development of the subpancreatic tunnel. The peritoneal attachments at the inferior border of the pancreas are incised
and a cleavage plane over the superior mesenteric vein and behind
the pancreas (the so-called "tunnel of love") is developed.
Development of the subpancreatic tunnel allows the surgeon to dissect posterior to the pancreatic neck and separate the tissues from
the underlying portal vein. It is vital that the portal vein be identified at this portion of the case to be certain it is not involved with
tumor. Note the clamp is behind the pancreas, over the SMV/PV

rior mesenteric vein should be identified and confirmed to be
free of tumor involvement. The peritoneal attachments at the
inferior border of the pancreas are incised and a cleavage
plane over the superior mesenteric vein and behind the pancreas (the so-called "tunnel of love") is developed Fig. 38.3.
Development of the subpancreatic tunnel will permit the
surgeon to continue dissecting behind the pancreas and over
the portal vein, to be certain it is not involved with tumor.

After the tumor is deemed resectable, irreversible steps
can be taken. The gallbladder should be removed to prevent
late complications from gallstone formation. Using electrocautery, the gallbladder is carefully dissected from the hepatic
fossa. Meticulous hemostasis, especially in the jaundiced

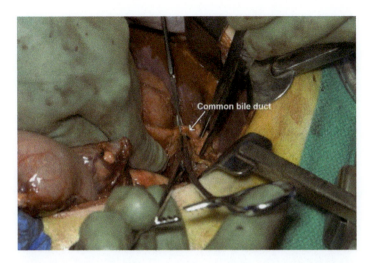

FIGURE 38.4 Identification and division of the common bile duct. The gallbladder should be removed to prevent late complications from gallstone formation. Using electrocautery, the gallbladder is carefully dissected from the hepatic fossa. Meticulous hemostasis, especially in the jaundiced patient, should be maintained within the liver bed. The cystic artery is identified, doubly clipped, and transected. Dissection should continue down the common bile duct, transecting it above the cystic duct

patient, should be maintained within the liver bed. The cystic artery is identified, doubly clipped, and transected. Dissection should continue to the common bile duct where it is encircled with a vessel loop for subsequent transection (Fig. 38.4). The surgeon then proceeds to ligate the blood supply necessary for antrectomy. The right gastric artery is identified, ligated with 2-0 silk sutures, and subsequently transected. Next, the gastroduodenal artery (GDA), passing inferiorly from the hepatic artery at the point where the portal vein passes posterior to the pancreas, should be suture ligated with 4-0 Prolene sutures. Just before ligating and dividing the GDA, the vessel should be occluded with a vessel loop or bulldog clamp to ensure adequacy of the hepatic artery pulse. At this point, important anatomic anomalies such as a replaced right hepatic artery originating from the superior mesenteric artery (SMA) or a replaced common hepatic artery off the SMA, should be evaluated by palpating for an arterial pulse behind the common bile duct through the foramen of Winslow. Following this, the right gastroepiploic vessels are ligated and tied.

The removal of the antrum greatly assists in the subsequent exposure of the more difficult portion of the resection. After an area is cleared on both the greater and lesser curvature of the stomach, an antrectomy is performed using a GIA stapler. Once the stomach is transected, the remainder of the resection is carried out. The common hepatic duct is sharply transected just above the cystic duct. This not only allows the surgeon to perform a hepaticojejunostomy during the reconstructive phase of the procedure but also allows him or her to adequately visualize the portal vein. Attention is now directed toward mobilization of the upper jejunum. The transverse colon is flipped superiorly, allowing for adequate visualization of the jejunum and its mesentery. The upper jejunum may be grasped with Babcock forceps and the bowel held up in order to adequately visualize the vascular arcades supplying the jejunum. The ligament of Treitz, in its avascular plane, is taken down with cautery Fig. 38.5. Utilizing incisions made in the avascular portions of the mesentery, the jejunum is divided with a GIA stapler. The jejunal arcades are divided and ligated to facilitate mobilization of the upper jejunum. A small opening is made in the mesocolon underneath the SMV and the mobilized upper jejunum is passed through the retrocolic window.

At this point, the only structure holding the specimen within the abdomen should be the pancreatic neck, which is now carefully divided. A surgical clamp may be carefully passed through the subpancreatic tunnel to protect the underlying portal vein and SMV while transecting the pancreas. Silk stay sutures are placed at the medial and lateral borders of the inferior and superior pancreas. Using a sharp scalpel, the pancreatic neck is divided Fig. 38.6. Sizable vessels may be encountered just above the pancreatic duct and care must be taken to ensure meticulous hemostasis.

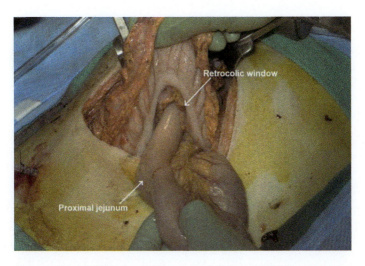

FIGURE 38.5 Mobilization of the upper jejunum. With the transverse colon flipped superiorly, the jejunum and its mesentery is clearly visualized. Utilizing incisions made in the avascular portions of the mesentery, the jejunum is divided with a GIA stapler. The jejunal arcades are divided and doubly ligated to facilitate mobilization of the upper jejunum. A small opening is made in the retrocolic mesocolon and the mobilized upper jejunum is passed through the window

Alternatively, if the pancreatic duct has been occluded by tumor and the gland is fibrotic, this division may be relatively bloodless. Should excessive bleeding be encountered, suture ligation with a 3-0 Vicryl suture is usually adequate to gain control of the offending blood vessel. The SMV and portal veins are then bluntly dissected off the uncinate process Fig. 38.7. Often, the superior pancreaticoduodenal vein, draining into the portal vein, and the first jejunal vein branch are encountered and must be doubly ligated and divided in order to remove the surgical specimen. The specimen, consisting of the gastric antrum, duodenum, proximal jejunum, gallbladder and distal biliary tree, and pancreatic head are then passed from the surgical field.

Attention is now turned to reconstructing gastrointestinal continuity. The jejunum, which has been passed into the lesser

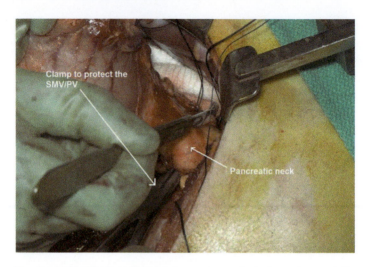

FIGURE 38.6 Dividing the pancreas. A surgical clamp is carefully passed through the subpancreatic tunnel to protect the underlying portal vein and SMV while transecting the pancreas. Silk stay sutures are placed at the medial and lateral borders of the inferior and superior pancreas. Using a sharp scalpel, the pancreatic neck is divided. Sizable vessels may be encountered just above the pancreatic duct and care must be taken to ensure meticulous hemostasis

sac through a retrocolic window, is allowed to lay in its usual fashion. The jejunal limb must be inspected to ensure adequate perfusion and the appropriate anastomotic sites for hepaticojejunostomy and pancreaticojejunostomy are identified. We typically perform the hepaticojejunostomy first, beginning with making a small enterotomy at least 5 cm distal to the proposed pancreaticojejunostomy site. The hepatic duct anastomosis is then carried out utilizing a single layer of 4-0 synthetic absorbable suture material placed in full-thickness fashion Fig. 38.8. Finally, the hepaticojejunostomy is inspected for leakage of biliary contents.

While the pancreaticojejunostomy may be performed in a variety of ways, all of which may be quite effective at reducing the incidence of pancreatic leaks, we prefer to invaginate the pancreatic remnant into the side of the jejunum using an

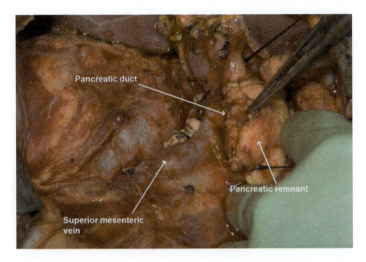

FIGURE 38.7 Anatomic relationships following pancreaticoduode-nectomy. Following transection of the pancreatic neck, the vascular structures deep to the proximal pancreas are evident

outer layer and a duct-to-mucosa anastomosis of the pancre-atic duct Fig. 38.9. This can be performed in many ways; the attached photographs document one technique for this anas-tomosis. Typically, we place a 10-French flat Jackson Pratt suction drain deep to the pancreatic and biliary anastomoses to monitor for a pancreatic or biliary leak. The jejunum, at the point in which it traverses the transverse mesocolon (retro-colic), may be secured to the mesocolon with 3-0 Vicryl suture to prevent undue traction on the above anastomoses.

Lastly, attention is turned to the final anastomosis consisting of an end-to-side gastrojejunostomy Fig. 38.10. To begin, the antecolic gastrojejunostomy is performed with an outer inter-rupted layer of 3-0 PDS placed in Lembert fashion. Once the outer posterior row of sutures has been placed and secured, a portion of the gastric staple line is excised and an appropriately-sized gastrotomy is made. The inner layer on the posterior row is a continuous suture of 3-0 synthetic absorbable suture mate-rial, which is subsequently continued onto the anterior row. The gastrojejunostomy is completed with an outer layer of inter-

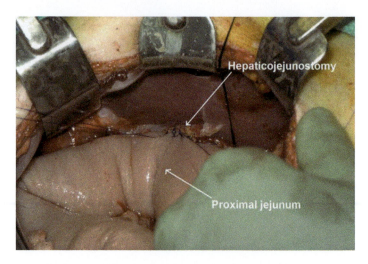

FIGURE 38.8 Completing the hepaticojejunostomy. When restoring gastrointestinal continuity, we typically perform the hepaticojejunostomy first, beginning with making a small enterotomy at least 5 cm distal to the proposed pancreaticojejunostomy site. The hepatic duct anastomosis is completed utilizing a single layer of 4-0 synthetic absorbable suture material placed in full-thickness fashion. Finally, the hepaticojejunostomy is inspected leakage of biliary contents

rupted 3-0 silk sutures at the anterior margin of the anastomosis. The surgeon should assess for patency and perfusion of the anastomosis at this point in the procedure.

Finally, the abdomen is irrigated and thoroughly inspected for hemostasis. The nasogastric tube should be flushed and secured in the appropriate position. The fascia is closed with a running #1 PDS suture in two layers. After irrigating the wound, the skin should be closed with surgical staples and the wound covered with a sterile surgical dressing.

Pylorus-Preserving Pancreaticoduodenectomy

The pylorus-preserving modification of the standard Whipple procedure has become the standard of care at many institutions. The procedure is nearly identical to PD with hemigas-

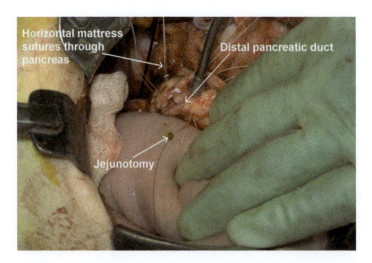

Figure 38.9 Performing the pancreaticojejunostomy. We prefer to invaginate the pancreatic remnant into the side of the jejunum. The duct-to-mucosa anastomosis is begun by placing an outer interrupted layer of horizontal mattress 3-0 Vicryl sutures through the posterior surface of the pancreas and then through the jejunum. A jejunotomy of the same size and adjacent to the pancreatic duct is then made. Then, to achieve the duct-to-mucosa anastomosis, interrupted 5-0 synthetic absorbable suture material is used as a posterior row of sutures passing from inside out on the pancreatic duct and outside in on the jejunal mucosa are placed. Once the posterior sutures are placed and secured, the anterior row of duct-to-mucosa sutures is placed. The outer anterior layer is then completed an using the preplaced 3-0 Vicryl horizontal mattress sutures, thus invaginating the pancreatic remnant and completing the anastomosis

trectomy; however, in this variation the antrum and pylorus are spared. To do this, the right gastric artery is spared. Rather than performing an antrectomy, the duodenum is transected 2–3 cm distal to the pylorus and is later anastomosed to the jejunal limb. Most often, the pylorus-preserving PD procedure is chosen for patients with benign disease (commonly chronic pancreatitis of the pancreatic head and/or neck) and is thought to portend a better long-term nutritional outcome, although prospective randomized trials have shown no difference in outcomes between standard and pylorus-preserving PD.

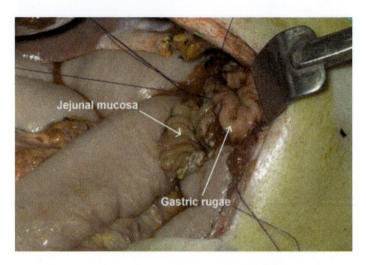

FIGURE 38.10 Antecolic gastrojejunostomy. The end-to-side gastro-jejunostomy is performed with an outer interrupted layer of 3-0 PDS placed in a Lembert fashion. Once the outer posterior row of sutures has been placed and secured, a portion of the gastric staple line is excised and an appropriately-sized gastrotomy is made. The inner layer on the posterior row is a continuous suture of 3-0 synthetic absorbable suture material, which is subsequently continued onto the anterior row. The gastrojejunostomy is completed with an outer layer of interrupted 3-0 silk sutures at the anterior margin of the anastomosis

Special Postoperative Considerations

Recent data have demonstrated rates of mortality of the order of 2–4 % for PD in the hands of experienced surgeons; unfortunately, postoperative morbidity continues to be much more significant [6, 7]. Delayed gastric emptying (DGE), anastomotic breakdown, marginal ulceration, intraabdominal abscess or infection, pancreatitis, and pancreatic leaks remain the common complications after PD. Accounting for the highest proportion of morbidity (15–40 %), delayed gastric emptying, while unpredictable, is thought to be related to the loss of motilin-secreting cells found throughout the duodenal mucosa. Anecdotal evidence supporting this theory is found in the favorable response rates seen in patients placed on erythromycin, an antibiotic with a similar structure to motilin. Though controversial, a recent metaanalysis suggests there is no difference in DGE for pylorus-preserving PD and classic pancreaticoduodenectomy [9]. Leakage from the pancreatic anastomosis is thought to occur in 15–20 % of patients. External drainage of these fistulas will usually facilitate resolution of symptoms within several weeks.

References

1. National Institutes of Health, National Cancer Institute Statistics. 2008. URL: http://www.cancer.gov. Accessed 16 July 2008.
2. Traverso LW, Peralta EA, Ryan JA, et al. Intraductal neoplasms of the pancreas. Am J Surg. 1998;175:426–32.
3. Paye F, Sauvanet A, Terris B, et al. Intraductal papillary mucinous tumors of the pancreas: pancreatic resections guided by preoperative morphological assessment and intraoperative extemporaneous examination. Surgery. 2000;127:536–44.
4. Bachellier P, Nakano H, Oussoultzoglou E, et al. Is pancreaticoduodenectomy with mesentericoportal venous resection worthwhile? Am J Surg. 2001;182:120–9.
5. Bold RJ, Charnsangavej C, Cleary KR, et al. Major vascular resection as part of pancreaticoduodenectomy for cancer: radiologic, intraoperative, and pathologic analysis. J Gastrointest Surg. 1999;3:233–43.
6. Yeo CJ, Cameron JL, Sohn TA, et al. Six hundred fifty consecutive pancreaticoduodenectomies in the 1990s: pathology, complications, and outcomes. Ann Surg. 1997;226:248–60.
7. Balcom JH, Rattner DW, Warshaw AL, et al. Ten-year experience with 733 pancreatic resections. Arch Surg. 2001;136:391–8.
8. Povoski SP, Karpeh Jr MS, Conlon KC, Blumgart LH, Brennan MF. Association of preoperative biliary drainage with postoperative outcome following pancreaticoduodenectomy. Ann Surg. 1999;230:131–42.
9. Diener MK, Heukaufer C, Schwarzer G, et al. Pancreaticoduodenectomy (classic Whipple) versus pylorus-preserving pancreaticoduodenectomy (pp Whipple) for surgical treatment of periampullary and pancreatic carcinoma. Cochrane Database Syst Rev. 2008;(2):CD006053.

Chapter 39
Distal Pancreatectomy

Nicholas A. Hamilton and William G. Hawkins

Abstract This chapter covers the surgical technique for distal pancreas including both open and laparoscopic approaches.

Keywords Distal pancreatectomy • left pancreatectomy

Indications

Distal pancreatectomy is the surgical procedure indicated for any pathology in the body or tail of the pancreas, as defined by being left of the portal vein. Disease processes include benign and malignant neoplasms, both primary and metastatic to the pancreas [1], pancreatic cysts [2], pseudocysts, or strictures from pancreatitis that have not spontaneously resolved [3] and benign inflammatory conditions. Patients sustaining a traumatic injury to the body or tail of the pancreas with suspicion or direct evidence of pancreatic

N.A. Hamilton • W.G. Hawkins (✉)
Department of General Surgery, Washington University,
St. Louis, MO, USA
e-mail: hawkinsw@wudosis.wustl.edu

H. Chen (ed.), *Illustrative Handbook of General Surgery*,
DOI 10.1007/978-3-319-24557-7_39,
© Springer International Publishing Switzerland 2016

duct disruption also should undergo a distal pancreatectomy [4].

Unlike diseases of the head or neck of the pancreas, diseases in the body or tail of the pancreas do not generally lead to jaundice, as they do not cause biliary obstruction. Symptoms usually include vague abdominal pain, weight loss, nausea, and early satiety. Rarely patients with neuroendocrine tumors may have symptoms such as dizziness, headaches, and palpitations as a result of hormonal activity.

Preoperative Preparation: Imaging Studies

Lesions requiring a distal pancreatectomy are usually found on computed tomographic (CT) imaging during the diagnostic process. Ultimately, a 3-phase fine-cut helical CT scan should be performed, especially in the case of suspected malignancy. Cystic [5] and solid lesions alike are amenable to biopsy during an endoscopic ultrasound, which can be performed both for tissue diagnosis as well as evaluation of locally advanced disease in the case of malignant tumors. In the case of pancreas adenocarcinoma, it is important to determine the extent of the disease, as patients with evidence of advanced regional disease or metastatic disease are not candidates for surgical resection. We recommend a bowel preparation, as a portion of the transverse colon may, on occasion, need to be resected.

Positioning and Anesthesia

Patients undergoing a distal pancreatectomy are most commonly placed in a supine position with their arms extended. General anesthesia is required. At the end of a laparoscopic distal pancreatectomy, local anesthesia is injected around the port sites for pain control in the initial postoperative period. The abdomen is prepped and draped from the nipples to the pubic symphysis.

Description of Procedure

The surgical technique for benign or premalignant pancreatic disease differs from that for malignant disease. For benign disease of the pancreatic body and tail, the resection approach can be from the spleen towards the body and neck of the pancreas (retrograde) or starting at the neck of the pancreas and working towards the tail (antegrade). In order to maximize the lymphatic dissection and improve the chance for a margin negative resection our group recommends that an antegrade resection should be performed when pancreatic cancer is suspected or proven [6].

Open Distal Pancreatectomy (RAMPS Procedure)

A staging laparoscopy is performed to rule out any peritoneal or liver metastases. Once it has been determined that there is no evidence of metastatic disease, a long, oblique, left upper quadrant incision that extends over the midline to the right and also vertically in the midline is made (a midline incision is an acceptable alternative, and may be preferable in thin patients). The greater omentum is dissected off of the colon using electrocautery and the short gastric vessels are divided close to the stomach using an ultrasonic or bipolar sealing device. Alternatively, the short gastric vessels can be individually clipped or ligated. The neck of the pancreas is then visualized by retracting the stomach superiorly. The pancreas is gently elevated off the superior mesenteric and portal veins inferiorly and superiorly. Dissection along the superior edge of the neck of the pancreas will reveal the common hepatic artery, which can be traced rightward to the gastroduodenal artery and leftward to the celiac confluence and identification of the splenic artery. The lymph nodes on the left border of the proper hepatic artery and portal vein as well as those anterior to the common hepatic artery are mobilized. The anterior surface of the portal vein is exposed by retracting the gastroduodenal artery to the right and the tunnel behind the neck of the pancreas is completed. The neck of the pancreas is then divided. We prefer a linear GIA stapler with a thick tissue load. This may be oversewn with interlocking figure of eight sutures. The celiac nodes are next dissected free by dividing the coronary vein near the lesser curve of the stomach and then dividing the peritoneum at the base of the caudate lobe, sweeping the fat and nodes inferiorly off the crus of the diaphragm. The fat and nodes anterior to the hepatic artery are then swept medially and the coronary vein is again divided, this time at the portal vein. The origin of the splenic artery from the inferior aspect of the celiac artery can now be seen and it is ligated near its origin. The splenic vein is next isolated at its junction with the superior mesenteric vein and divided. The dissection now proceeds vertically until the superior mesenteric artery is encountered. The artery is followed posteriorly and superiorly on its left side to the aorta. The lymph nodes anterior to the aorta between the celiac artery and superior mesenteric artery and those anterior to the left of the superior mesenteric artery are taken. If preoperative imaging suggests posterior invasion the dissection can easily be extended posteriorly to include the adrenal gland superiorly and Gerota's fascia inferiorly. The superior and inferior attachments of the pancreas are divided as the dissection proceeds to the left and the inferior mesenteric vein is ligated and transected and the lienorenal ligament is divided. Once the lienorenal ligament is divided, the specimen is removed *en bloc*. The abdomen is irrigated and hemostasis is obtained. A drain is placed in the resection bed, exiting the skin in the left upper quadrant. The incision is closed using number 1 Prolene sutures in a running fashion starting laterally and tied to each other medially. The skin is closed with staples and a sterile dressing is applied [6].

Laparoscopic Distal Pancreatectomy

An infraumbilical incision is made and a 10–12-mm trocar is inserted. The abdomen is insufflated and the following additional trocars are placed in the upper abdomen; one 5-mm

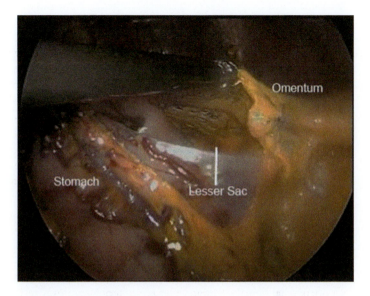

FIGURE 39.1 Entering the lesser sac

and one 10-mm port just to the right of midline and two 5-mm ports in the left upper abdomen. A four-quadrant examination of the abdomen is undertaken, paying particular attention to any nodules or irregularities of the liver or the peritoneum. The stomach is mobilized from the transverse mesocolon and the lesser sac is entered (Fig. 39.1). The splenic flexure of the colon is mobilized using the ultrasonic dissector or 5-mm ligaSure. This can be aided by tilting the operating table so the patient's left side is elevated 30–45°. This is carried towards the inferior margin of the spleen. If the spleen is to be removed, all short gastric arteries to it are taken down with the ultrasonic dissector or with hemoclips (Fig. 39.2). The dissection then proceeds toward the gastroesophageal junction, making sure to stay on the inferior aspect of the gastroepiploic vessels. Filmy attachments between the pancreas and the posterior stomach are dissected (Fig. 39.3). A fixed retractor is utilized to elevate the stomach and left liver anteriorly and cephalad to expose the entire length of the pancreas. The superior aspect of

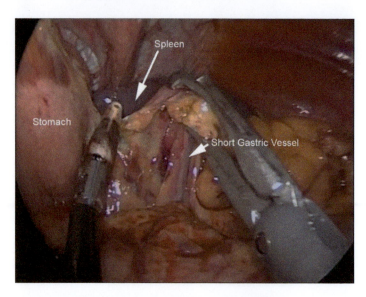

FIGURE 39.2 Taking down the short gastric vessels

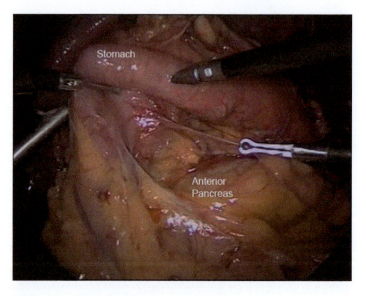

FIGURE 39.3 Exposing the anterior pancreas

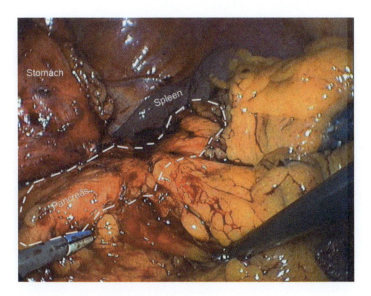

FIGURE 39.4 The pancreas in situ

the pancreas is then mobilized toward the portal vein along the hepatic artery. The hepatic artery is then traced back to the confluence of the celiac artery and the left gastric artery. The inferior aspect of the pancreas is next mobilized toward the spleen (Figs. 39.4 and 39.5). If the spleen is to be preserved, the splenic vein is dissected free of the posterior pancreas. Hemostasis is achieved with the ultrasonic dissector and the application of hemoclips. The pancreas is elevated superiorly to allow for retroperitoneal pancreatic access and a tunnel is then created underneath the pancreas to expose the portal vein. The pancreas is then transected using an endo GIA stapler (Figs. 39.6 and 39.7). The staple line can be reinforced by using buttress material, as seen in the figures. The use of buttress material to reinforce the staple line may or may not reduce the postoperative fistula rate [7]. The splenic artery is identified (Fig. 39.8) and stapled with a vascular load of a GIA Endo stapler if it is to be removed. The portal-splenic confluence is identified by

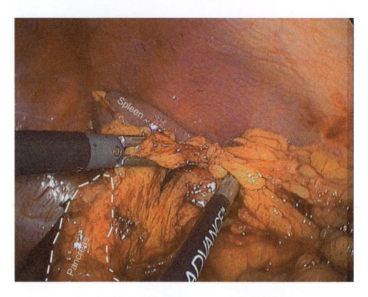

FIGURE 39.5 Mobilizing the inferior pancreas near the spleen

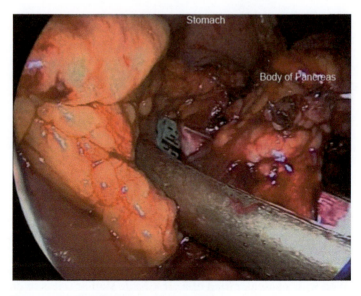

FIGURE 39.6 Stapling across the pancreas

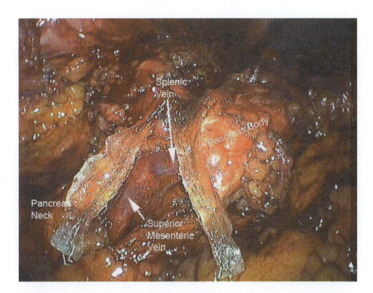

FIGURE 39.7 The transected pancreas

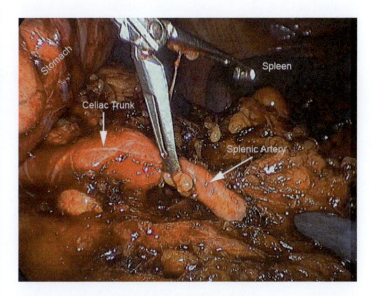

FIGURE 39.8 Identification of the splenic artery

retracting the resected pancreas laterally (Fig. 39.9). The splenic vein is then stapled here (Fig. 39.10), if the spleen is to be removed. The specimen is placed into a specimen bag (Fig. 39.11). The upper midline port incision is extended and the specimen is delivered from the small upper midline incision (Fig. 39.12). Hemostasis is assured and a drain is placed at the pancreatic transection line, coming out of the left upper quadrant. The trocar sites and the specimen extraction sites are closed with absorbable sutures and the skin is closed with a subcuticular monofilament suture and a sterile dressing is applied.

Postoperative Care

The complication rate following distal pancreatectomy is approximately 30 %. The most common complications encountered are pancreatic leak or fistula (5–29 %) [8, 9], new-onset insulin-dependent diabetes (9 %) [9], intraabdominal abscess (4 %), small bowel obstruction (4 %), and postoperative hemorrhage (4 %) [8]. Postoperative care is targeted to avoid or minimize these complications.

Postoperatively uncomplicated patients are admitted to a general ward for 2–3 days. Perioperative pain may be managed by intravenous narcotics or epidural catheters. One of the most critical aspects of their recovery is the diligent use of an incentive spirometer to encourage deep breathing and to prevent atelectasis and pneumonia. It is also important to routinely monitor blood glucose levels, as removing part of the pancreas can make a patient either temporarily or permanently diabetic [10]. Another aspect of patient management that should not be overlooked is adequate venous thrombosis prophylaxis, particularly in patients with malignancies. Patients should be encouraged to ambulate as soon and as often as possible. The Foley catheter is discontinued once the patient demonstrates that they are adequately volume resuscitated. In most patients the nasogastric tube is discontinued on postoperative day 1. The diet is advanced from clear liquids to a regular diet as tolerated by the patient. When an oral

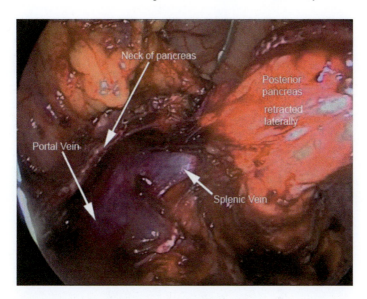

FIGURE 39.9 Portosplenic confluence exposed

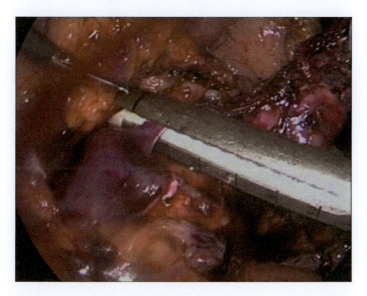

FIGURE 39.10 Dividing the splenic vein

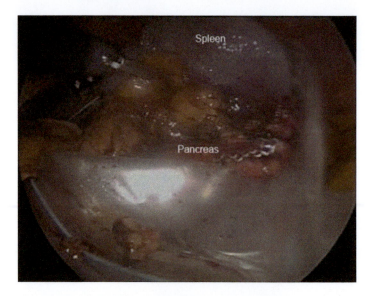

FIGURE 39.11 The final specimen in the specimen bag

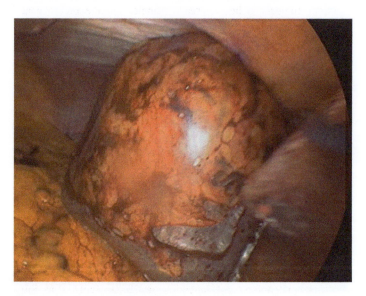

FIGURE 39.12 The specimen being removed

diet is resumed, medications are changed from intravenous to oral. If there is a change in the abdominal drain output, volume or quality, drain fluid amylase and lipase are sent in conjunction with a patient's serum amylase and lipase. If the drain amylase or lipase is greater than three times that of the serum, the patient has a pancreatic leak and is discharged home with the drain in place. When the patient demonstrates the ability to maintain an oral intake to keep himself adequately hydrated and has significant pain control on oral pain medication, he may be discharged from the hospital. Patients are seen back in the surgeon's clinic in 2 weeks for a routine postoperative visit. If there was a leak at the time of discharge, the drain fluid is again analyzed and may be removed if it has normalized.

References

1. Crippa S, Angelini C, Mussi C, et al. Surgical treatment of metastatic tumors to the pancreas: a single center experience and review of the literature. World J Surg. 2006;30:1536–42.
2. Garcea G, Ong SL, Rajesh A, et al. Cystic lesions of the pancreas. Pancreatology. 2008;8:236–51.
3. Aghdassi A, Mayerle J, Kraft M, et al. Diagnosis and treatment of pancreatic pseudocysts in chronic pancreatitis. Pancreas. 2008;36:105–12.
4. Degiannis E, Glapa M, Loukogeorgakis SP, et al. Management of pancreatic trauma. Injury. 2008;39:21–9.
5. Sugiyama M, Suzuki Y, Abe N, et al. Management of intraductal papillary mucinous neoplasm of the pancreas. J Gastroenterol. 2008;43:181–5.
6. Strasberg SM, Drebin JA, Linehan D. Radical antegrade modular pancreatosplenectomy. Surgery. 2003;133:521–7.
7. Thaker RL, Matthews BD, Linehan DC, et al. Absorbable mesh reinforcement of a stapled pancreatic transection line reduces the leak rate with distal pancreatectomy. J Gastrointest Surg. 2007;11:59–65.
8. Lillemoe KD, Kaushal S, Cameron JL, et al. Distal pancreatectomy: indications and outcomes in 235 patients. Ann Surg. 1999;229(5):693–700.

9. Ferrone CR, Warshaw AL, Rattner DW, et al. Pancreatic fistula rates after 462 distal pancreatectomies: staplers do not decrease fistula rates. J Gastrointest Surg. 2008;12(10):1691–7.
10. King J, Kazanjian K, Matsumoto J, et al. Distal pancreatectomy: incidence of postoperative diabetes. J Gastrointest Surg. 2008;12(9):1548–53.

Chapter 40
Surgical Treatment of Chronic Pancreatitis

Matthew R. Porembka, William G. Hawkins, and Steven M. Strasberg

Abstract This chapter covers the surgical management of chronic pancreatitis including indications, perioperative workup, procedure selection, surgical techniques, post-operative care and outcomes.

Keywords Chronic pancreatitis • Surgical management • Review

Background

Chronic pancreatitis is characterized by progressive parenchymal fibrosis resulting in loss of pancreatic exocrine and endocrine function. The pathogenesis of chronic pancreatitis

M.R. Porembka
Section of HPB Surgery, Department of Surgery,
University of Texas Southwestern, St Louis, MO, USA

W.G. Hawkins (✉) • S.M. Strasberg
Section of HPB Surgery, Department of Surgery,
Washington University in St Louis, St Louis, MO, USA
e-mail: hawkinsw@wudosis.wustl.edu

H. Chen (ed.), *Illustrative Handbook of General Surgery*,
DOI 10.1007/978-3-319-24557-7_40,
© Springer International Publishing Switzerland 2016

is unclear, but is thought to be secondary to repeated parenchymal injury. Common etiologies include alcoholic pancreatitis, autoimmune pancreatitis, and pancreatic duct obstruction caused by pancreatic divisum or stricture. The disease affects all elements of the gland; exocrine dysfunction can occur early in the disease process followed by subsequent endocrine dysfunction. Parenchymal fibrosis often causes pancreatic duct strictures resulting in distal pancreatic duct dilation. Intraparenchymal calcification and intraductal calcium calculi are common.

The presentation of chronic pancreatitis is variable, however, patients most commonly present with severe, recurrent abdominal pain. Although several mechanisms have attempted to explain how chronic pancreatitis causes abdominal pain, the exact etiology remains unknown [1].

The treatment of chronic pancreatitis can be difficult and requires multidisciplinary treatment by general practitioners, gastroenterologists, radiologists, and surgeons. Initial treatment is nonoperative and includes pain control with oral analgesics. Frequently, patients require escalation to narcotic pain medicines and referral to pain management specialists. Endoscopic treatments aimed at reliving the chronic pain associated with chronic pancreatitis have been developed and include celiac axis block, pancreatic sphincterotomy, and pancreatic duct stenting. The published results of these interventions have demonstrated varying efficacy and durability [2, 3, 15]; their discussion is beyond the scope of this chapter.

Indications for Surgical Therapy

Although initial treatment of chronic pancreatitis is nonoperative, the indications which require surgical treatment are listed in Table 40.1. The most frequent indication for surgery in patients with chronic pancreatitis is intractable pain.

TABLE 40.1 Indications for surgery in chronic pancreatitis

Pain refractory to medical therapy

Recurrent pancreatitis secondary to pancreatic duct stenosis

Bile duct stenosis

Gastric outlet obstruction/duodenal obstruction/colonic obstruction

Pancreatic fistula

Pseudocyst

Pancreatic carcinoma

Preoperative Preparation

Preoperative Workup

Just as in all major intraabdominal surgeries, thorough preoperative cardiac risk evaluation should be carried out [5]. In addition, patients with chronic pancreatitis should be screened for ongoing alcohol abuse and referred to a treatment program, if necessary, before undergoing elective resection. In a recent review, 20 % of patients undergoing surgery for chronic pancreatitis retrospectively reported active alcohol abuse at the time of surgery [10].

In cases in which sequelae of chronic pancreatitis have resulted in severe malnutrition (albumin <2), consideration should be given to nutrition supplementation. Enteral feeding is preferable to total parenteral nutrition [9]. Pancreatic enzyme therapy is often required for adequate digestion of food. All patients should receive a bowel regimen such as magnesium citrate the night before surgery to facilitate the creation of a Roux loop, if necessary.

Imaging Studies

Imaging studies are crucial for fully evaluating the extent of disease and for surgical planning. It provides confirmation of

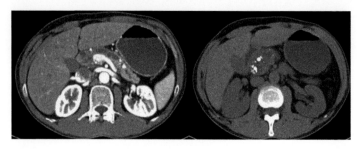

FIGURE 40.1 Preoperative CT scan demonstrating dilated pancreatic duct on contrast scan and severely calcified and diseased pancreatic head on non-contrast images

chronic pancreatitis, assessment of pancreatic duct diameter, definition of pancreatic anatomy, and the determination of associated disease or malignancy.

Triple-phase contrast-enhanced, fine-cut, computed tomography is the preferred modality for the evaluation of chronic pancreatitis. The sensitivity of CT scan is almost 100 % for diagnosing advanced disease and readily detects the common sequelae of pancreatitis including the presence of an inflammatory mass, pancreatic pseudocyst, bile duct stricture, pancreatic ductal dilation, and gastric outlet obstruction (Fig. 40.1). In patients with an inflammatory mass, it is crucial to rule out pancreatic adenocarcinoma. If the diagnosis is unclear on axial imaging, additional studies may be required to completely evaluate the patient. Endoscopic retrograde cholangiopancreatogram (ERCP), endoscopic ultrasound (EUS) with biopsy, magnetic resonance imaging (MRI), and magnetic resonance cholangiopancreatogram (MRCP) can provide valuable information in difficult cases. Definitive oncologic resection is indicated if the presence of malignancy is suspected and cannot be ruled out.

ERCP is the gold standard for examination of pancreatic ductal anatomy. In chronic pancreatitis, the pancreatic duct displays an irregular contour with multifocal strictures, dilations, and stones. MRCP provides similar images without the invasiveness of an endoscopy, but is less precise. EUS easily defines pancreatic anatomic relationships and allows for non-invasive tissue sampling under ultrasound guidance [13].

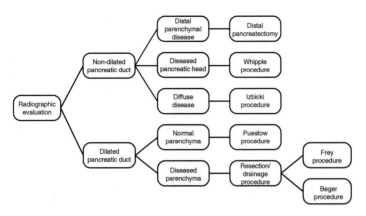

FIGURE 40.2 Treatment algorithm for the surgical management of chronic pancreatitis

Procedure Selection

The choice of operation is dependent on pancreatic ductal anatomy and the extent of disease throughout the gland. Operations to palliate abdominal pain either (1) drain a dilated pancreatic ductal system or (2) resect diseased pancreatic parenchyma in cases in which the duct is of normal diameter. The main pancreatic duct normally measures 4–5 mm in the head of the pancreas and gently tapers throughout the body (3–4 mm) and tail (2–3 mm).

Patients with a dilated main pancreatic duct (>7 mm in the body of the gland) are best treated with procedures to decompress and drain the dilated duct (longitudinal pancreaticojejunostomy – Puestow procedure, or longitudinal pancreaticojejunostomy with coring of the head – Frey procedure). On the other hand, patients with a diseased gland and normal pancreatic duct diameter may require resection of the diseased gland. The choice of resection (distal pancreatectomy, pancreaticoduodenectomy, Beger procedure, Izbicki procedure) is dependent on surgeon's preference and the anatomical extent of disease. Some of these operations (Frey, Beger, Izbicki) have elements of resection and drainage (Fig. 40.2).

Surgical Procedures for Chronic Pancreatitis

Drainage Procedures

Longitudinal pancreaticojejunostomy (Puestow procedure) is performed for the drainage and decompression of a dilated pancreatic duct. Despite providing temporary pain relief, the procedure is associated with approximately 50 % of patients developing recurrent abdominal pain within 5 years. Failure is due to the fact that the procedure may inadequately decompress ducts in the head and uncinate process.

Resection for Chronic Pancreatitis

Patients with parenchymal disease and a normal diameter or narrowed pancreatic duct are candidates for pancreatic resection. The extent of resection is dependent upon the location and extent of disease. Pancreaticoduodenectomy (Whipple resection) may be indicated in patients with an enlarged pancreatic head, containing multiple cysts or calcifications. Distal pancreatectomy is indicated in patients with a normal pancreatic duct and disease confined to the distal gland. However, resection is associated with an increased incidence of postoperative endocrine and exocrine dysfunction.

Combined Resection and Drainage Procedures

Procedures that involve limited pancreatic resection and pancreatic duct drainage attempt to provide permanent pain relief, while avoiding exocrine and endocrine dysfunction. Variations exist based on the method of pancreatic head resection. The Frey procedure combines limited resection by coring of the pancreatic head with unroofing of the dilated pancreatic duct and lateral pancreaticojejunostomy. The Beger procedure is a duodenal-sparing resection of the pancreatic head; drainage is accomplished through a Roux limb to the periampullary pancreas and the remaining tail, either through an end-to-end anastomosis or lateral pancreaticojejunostomy. Both procedures are indicated in severe chronic pancreatitis with an enlarged pancreatic head.

Table 40.2 illustrates the salient differences between the operations employed to treat chronic pancreatitis.

Positioning and Anesthesia

The patient is positioned supine on the operating table with arms extended. The level of intraoperative monitoring is dependent on the patient's general health status. All patients require adequate peripheral intravenous access, should thevneed for rapid fluid replacement arise. Arterial monitoring is often performed to obtain realtime hemodynamic monitoring. Central venous cannulation should not be routinely employed, but reserved for patients whose peripheral intravenous access is inadequate or preexisting medical conditions, which require close attention to cardiac preload or fluid status.

General anesthesia and adequate muscle relaxation is required in all patients to facilitate exposure. Frequently, a self-retaining retractor system is employed. All patients should have a nasogastric tube placed for gastric decompression.

Description of the Procedure

Although several different operations for chronic pancreatitis exist, the Frey procedure, which combines a limited pancreatic head resection and a lateral pancreaticojejunostomy, will be described in detail here. The surgery can be divided into three parts: exposure and complete pancreatic evaluation, resection of pancreatic parenchyma facilitating pancreatic duct decompression, and construction of a Roux loop to drain the decompressed duct.

Table 40.2 Comparison of various procedures for chronic pancreatitis [4, 6–8, 11, 12, 14, 16]

Procedure	Mortality	Endocrine insufficiency	Exocrine insufficiency	Pain relief	Fistula	Comments
Puestow procedure	<3 %	Minimal	Unchanged	85 %	2 %	Recurrent pain occurs in 40–50 % of patients within 5 years
Whipple procedure		40 %	55 %	85 %	7 %	
Distal pancreatectomy		35 %	30 %	60 %	5 %	
Frey procedure		<10 %	15 %	90 %	3 %	
Beger procedure		20 %	20 %	70 %	<1 %	

Table comparing the various procedures performed for chronic pancreatitis. Specifically, procedure related mortality, incidence of new-onset endocrine and exocrine dysfunction, pancreatic fistula, and pain relief were compared

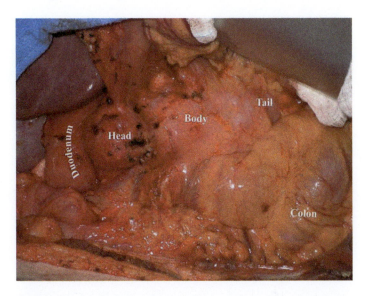

FIGURE 40.3 Normal anatomy of the pancreas after entering the lesser sac

Exposing the Pancreas

A laparotomy is performed through a "Mercedes-Benz", chevron, or midline incision. Access to the lesser sac is obtained through the gastrocolic ligament and the posterior attachments of the stomach are released (Fig. 40.3).

An extensive Kocher maneuver with hepatic flexure mobilization is performed to expose the pancreas. Once complete, the right gastroepiploic vein is divided close to its union with the middle colic vein. The right gastroepiploic artery is divided where it originates from the gastroduodenal artery on the anterior surface of the pancreas. The gastroduodenal artery, which runs from superior to inferior across the neck of the pancreas, is ligated above and below the planned line of incision in the pancreas. Using ultrasound guidance, a needle is navigated into the dilated pancreatic duct. Fine-tipped cautery is used to trace the path of the needle and enter the duct. The parenchyma overlying the duct is excised to unroof the

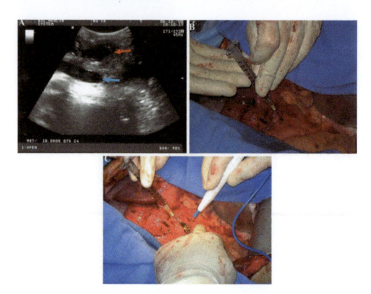

FIGURE 40.4 Locating the pancreatic duct using ultrasound guidance and a syringe. (**a**) The *red arrow* indicates the dilated pancreatic duct and the *blue arrow* highlights the superior mesenteric vein. (**b**) Note the presence of pancreatic ductal hypertension as pancreatic fluid spontaneously decompresses into the syringe. (**c**) Bovie cautery is used to unroof the pancreatic duct

dilated duct and permit adequate decompression (Fig. 40.4a–c).

Resection of the Pancreatic Parenchyma

Resection of the overlying pancreatic tissue is required to facilitate decompression of the duct. Normally the duct in the body and tail is exposed first. A trough is created by resecting the overlying pancreatic tissue, with the pancreatic duct at the base. Enough pancreatic issue is left at the upper and lower borders of the pancreas to provide a margin to attach the Roux loop. Frequently, large pancreatic duct stones are encountered and are easily extracted.

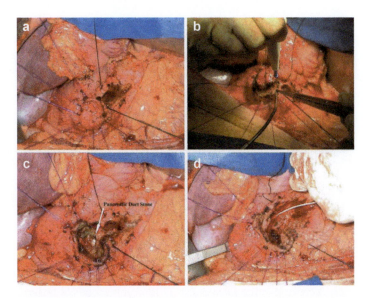

FIGURE 40.5 Parenchymal resection. (**a**) Stay sutures are placed around the head of the pancreas to maintain hemostasis during resection. (**b**) The parenchyma is excised in layers. (**c**) A pancreatic duct stone is encountered in the remnant pancreatic duct. (**d**) After resection is complete, open communication between the duct and the duodenum is demonstrated by inserting a Fogarty catheter through the ampulla

To prepare for head coring, a series of 3-0 synthetic absorbable sutures is placed around the pancreatic head at the border of the duodenum to maintain hemostatic control during parenchymal resection. The incision in the pancreatic duct is carried into the head and all tissue anterior to the duct is excised in layers. Resection proceeds until approximately a thin, 1 cm margin of pancreas remains along posterior, lateral, superior, and inferior aspects. A biliary balloon catheter or sound is placed through the papilla into the duodenum to demonstrate unobstructed communication and to determine the right lateral resection margin (Fig. 40.5a–d). The surgeon must maintain awareness of the position of the portomesenteric veins and the posterior surface of the pancreas, the latter by manual palpation of the mobilized duodenum. Excised tissue is sent for pathologic evaluation for occult pancreatic cancer.

Pancreaticojejunostomy

A Roux-en-Y pancreaticojejunostomy is used to drain the decompressed pancreatic duct. The Roux loop is created by transecting the small bowel approximately 20 cm distal to the ligament of Treitz. A functional end-to-end, side-to-side enteroenterostomy is created 60 cm downstream from the stapled end of the jejunum.

The free, stapled end of the jejunum is used to fashion the pancreaticojejunostomy (Fig. 40.6a–c). The Roux loop is brought into the lesser sac in a retrocolic fashion through a defect created in the mesocolon. Different methods of fashioning the side-to-side anastomosis have been described. In cases where the remaining pancreas is firm and can hold suture easily, the anastomosis is created using single-layer, running monofilament synthetic suture (3-0 polydioxanone, PDS). However, when the pancreas is soft, a two-layered closure can be performed with an inner layer of continuous monofilament suture and an outer layer of interrupted 3-0 silk sutures to anchor the small bowel to the surface of the pancreas.

After the anastomosis is completed, the defect in the mesocolon is approximated around the Roux loop. The field is thoroughly irrigated and hemostasis is confirmed. Closed suction drains are placed around the anastomosis before closing the abdomen.

Postoperative Care

Patients undergoing surgery for chronic pancreatitis require attentive care in the postoperative period, to assure optimal outcomes. Postoperative pain control can be difficult as many patients are dependent on narcotic pain medications. Epidural

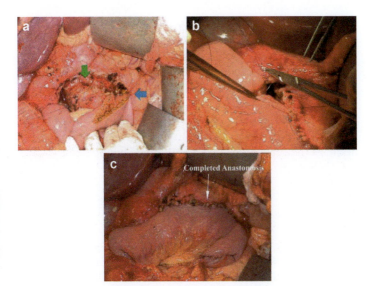

FIGURE 40.6 Fashioning the pancreaticojejunostomy. (**a**) The small bowel enterotomy is considerably smaller than the length of the exposed duct, as the bowel wall is fairly elastic. The anastomosis is fashioned using a single layer of continuous running 3-0 polydioxanone (PDS) synthetic monofilament suture. The posterior anastomosis is created first (*blue arrow*); pancreatic duct (*green arrow*). (**b**) The superior aspect of the anastomosis is complete. (**c**) The finished pancreaticojejunostomy is shown

and patient-controlled analgesia are useful methods; the latter allows titration of pain medication to obtain adequate pain relief. All patients require monitoring for symptoms of alcohol withdrawal including autonomic instability (tachycardia, hypertension, and hyperthermia), insomnia, emotional irritability, and diaphoresis. Prophylaxis with benzodiazepines is indicated if symptoms of withdrawal of alcohol appear or alcohol dependence is suspected in order to prevent life-threatening complications such as delirium tremens and seizure.

The appearance of gland dysfunction may begin to present in the early postoperative period. Fasting blood glucose levels should be monitored; if needed, insulin replacement therapy and diabetic counseling are implemented. Patients should be monitored for malabsorption and steatorrhea. Malabsorption should be treated with pancreatic enzyme replacement (30,000 units of lipase with each meal). Restriction of dietary fat intake should improve steatorrhea.

Patients require routine follow up once discharged from the hospital. Recurrent pain should prompt a thorough evaluation, as the recurrence may herald the development of pancreatic cancer.

References

1. Anaparthy R, Pasricha PJ. Pain and chronic pancreatitis: is it the plumbing or the wiring? Curr Gastroenterol Rep. 2008;10(2):101–6.
2. Arslanlar S, Jain R. Benign biliary strictures related to chronic pancreatitis: balloons, stents, or surgery. Curr Treat Options Gastroenterol. 2007;10(5):369–75.
3. Cahen DL, Gouma DJ, et al. Endoscopic versus surgical drainage of the pancreatic duct in chronic pancreatitis. N Engl J Med. 2007;356(7):676–84.
4. Diener MK, Rahbari NN, et al. Duodenum-preserving pancreatic head resection versus pancreatoduodenectomy for surgical treatment of chronic pancreatitis: a systematic review and meta-analysis. Ann Surg. 2008;247(6):950–61.
5. Fleisher LA, Beckman JA, et al. ACC/AHA 2007 guidelines on perioperative cardiovascular evaluation and care for noncardiac surgery: executive summary: a report of the American College of Cardiology/American Heart Association Task Force on Practice Guidelines (Writing Committee to Revise the 2002 Guidelines on Perioperative Cardiovascular Evaluation for Noncardiac Surgery) Developed in Collaboration With the American Society of Echocardiography, American Society of Nuclear Cardiology, Heart Rhythm Society, Society of Cardiovascular Anesthesiologists, Society for Cardiovascular Angiography and Interventions, Society for Vascular Medicine and Biology, and Society for Vascular Surgery. J Am Coll Cardiol. 2007;50(17):1707–32.
6. Hutchins RR, Hart RS, et al. Long-term results of distal pancreatectomy for chronic pancreatitis in 90 patients. Ann Surg. 2002;236(5):612–8.

7. Jalleh RP, Williamson RC. Pancreatic exocrine and endocrine function after operations for chronic pancreatitis. Ann Surg. 1992;216(6):656–62.
8. Riediger H, Adam U, et al. Long-term outcome after resection for chronic pancreatitis in 224 patients. J Gastrointest Surg. 2007;11(8):949–59; discussion 959–60.
9. Schnelldorfer T, Adams DB. The effect of malnutrition on morbidity after surgery for chronic pancreatitis. Am Surg. 2005;71(6):466–72; discussion 472–3.
10. Schnelldorfer T, Adams DB. Surgical treatment of alcohol-associated chronic pancreatitis: the challenges and pitfalls. Am Surg. 2008;74(6):503–7; discussion 508–9.
11. Schnelldorfer T, Lewin DN, et al. Operative management of chronic pancreatitis: longterm results in 372 patients. J Am Coll Surg. 2007;204(5):1039–45; discussion 1045–7.
12. Schnelldorfer T, Mauldin PD, et al. Distal pancreatectomy for chronic pancreatitis: risk factors for postoperative pancreatic fistula. J Gastrointest Surg. 2007;11(8):991–7.
13. Sica GT, Braver J, et al. Comparison of endoscopic retrograde cholangiopancreatography with MR cholangiopancreatography in patients with pancreatitis. Radiology. 1999;210(3):605–10.
14. Sohn TA, Campbell KA, et al. Quality of life and long-term survival after surgery for chronic pancreatitis. J Gastrointest Surg. 2000;4(4):355–64; discussion 364–5.
15. Tringali A, Boskoski I, et al. The role of endoscopy in the therapy of chronic pancreatitis. Best Pract Res Clin Gastroenterol. 2008;22(1):145–65.
16. Warshaw AL, Popp Jr JW, et al. Long-term patency, pancreatic function, and pain relief after lateral pancreaticojejunostomy for chronic pancreatitis. Gastroenterology. 1980;79(2):289–93.

Part X
Office-Based Procedures

Sarah C. Schaefer

Chapter 41
Vascular Access for Hemodialysis

David M. Melnick

Abstract General, vascular and transplant surgeons all perform operations for vascular access. The arteriovenous fistula, when compared with an external catheter or a non-autogenous graft, has the best outcome for vascular access among many patients with end stage renal disease. Professional and governmental organizations emphasize the importance of using autogenous fistulas when appropriate. This chapter will describe the preoperative evaluation, surgical techniques and postoperative care for performing radiocephalic and brachiocephalic arteriovenous fistulas and the basilic vein transposition.

Keywords Hemodialysis • Vascular access • Arteriovenous fistula • Basilic vein transposition

D.M. Melnick, MD, MPH, FACS
Department of Surgery, University of Wisconsin School of Medicine and Public Health, One South Park Street, Madison, WI 53715, USA
e-mail: melnick@surgery.wisc.edu

H. Chen (ed.), *Illustrative Handbook of General Surgery*,
DOI 10.1007/978-3-319-24557-7_41,
© Springer International Publishing Switzerland 2016

747

Indications

The arteriovenous fistula [AVF], when compared with an external catheter or a non-autogenous graft in multiple non-randomized, non-controlled studies, has the best outcome for vascular access among patients with end stage renal disease [1]. The National Kidney Foundation Kidney Disease Outcomes Quality Initiative (KDOQI) and the Society for Vascular Surgery each have excellent guidelines for the surgeon performing vascular access operations [2, 3]. The Fistula First Initiative, instituted in 2004 and sponsored in part by the Center for Medicare Services, strongly promotes the use of native AV fistulas for access. The initiative's name has changed to "Fistula First, Catheter Last," to promote the primary goal of avoiding catheters, and to recognize the idea that some patients such as the elderly and others may have better outcomes with grafts rather than fistulas. This review will describe the surgical techniques for radiocephalic and brachiocephalic arteriovenous fistulas and the one stage basilic vein transposition [BVT].

Preoperative Care

A successful access requires good arterial inflow and good venous outflow, including patency of the central veins. Important aspects of history specific to vascular access include hand dominance, history of central lines and pacemakers, and history of radial artery operations for coronary artery bypass surgery. If both arms have adequate veins, use the non-dominant arm for access. The patient will then have more mobility of their dominant hand during dialysis. A history of central lines would prompt you to consider evaluation for central venous stenosis with a venogram. The presence of a pacemaker in the ipsilateral subclavian vein predicts a higher risk of complications including subclavian vein thrombosis after AV fistula placement in that arm. History of radial artery excision would preclude a wrist fistula. On physical exam, evaluate for pulse quality at the radial artery at the wrist and the brachial artery at the elbow. Perform an Allen's test to evaluate the palmer arch prior to consideration of performing a radial-cephalic wrist fistula, to ensure that the ulnar artery will adequately perfuse the hand. Inspect for collateral veins in the upper arm and around the shoulder to evaluate for sequalae of central venous stenosis.

The ultrasound is an excellent instrument you can use in the office to evaluate artery and vein size and course to plan an appropriate operation (Fig. 41.1).

In most cases, a vein 2.5–3 mm or larger would be appropriate to attempt an operation, while an artery 2–2.5 mm at a minimum may work, although larger vessels size will predict a greater likelihood of success [4]. You can gain more information and detail by performing the ultrasound yourself rather than depending upon a radiology report. In patients with a history of multiple failed attempts at access, a concern for central venous stenosis, or other factors that may make the access more likely to fail, a venogram with iodinated contrast or CO_2 may also help delineate the anatomy of the venous system including the central venous system to plan the operation (Fig. 41.2).

Positioning and Anesthesia

You can perform the operations utilizing local anesthesia with sedation (or sometimes without sedation,) monitored anesthesia care, or a regional block. Place the operative arm in the abducted position on an arm board and prep and drape appropriately.

Description of the Procedure

Wrist Fistula (Radiocephalic Fistula)

Dr. Kenneth Appel, a general surgeon in The Bronx in New York City, performed the first radiocephalic wrist fistula

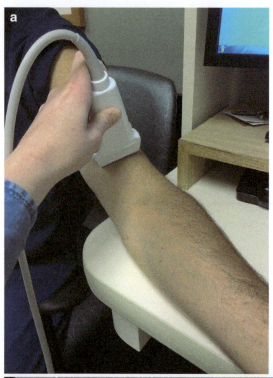

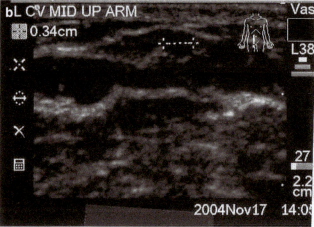

FIGURE 41.1 (**a**, **b**) Ultrasound mapping of veins, performed in the office (Courtesy of David Melnick, MD)

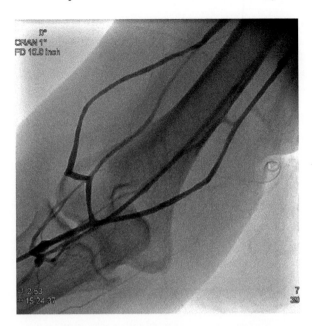

FIGURE 41.2 Right upper arm venogram using iodinated contrast demonstrating the cephalic vein (*upper left*) brachial vein (*middle*) and basilic vein (*lower right*) (Courtesy of Amanda Valliant, MD)

(also known as the Brescia-Cimino-Appel fistula) in 1963 [5]. He improved upon the other option at that time, the Scribner Shunt, an external metallic shunt placed in the forearm associated with significant major complications. The patient should have a normal Allen's test to prevent ischemic complications to the hand. A preoperative ultrasound can sometimes identify an area more proximal than the wrist where the vein and/or artery may have a larger diameter and be easier to work with. After prepping, draping, and anesthetizing, incise the skin longitudinally between the cephalic vein and the palpable radial artery in the distal forearm. Develop a lateral skin flap to expose the cephalic vein. Mobilize it for a distance of 4–5 cm and control it with vessel loops. To expose the radial artery, palpate it or use a Doppler to identify it then incise the overlying fascia. Preserve the superficial branch of the radial nerve lying lateral to the artery as it supplies sensation to the thumb. Mobilize the artery and gain proximal and distal control with vessel loops. Depending on the quality and location of the vein, you can perform either a side to side or end vein to side artery anastomosis. The initial description of this procedure by Appel utilized a side to side anastomosis, but this chapter will describe an end vein to side artery anastomosis. Divide the vein distally at the appropriate point to prepare for the anastomosis. Locally heparinize the vein and sequentially dilate to 4–5 mm with vessel dilators to ensure lack of stenosis, then heparinize again and place a bulldog on the vein. Some authors recommend a different approach, limiting trauma to the vein and artery by minimizing the contact with them around the area of the anastomosis.

Elbow Fistula (Brachiocephalic Fistula)

After prepping and draping, anesthetize the skin just distal to the antecubital crease and incise the skin transversely at that location. Dissect though the subcutaneous fat to expose the cephalic vein and mobilize it proximally and distally. Often you will find the cephalic vein anastomosing to the basilic vein in an arch formation, with distal venous branches. Using a branch point of the cephalic vein can help with an easier anastomosis. After exposing the vein, palpate or Doppler medially to find the brachial artery and brachial veins then incise the overlying bicipital aponeurosis (*lacertus fibrosus*) to expose them. Mobilize the artery and gain control with vessel loops. You can expose distally and gain control of the proximal radial artery to perform the anastomosis there, with the potential advantage of a lower risk of steal syndrome, or use the main brachial artery for the anastomosis. Ligate and divide small arterial branches to prevent avulsion. Gain proximal and distal control of the artery with vessel loops. Divide the vein distally at the appropriate point to prepare for the anastomosis. Locally heparinize the vein and sequentially dilate to 4–5 mm with vessel dilators to ensure lack of stenosis, then heparinize again and place a bulldog on the vein.

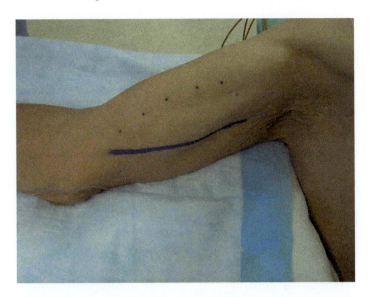

FIGURE 41.3 Preoperative ultrasound mapping of basilic vein (*solid line*). The *dotted line* is the planned tunneled path of the transposed basilic vein (Courtesy of David Melnick, MD)

Basilic Vein Transposition

The BVT may be performed in one stage or two stages. The first stage of the two stage approach involves performing a brachio-basilic AVF at the antecubital fossa or distal upper arm. The transposition is then performed at a later date after the fistula has been evaluated and is working. The one stage approach will be described here. After the patient is positioned with the ipsilateral arm abducted on an arm board, map out the course of the vein using the ultrasound and a marker to aid in dissection (Fig. 41.3).

After mapping out the course of the vein, prep and drape. Anesthetize as appropriate and incise the skin in the distal upper arm where you marked out the course of the vein. Dissect through the subcutaneous fat to expose the vein and control it with a vessel loop. Then sequentially incise the skin and mobilize the vein, tying off and dividing side branches all the way up the arm to the axilla. Doubly ligate the venous branches coming off the basilic vein to prevent postoperative hemorrhage. Curve the distal end of the skin incision laterally as you approach the antecubital crease to aid with exposure of the brachial artery. After the vein is completely mobilized, expose the artery. Palpate or use doppler to find the artery medially, then incise the overlying fascia to find it. Dissect the brachial veins off the artery and place a vessel loop around the artery. Mobilize the artery for two to three centimeters so you have enough room to perform the anastomosis.

Divide the basilic vein and ligate it distally. Use a marker to indicate the anterior surface of the vein along its course to aid in orienting the vein so it does not get twisted during tunnelling. Locally heparinize the vein and dilate it if appropriate. Secure the vein to a Kelly-Wick tunneller, then tunnel the vein from the axilla, laterally and subcutaneously, to the area around the exposed artery. The more lateral the tunnel, the easier time the vascular access nurses will have cannulating the vein. Cut the stitch securing the vein to the tunneller and locally heparinize the vein, ensuring that it is not twisted.

The Anastomosis

If you have access to a venous bifurcation, divide the vein just distal to that and spatulate the anastomosis by using a right angle Potts scissor to enter one branch and come out the other, then cut to open up the vein. Alternatively, using a right angle Potts scissors make an incision in the vein at the "heel" if needed to make a wider anastomosis. Use a small bulldog to prevent back-bleeding from the vein. Bring the artery and vein next to each other and gain control of the inflow and outflow of the artery with double vessel loops or vascular clamps.

Make an arteriotomy with an 11 blade and extend it with right angle Pott's scissors. Some surgeons use a vascular punch instead of the scissors. Place a 7–0 polypropylene

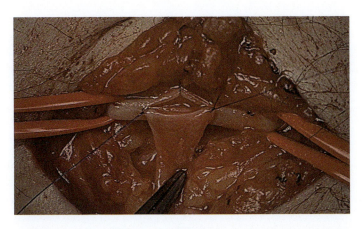

FIGURE 41.4 Preparation for radiocephalic arteriovenous wrist fistula (Courtesy of David Melnick, MD)

suture as a "stay" suture in the center of one wall of the artery to assist in retraction of the wall for exposure. Locally heparinize the artery proximally and distally. Use double armed 6–0 or 7–0 polypropylene sutures for the anastomosis.

Approximate the artery and vein at the "heel" of the anastomosis (located proximally on the arm) with the polypropylene suture and tie that down. Use another suture to bring the "toe" together so now the artery and vein are set up for the anastomosis (Fig. 41.4).

The needle typically travels outside to inside on the vein, and inside to outside on the artery to avoid raising an arterial intimal flap. Close the posterior layer first with one of the "heel" needles, traveling outside to inside on the vein for the first bite. Then travel inside to outside on the artery, then outside to in again on the vein. This will be easy if the anastomosis is set up correctly. Continue with that same suture past the "toe" and around halfway up the anterior anastomosis (Fig. 41.5).

Then change to the other "heel" needle and finish the anastomosis. Prior to tying the sutures, make sure the anastomosis is patent and you have good flow in the vein. If not, you

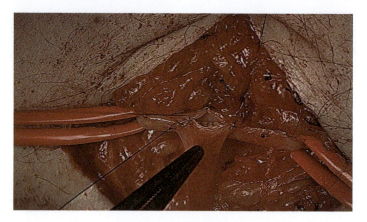

FIGURE 41.5 Completing the radiocephalic anastomosis (Courtesy of David Melnick, MD)

can explore the anastomosis for technical problems prior to tying the suture. With small vessels, less than 3 mm, you may not appreciate a thrill immediately but only hear a good signal by Doppler demonstrating flow. If the vein had a side branch that you ligated prior to the anastomosis, you can cut that stitch and use the sidebranch to interrogate the anastomosis by passing dilators, thrombectomy catheters, and instilling heparinized saline.

Palpate or doppler the pulse distally to ensure adequate hand perfusion. Ensure hemostasis then close the wound.

Postoperative Care

Evaluate the patients in around two weeks to assess the quality of the AVF. Along with examining for a thrill, use ultrasound if available to assess the size and depth of the fistula. If the thrill is not robust or the size of the vein seems small, you can send the patient for a fistulagram to assess for stenosis and potential balloon angioplasty. It should be apparent within 2–4 weeks whether the fistula will have enough flow to cannulate successfully for dialysis; the patient should not have to wait months for the fistula to mature. In Appel's original series of 16 patients, aged 28–54 years old and all with end stage renal disease caused by glomerulonephritis, dialysis utilizing the fistula was attempted on postoperative day one. If there is a concern about fistula maturation, obtain a fistulagram and if necessary evaluate for revision or a new site.

Acknowledgment Thank you to Marge Hunter for assisting as a scrub tech in hundreds of these cases.

References

1. Murad MH, Elamin MB, Sidawy AN, et al. Autogenous versus prosthetic vascular access for hemodialysis: a systematic review and meta-analysis. J Vasc Surg. 2008;48(5 Suppl):34S–47.
2. National Kidney Foundation [internet.] Updates clinical practice guidelines and recommendations. 2006 [cited 13 Aug 2014]. Available from http://www.kidney.org/professionals/KDOQI/guideline_upHD_PD_VA/index.htm.
3. Sidawy AN, Spergel LM, Besarab A, et al. The society for vascular surgery: clinical practice guidelines for the surgical placement and maintenance of arteriovenous hemodialysis access. J Vasc Surg. 2008;48(5 Suppl):2S–5.
4. Lauvao LS, Ihnat DM, Goshima KR, et al. Vein diameter is the major predictor of fistula maturation. J Vasc Surg. 2009;49(6): 1499–504.
5. Brescia MJ, Cimino JE, Appel K, Baruch J. Chronic hemodialysis using venipuncture and a surgically created arteriovenous fistula. N Engl J Med. 1966;275(20):1089–92.

Chapter 42
Drainage of Abscess

Sarah E. Smith

Abstract Drainage of an abscess is indicated as primary treatment for purulent skin infections. The need for incision and drainage may be based on physical exam or with ultrasonography. If indicated, this may be done with local anesthetic. With consideration given to access to abscess, patient comfort and provider ergonomics, prep skin with cleansing agent. Using local anesthetic, inject intradermally. Incision should be across the abscess and once purulence is drained and irrigated, pack wound, covering with gauze. If systemic symptoms such as fever are present, oral antibiotic may be necessary in conjunction with procedure.

Keywords Abscess • Incision • Drainage • Wound • Packing • Infection

With increasing awareness of overuse of antibiotic therapy and surge in prevalence of antibiotic resistant bacteria, the place for incision and drainage of abscess is well established.

S.E. Smith, RN, MS, ANP-BC, APNP
Department of General Surgery, University of Wisconsin,
University of Wisconsin-Madison, 1 South Park Street,
53715 Madison, WI, USA
e-mail: smiths@surgery.wisc.edu

H. Chen (ed.), *Illustrative Handbook of General Surgery*,
DOI 10.1007/978-3-319-24557-7_42,
© Springer International Publishing Switzerland 2016

The Center for Disease Control and Prevention continues to rely on incision and drainage as primary therapy for treatment of abscesses as well as recommendations from the Infectious Diseases Society of America [1].

Indications

Indications for incision and drainage of an abscess are determined on the basis of purulent versus non-purulent infections. On exam, a purulent infection will likely have an area of fluctuance surrounded by induration. Generally speaking, the area of fluctuance correlates with the most painful and erythematous location as well. The majority of the time determining purulence can be done solely by physical exam.

If no purulence is present, then surgical intervention is likely not appropriate and oral antibiotics may be effective. However, in some situations, incision and drainage may be indicated further along the course of infection.

Pre-procedure Evaluation

Physical exam- This is generally sufficient to identify a simple abscess. Presence of swelling, pain, erythema, and fluctuance can confirm an abscess as can spontaneous purulent drainage.

Bedside/ in-office ultrasonography- This method may be used in conjunction with physical exam to evaluate for fluid collection, dimensions and rough size and expectations for drainage. It may also aid in locating the most appropriate area to make incision [1]. This is illustrated in Fig. 42.1. Aspiration of an abscess with US guidance has found to be successful only 25 % of the time [2].

Contraindications to bedside or in-office drainage of an abscess would include the following and require specialization or additional anesthesia: Large size of abscess, location requiring specialization (face, eyes, hands, feet), extensive

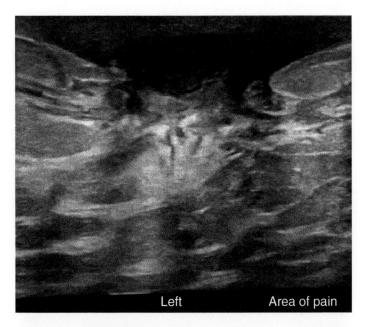

Left   Area of pain

FIGURE 42.1 Ultrasound of abscess demonstrating fluid present (Courtesy of Sarah Smith)

cellulitis without fluid collection, and conditions that require pre-medication such as anti-coagulation or pre-operative antibiotics [3].

Positioning and Anesthesia

Positioning for drainage of an abscess is based on abscess location and patient's tolerance and comfort as well as ergonomics of the provider.

Anesthesia for abscess drainage can generally be achieved with local anesthetic using 1 % Lidocaine with epinephrine to minimize bleeding. If area to be anesthetized is at genitalia, the nipple/areolar complex or an area with low vascularity, it is appropriate to forgo the epinephrine. With purulent infections, complete anesthetization is challenging, as the uptake of anesthetic is reduced due to purulence. Progressive anesthesia throughout the procedure may be indicated.

In the event the patient does not tolerate complete drainage of the abscess due to incomplete anesthesia, it may be necessary to have patient to return in 1–2 days as with drainage, some inflammation may decrease and allow for tolerable debridement.

Description of the Procedure

(a) Gather appropriate personal protective equipment and instruments for procedure (Table 42.1).
(b) Obtain informed consent and disclose potential risks of bleeding, pain, and scar formation

TABLE 42.1 Protective equipment

Personal protective equipment	Procedure equipment
Face shield	Skin cleansing agent
Fluid resistant gown	Local anesthetic
Sterile gloves	5–10 ml syringe
Mask	25–30 gauge needle
	Sterile gauze
	Scalpel
	Small curved hemostat
	Normal saline and sterile bowl
	Large syringe
	Culture swabs
	Packing material
	Scissors
	Tape

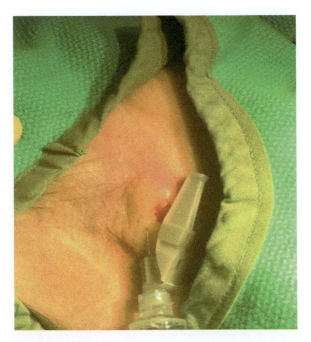

FIGURE 42.2 Blanching of skin created by intradermal injection (Courtesy of Sarah Smith)

(c) Skin preparation – Proceed with skin preparation using skin cleansing agent such as chlorhexidine. Start at the center of the abscess.

(d) Anesthetization – Prepare the patient. This may be the most painful part of the procedure. This is due to the pH difference of the anesthetic and body tissues. Using a 25–30 gauge needle, inject anesthetic into the intradermal tissue above the abscess cavity, which will create blanching of the skin as illustrated in Fig. 42.2. Injecting slowly will minimize discomfort the patient will experience. Give time for the anesthetic to take effect and re-anesthetize if necessary.

(e) Incision – Using the scalpel, make an incision across the area of abscess. No drainage will be present until the abscess cavity is entered as illustrated in Fig. 42.3.

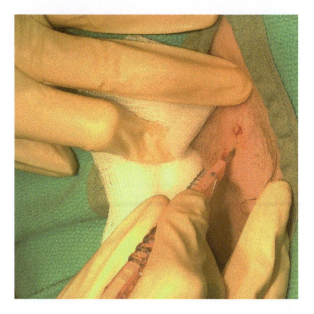

FIGURE 42.3 Incision of abscess cavity (Courtesy of Sarah Smith)

(f) Allow the wound to drain. Break up loculations inside the cavity. This is best done in a circular motion as diagramed in Fig. 42.4. Additional drainage will most likely result. It may be necessary to add additional anesthetic during this process. If indicated, this is also an appropriate time to swab the wound for culture. In uncomplicated abscesses, this is unnecessary as those infections caused by community-acquired MRSA have a cure rate of 85–90 % [4].

(g) Irrigate the wound until clear drainage present.

(h) Pack the wound with packing material in a circular direction as illustrated in Fig. 42.5. Be careful not to overpack, as tension could cause tissue ischemia or prevent drainage. In a small study, packing was found to cause more pain and did not improve healing than just covering with gauze [4]. This is ultimately left up to the provider [5].

(i) Cover with sterile gauze and secure with tape.

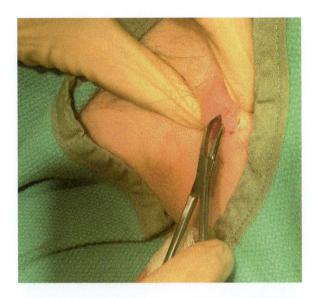

FIGURE 42.4 Breaking up loculations of abscess cavity (Courtesy of Sarah Smith)

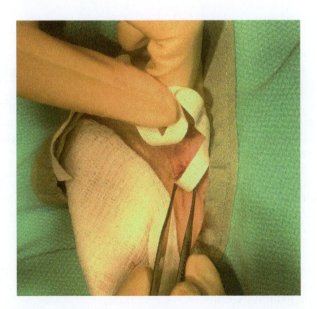

FIGURE 42.5 Packing abscess cavity (Courtesy of Sarah Smith)

Post-procedure Instructions

Review care instructions with patient and schedule return visit to remove packing in 2–3 days. If continued drainage, wound may require repacking of site. Review symptoms that would warrant earlier return such as worsening redness, fever, increased pain or bleeding. Depending on size and location of abscess, additional pain medication may be necessary.

Complications

Complications of the procedure could include worsening infection despite incision and drainage. If this would occur, antibiotic therapy may be necessary [1]. If recurrent infections would occur, further work up should be completed for conditions such as diabetes or autoimmune disorders. Referral to Infections Disease may also be warranted.

References

1. Stevens DL, Bisno AL, Chambers HF, Dellinger EP, Goldstein EJ, Gorbach SL, et al. Practice guidelines for the diagnosis and management of skin and soft tissue infections: 2014 update by the infectious diseases society of america. Clin Inf Dis. 2014;59: e10–52.
2. Singer AJ, Talan DA. Management of skin abscesses in the era of methicillin-resistant *Staphylococcus aureus*. N Engl J Med. 2014;370(11):1039–47.
3. Fitch MT, Manthey DE, McGinnis HD, Nicks BA, Pariyadath M. Videos in clinical medicine: abscess incision and drainage. N Engl J Med. 2007;357, e20.
4. Abrahamian FM, Talan DA, Moran GJ. Management of skin and soft tissue infections in the emergency department. Infect Dis Clin N Am. 2008;22:89–116.
5. May L, Harter K, Yadav K, Strauss R, Abualenain J, Keim A, et al. Practice patterns and management strategies for purulent skin and soft-tissue infections in an urban academic ED. Am J Emerg Med. 2012;30:302–10.

Chapter 43
Biopsy of Skin Lesions

Mary Beth Henry

Abstract This chapter discusses the complexity of issues to consider when determining to do a relatively easy and inexpensive procedure – punch biopsy. Reviewed are lesions appropriate to diagnose with punch, and absolute contraindications to punch, which are few but serious. Review of data and consensus guidelines are clear regarding pigmented lesions highly suspicious for melanoma but there is no clear cut recommendation for type and size of biopsy for a myriad of other lesions. How to obtain a full thickness tissue sample, closure and wound care is outlined. General points of discussion to be reviewed with patients regarding the goal of the procedure and individual considerations are made.

Keywords Punch biopsy • Suspected melanoma • Incisional • Excisional • Wound closure • Full thickness skin biopsy

M.B. Henry, RN, MS, CS, APNP
Department of Surgical Oncology, University of Wisconsin
Health System, 600 Highland Avenue K4/755 CSC,
53792-7375 Madison, WI, USA
e-mail: henry@surgery.wisc.edu

H. Chen (ed.), *Illustrative Handbook of General Surgery*,
DOI 10.1007/978-3-319-24557-7_43,

Indications

Punch biopsies are a simple, practical and inexpensive diagnostic tool. Compared with excisional biopsies, very little training and experience is needed to do a skin punch biopsy well. However, choosing which biopsy technique and which lesion to biopsy is a complex decision. There are few evidence- based or best practice consensus guidelines to direct which type of biopsy to perform and how big the tissue specimen should be. National Comprehensive Cancer Network (NCCN) guidelines and an overwhelming amount of data recommend an excisional biopsy with a 1–3 mm margin for pigmented lesions worrisome for melanoma. However, for patients presenting with a variety of symptomatic lesions or worrisome dermatoses, early and rapid diagnosis is essential and a punch biopsy is often the preferred approach. Skin cancer is the most common of all cancers. Early detection and treatment can lead to cure even if a lesion is malignant and early biopsy is critical to diagnosis. Once the decision to perform a punch biopsy is made, it is essential to clearly explain to the patient the indication for the procedure, the technique and the potential complications including missed diagnosis due to sample error or need for further surgery to definitively treat the lesion.

Excisional biopsies are expensive and time consuming procedures which require visits for both the procedure and the subsequent suture removal. They also create bigger defects, more scarring and potentially conflict with the surgeon's intended approach in cases where a wide local excision and sentinel node biopsy are required. Draining lymph basins can potentially be obscured with larger biopsies. Excisional biopsies also have the potential for poorer cosmesis [1]. Punch biopsies are a perfect diagnostic tool for inflammatory lesions or for small pigmented lesions. All the layers of the skin including the epidermis, dermis and upper parts of the subcutis are included in a punch specimen.

An estimated 76,100 new cases of invasive melanoma will be diagnosed in the US in 2014 [2]. In 2015, 1 in 50 Americans will develop melanoma and 1 in 5 Americans will develop basal cell carcinoma or squamous cell carcinoma [3]. Many cancers can be cured by early excision. Despite the possible interference with T-staging a malignant lesion, errors from failing to biopsy due to time and healthcare cost constraints are worse than using the non-excisional (punch) technique to diagnosis possible malignancy.

Non-excisional biopsy may result in inadequate histology. However, a review of nine studies demonstrates that non-excisional biopsy of primary lesions with poor prognostic indicators has no effect on prognosis [4]. The type of biopsy performed does not influence survival rates in patients with melanoma [5]. Partial biopsies may result in misdiagnosis and inaccurate microstaging [6]. For patients presenting with large lesions which are obviously malignant melanoma, complete excision with 1–3 mm margins is often impractical or too morbid. If complete excision cannot be performed as a primary procedure, then a punch of the most suspicious or thickest area should be done [5]. Moreover, if the initial tissue obtained is inadequate, additional biopsy is recommended.

Preoperative Care

Site Selection of Lesion

Punch biopsy is indicated with all suspected neoplastic lesions, lesions that require evaluation of the deeper dermis, all bullous disorders and to clarify a diagnosis when the differential list is limited [4]. For inflammatory lesions, biopsy the newer lesions with erythema. If possible take samples from several representative stages of the process. For blistering lesions, biopsy the newest vesicles and blisters first, within 48 h of onset. Older lesions may yield obscured pathological information. For very large lesions, biopsy the center or the most abnormal area or the thickest area [4]. For vesicles, biopsy them intact when possible, with some adjacent normal skin [4]. For bullae/circumscribed fluid filled lesions >1 cm in diameter, biopsy the edge to include a part of the blister with adjacent intact skin [4].

Contraindications

Avoid face and distal lower extremities and over the tibia if possible to avoid cosmetic problems and delayed healing. Lesions on the distal lower extremities can show histological signs of stasis. Also avoid axilla and groin if possible to avoid secondary infection [1]. There are rare absolute contraindications to punch biopsy. Use caution with patients on anticoagulation therapy and carefully consider the site. Take particular care when working near large pulsatile vessels in the trunk or head and neck [7]. Warfarin/Coumadin, Plavix/clopidogrel and aspirin should not be discontinued for a simple punch. A punch site on limbs with a bypass graft, near large vessels or articular capsules is contraindicated. One case study reports a massive arterial bleed from a 5 mm punch biopsy causing an arteriotomy to right femoral to anterior tibial artery Teflon bypass graft located at the distal right lateral thigh [8]. Allergic reactions to anesthesia are rare. Use caution when using lidocaine with cardiac patients. Anaphylactic reactions or arrhythmias may occur, therefore, it is important to be ready to perform basic resuscitation if needed [7]. If a full thickness excision with punch is inappropriate due to large size of the lesion or location, such as: face, or near a vessel graft, then modification of the approach is reasonable and warranted [9].

Review medications, allergies, recent treatments of the lesion and concomitant illnesses. Obtain informed consent. Discussion should include the risk of infection, bleeding and potential scarring. Tissue sampling error and a caveat that more complicated surgery or diagnostic tests are a possibility should be discussed.

Positioning and Anesthesia

Skin Preparation

Use chlorhexidine to cleanse the skin. It is effective against gram negative and positive bacteria and lasts for several hours. Alcohol provides poor coverage against gram negative

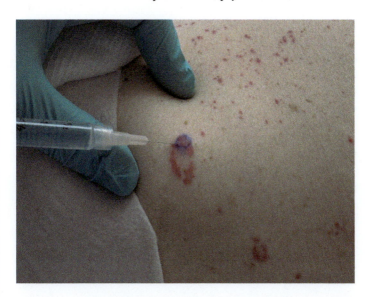

FIGURE 43.1 Inject anesthetic (Courtesy of Andrew M. Swanson MD)

bacteria but it can be used if chlorhexidine is not available. Povidone-iodine is also acceptable to prepare the site.

Anesthetic

Outline the clinical margins of the lesion in indelible ink, preferably using a sterile pen, after adequate skin preparation but before instillation of anesthetic fluid (See Fig. 43.1).

Use 1 or 2 % lidocaine with epinephrine. An allergy to procaine (Novacain) is not a contraindication to the use of lidocaine [1]. Buffer the sting with lidocaine (A 10:1 ratio of lidocaine: sodium bicarbonate 8.4 % $NaHCO_3$) will minimize the pain (1 mL of $NaHCO_3$ with 9 mL of lidocaine) [10]. Use a small long needle: ½inch/gauge 27 or 26 or 5/8 inch/gauge 25. Warm the solution by gently rolling the vial between your hands. Inject perpendicular (90°) to the skin. Sensory nerve endings branch out like a tree and if the skin is penetrated at a 90° angle then the needle intersects fewer nerves [11]. The

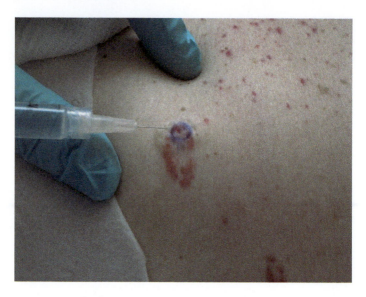

FIGURE 43.2 Make a wheal injecting at 45° (Courtesy of Andrew M. Swanson MD)

first 0.2–0.5 mL should be injected intra-dermally, to form a wheal beneath the skin. Then change the angle and slowly inject more anesthetic (See Fig. 43.2).

Keep 0.5 mL of palpable anesthetic ahead of the tip of the needle. This will anesthetize subdermal nerve endings in front of the tip of the needle [10]. Wait about 5 min for the effect of the lidocaine with epinephrine to take effect. You can use this time to fill out forms and discuss wound care with the patient. Epinephrine is absolutely contraindicated in digital and penile blocks because it may compromise blood flow [10].

Description of the Procedure

This is a clean, not sterile procedure. If the patient is at risk of infection, or immunocompromised, it should be done with sterile technique.

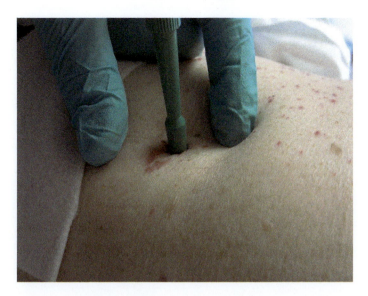

FIGURE 43.3 Pull skin perpendicular to Langer's lines (Courtesy of
Andrew M. Swanson MD)

- Non-sterile gloves
- 3 ml syringe filled with lidocaine with epinephrine (hemostasis is improved but may cause blanching and obscure
  outline of lesion)
- 30 g needle 0.5 or 1 inch
- Punch biopsy circular blades are available in 2–8 mm
  diameters. A 4 mm punch tool is usually used.
- Scissor
- Labeled formalin containers
- 4–0, 5–0 or 6–0 nylon suture
- Needle driver
- Tissue forceps to close wound not to pick up the specimen

Clean the skin, mark with a sterile skin marker. The lesion
should be outlined in case of blanching due to epinephrine
with lidocaine. Stretch the skin perpendicular or 90° to the
Langer's lines. Langer's lines are the tension lines and they
usually run perpendicular to the underlying musculature but
can vary within individuals (See Fig. 43.3).

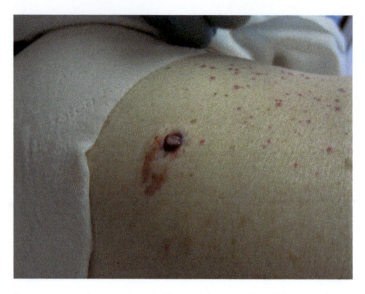

FIGURE 43.4 Remove the disposable punch without twisting (Courtesy of Andrew M. Swanson MD)

To find the Langer's lines, gently pinch the skin and look for parallel lines, hold tension in the opposite direction of the Langer's lines when the punch is being performed. This will turn the round punch hole into a more elliptical defect that parallels the skin's natural tension lines. This procedure will allow for a more oval shape and can be closed more easily with a suture. Place the circular blade on the skin at a 90° angle and twist back and forth until you feel a 'give' in the skin- you know you are in the fat when the tugging sensation is gone. Do not pull the punch tool in and out of the wound to check progress (See Fig. 43.4).

When you feel the 'give' of the fat then remove the punch and depress the skin around the defect and use the injection needle to pierce the core specimen and place in container (See Fig. 43.5).

You may need to use a scissors to cut the base of the specimen to free it up. Avoid using forceps to remove the tissue form the defect as they can cause crush artifact of the specimen (See Fig. 43.6).

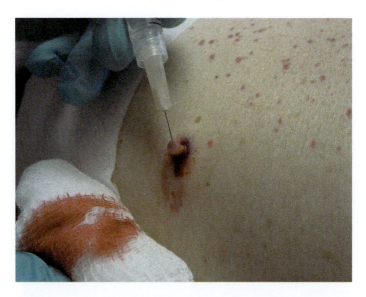

FIGURE 43.5 Avoid crush artifact by removing tissue with injection needle (Courtesy of Andrew M. Swanson MD)

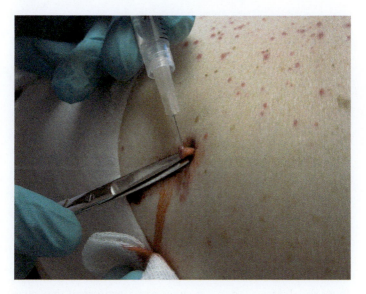

FIGURE 43.6 Cut the base of the specimen with a scissors (Courtesy of Andrew M. Swanson MD)

Apply pressure over the defect with gauze. Cover with white petrolatum. It is a safe wound care ointment for ambulatory surgery procedures and decreases the risk of allergic reactions and gram-negative bacterial superinfections [5]. Cover the petroleum with dry sterile gauze.

Wound Closure with Suture

Defects >4 mm close with 1–2 interrupted sutures (See Fig. 43.7).

Secondary intention healing and suturing have similar cosmetic results for lesions 1–4 mm in diameter [5]. Use 4–0 or 5–0 monofilament nylon suture. Unbraided nylon will decrease infection but may be more difficult to use. Use a cutting needle. C-17 needles were made to close punch biopsy defects. The higher the number of the needle, the larger the body and length of the needle is. Grab the needle at about 1/3 from the eye and insert in the skin perpendicular to the skin about 2 mm from the edge of the wound (See Fig. 43.8).

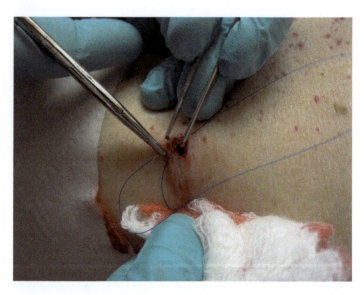

FIGURE 43.7 Use a cutting needle to suture (Courtesy of Andrew M. Swanson MD)

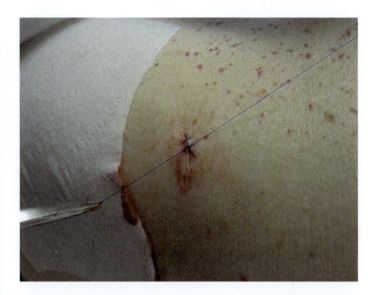

FIGURE 43.8 Close the defect with 1 or 2 interrupted sutures (Courtesy of Andrew M. Swanson MD)

Specimen

Label the specimen and provide as much clinical information as you can –site, size of punch, history of lesion, treatment of lesion prior to biopsy and concomitant diseases if applicable. Place the specimen in formalin and send to a dermatopathologist.

Postoperative Care

Remove the gauze in 24 h. If sutured, remove sutures in 7–10 days.

Complications

Complications are rare but include bleeding or infection. If bleeding occurs it can be controlled with pressure dressings or with sutures. Infection will likely occur within 2 or 3 days after biopsy. Watch for redness, swelling, change in drainage color, warmth to area, or fevers. Infections can be treated with oral antibiotics.

Conclusion

It is important to remember that, except for lesions in regions which make excisional biopsies an impractical solution, punch biopsies are not ideal for lesions suspected for melanoma. Nonetheless, the punch biopsy is a very helpful tool to diagnose many types of skin lesions and its comparative simplicity and relative low cost make the punch biopsy the most efficacious procedure in many instances. In fact, for certain lesions, punch biopsies can even serve as the treatment.

References

1. Achar S. Principles of skin biopsies for the family physician. Am Fam Physician. 1996;54(8):2411–8.
2. Skin Cancer Foundation [internet.] Skin cancer information. 2014. [cited 29 June 2014]. Available from http://www.skincancer.org/skin-cancer-information.
3. Halloran L. Here comes the sun: addressing skin cancer. J Nurs Pract. 2014;10(6):439–40.
4. Alguire PC, Mathes BM. Skin biopsy techniques for the internist. J Gen Intern Med. 1998;13(1):46–54.
5. Pickett H. Shave and punch biopsy for skin lesions. Am Fam Physician. 2011;84(9):995–1002.
6. Egnatios GL, Dueck AC, Macdonald JB, Laman SD, Warschaw KE, DiCaudo DJ, et al. The impact of biopsy technique on upstaging, residual disease, and outcome in cutaneous melanoma. Am J Surg. 2011;202(6):771–7; discussion 7–8.
7. Llamas-Velasco M, Paredes BE. Basic concepts in skin biopsy. Part I. Actas Dermosifiliogr. 2012;103(1):12–20.
8. Fite LP, Butler DF, Fiala K. Potential exsanguination from a punch biopsy. J Am Acad Dermatol. 2013;69(4):e197–8.
9. Geisse JK. Biopsy techniques for pigmented lesions of the skin. Pathology (Phila). 1994;2(2):181–93.

10. AlGhamdi KM, AlEnazi MM. Versatile punch surgery. J Cutan Med Surg. 2011;15(2):87–96.
11. Strazar R, Lalonde D. Minimizing injection pain in local anesthesia. CMAJ. 2012;184(18):2016.

Chapter 44
Excisional Biopsy of Dermal and Subcutaneous Lesions

Jennifer B. Wilson

Abstract The removal of dermal and subcutaneous lesions is one of the most common procedures performed in the outpatient setting. General surgeons and surgical advanced practice providers along with primary care specialists all perform excisional biopsies. This chapter will describe the preoperative evaluation, surgical techniques, and postoperative care for performing excisional biopsy, specifically the linear and elliptical technique.

Keywords Excisional biopsy • Dermal lesions • Subcutaneous mass • Lipoma • Epidermoid cyst

Information and Indications

The removal of dermal or subcutaneous lesions is one of the most common procedures performed in the outpatient clinic. Typical reasons for removal are concern for malignancy, pain

J.B. Wilson, PA
Department of General Surgery, University of Wisconsin Hospital and Clinics, 600 Highland Avenue, Madison, WI 53792, USA
e-mail: wilsonj@surgery.wisc.edu

H. Chen (ed.), *Illustrative Handbook of General Surgery*,   781
DOI 10.1007/978-3-319-24557-7_44,
© Springer International Publishing Switzerland 2016

and discomfort, change or growth of the lesion, discharge from the lesion, previous or recent infection or inflammation of the lesion, cosmetic concerns, and clinical diagnosis of the mass especially in ones that are difficult to differentiate from lymph nodes or solid tumors [1].

Lipomas and epidermoid cysts are the most common lesions removed in an outpatient clinic. Lipomas are soft tissue mesenchymal tumors located subcutaneously and consist of mature fatty tissue [2]. Epidermoid cysts are also known as epidermal inclusion cysts or epidermal cysts, which are discrete nodules [1, 3]. They are often called sebaceous cysts, which is a misnomer because they are not actually made of sebum [1]. The cyst walls consist of normal epidermis that produces keratin [3].

Preoperative Care

Important aspects to the history include onset, related symptoms, history of infection or previous surgical procedures to area, and/or similar masses on the body. On physical exam, one evaluates for skin involvement, mobility, vascularity and borders. Cysts have a central pore, round and smooth, and tend to be tenser than lipomas [1–3]. Lipomas are soft, irregular, rubbery, and move freely [1–3]. Cysts are more likely to be superficial whereas lipomas can be superficial or deep into the fascia [1–3] (Figs. 44.1 and 44.2).

Imaging, such as ultrasound and magnetic resonance imaging (MRI), can be used when the history and physical is in question. MRI may help differentiate between benign and malignant lesions, such as liposarcomas [1, 4]. Lesions directly over the spine can be imaged with an MRI to see if there is any communication with the nervous system [1, 4, 5].

Contraindications

Infected epidermoid cysts should be incised and drained (I&D) and time allotted for the infection to resolve. If the walls of an epidermoid cyst rupture, which is usually associ-

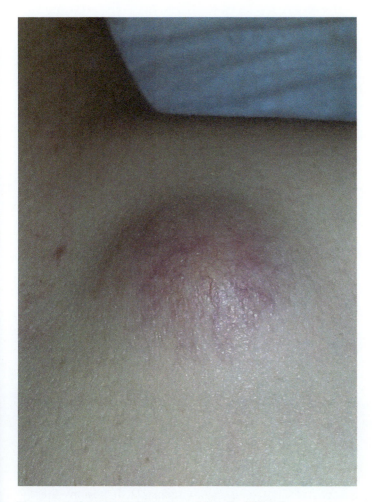

FIG. 44.1 Inflamed cyst (Courtesy of Jennifer Wilson)

ated with trauma, the contents within come in contact with the surrounding soft tissue, causing an inflammatory response indicated by symptoms including erythema, warmth, and mild discomfort [1]. Treatment of an inflamed cyst is not necessary unless requested by the patient or it progresses to an abscess. Inflamed epidermoid cyst walls are friable making successful remove of the entire cyst wall difficult. The use of curette to

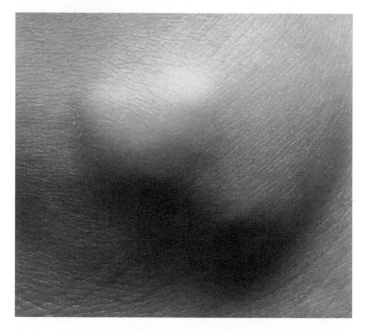

Fɪɢ. 44.2 Lobulated lipoma pre-excision (Courtesy of Jennifer Wilson)

scrape the walls of an inflamed cyst may be necessary to remove all wall remnants. Recurrence is less likely if the cyst is removed when not inflamed. There is increase risk of cellulitis with I&D of an inflamed, non-infected cyst [1, 4, 5] (Fig. 44.3).

Positioning and Anesthesia

The location of the lesion requiring excision will determine the positioning of the patient. Proper positioning provides access for the clinician while providing comfort for the patient. The surgical site should be prepped and draped

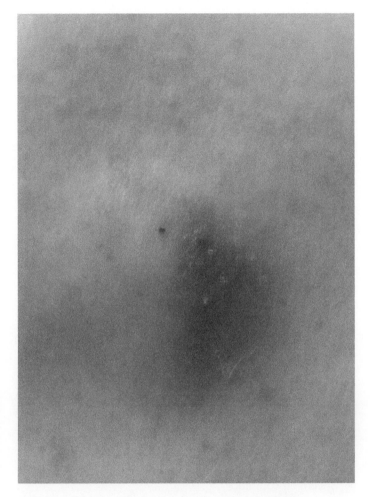

FIG. 44.3 Cyst pre-excision (Courtesy of Jennifer Wilson)

appropriately. Local anesthetic can be utilized in most instances. Monitored or general anesthesia may be appropriate in some cases with large lesions where proper positioning requires the patient to be sedated.

Description of Procedure

Personal Protective Equipment

- Face shield or eye protection
- Mask
- Gown
- Sterile gloves

Equipment

- Sterile gauze
- Surgical marking pen with ruler
- 10 ml syringe
- Scalpel
- Needles of various gauges
- Local anesthetic
- Skin cleaning agent for topical antiseptic
- Sterile towels
- Towel clamps
- Needle driver
- Iris, curved and straight scissors
- Adson forceps
- Hemostats
- Skin retractors
- Sutures
- Electrocoagulation unit
- Normal saline
- Specimen container
- Outer dressing

Technique of Procedure

Review the risks and benefits of the procedure with the patient. Risks include pain, bleeding, infection, seroma or hematoma formation, scarring, change in pigmentation, delayed healing, change in appearance, skin indentation, skin protrusion, local nerve damage/numbness, loss of muscle function, and need for further treatment [1, 5, 6]. After discussing with the patient the risk and benefits of the procedure, informed consent is obtained.

Dermal and subcutaneous lesions can be removed with multiple techniques. The most common methods are by linear excision, elliptical excision, and punch biopsy. For very small or superficial lesions, a punch biopsy may be indicated [2, 5]. The linear excision is used more for the removal of lipomas. Elliptical excision is used more for cyst removal when it is important to ensure the entire cyst sac is excised to prevent recurrence [2, 5].

The patient is placed in a position on the table that provides adequate access to the lesion. The patient is padded and draped appropriately to ensure comfort during the procedure. Prep the surgical site with a topical antiseptic and drape in a sterile field. Infiltration with local anesthetic may make the mass difficult to find. Outlining the area prior to the administration of the anesthetic can be helpful in locating the lesion before excision. Anesthetize the skin and subcutaneous tissue around the lesion. Make a linear or elliptical incision. The incision should be made over the top of the lesion in the direction of the skin tension line also known as Langer's lines (Fig. 44.4).

Gently use the forceps to grasp skin edges. Dissect through the subcutaneous fat if needed to expose the lesion, freeing it from any surrounding structures. Perform sharp or blunt dissection using a scalpel, iris scissors or hemostat (Fig. 44.5).

Continue to gently dissect the tissue surrounding the lesion until it is completely excised. Inspect the area to ensure that no remnants of the lesion remain. Provide wound hemostasis whether by direct pressure, cautery, or suture. Close the wound in a layered fashion. The skin edges can be approximated and closed using sutures. Apply an outer dressing if indicated (Fig. 44.6).

Postoperative Care

Review instructions with the patient and arrange follow up if needed. Review signs and symptoms of infection such as erythema, drainage, warmth, tenderness, edema, fever and/or

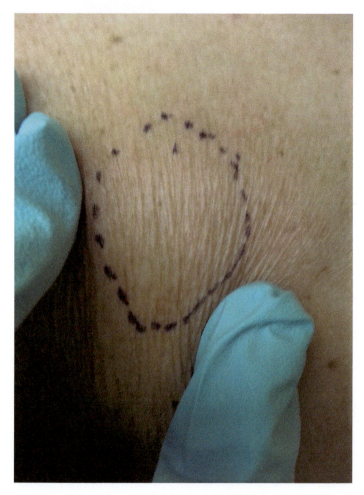

Fɪɢ. 44.4 Marked incision showing Langer's lines (Courtesy of Jennifer Wilson)

chills. Complications are rare, but include bleeding, infection, seroma, hematoma, and/or wound dehiscence.

Advantages to performing this procedure in an outpatient clinic include the need for fewer instruments and staff, a decreased cost for patients, convenience of same day treat-

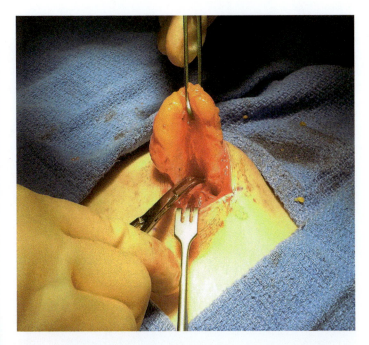

FIG. 44.5 Dissection of a lipoma (Courtesy of Jennifer Wilson)

ment, and often negates the need for a second appointment for suture removal and post-operative check [1].

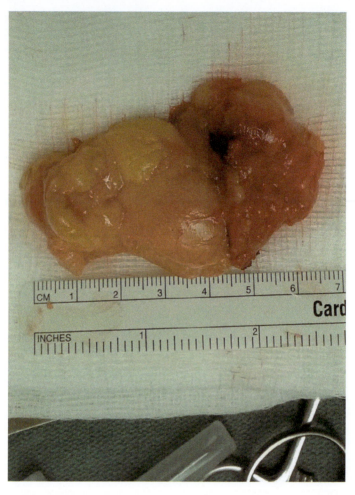

FIG. 44.6 Lipoma post-excision by ruler (Courtesy of Jennifer Wilson)

References

1. Usatine RP, Pfenninger JL, Stulberg DL, Small R. Dermatologic and cosmetic procedures in office practice. Philadelphia: Elsevier; 2012. p. 133–45.
2. McTighe S, Chernev I. Intramuscular lipoma: a review of the literature. Orthop Rev. 2014;6(5618):156–63.
3. Goldstein B, Goldstein A. Overview of benign lesions of the skin. UpToDate. 2014. Available: http://www.uptodate.com/contents/overview-of-benign-lesions-of-the-skin?source=search. Accessed 16 Feb 2015.
4. Matsumoto K, Hukuda S, Ishizawa M, Chano T, Okabe H. MRI finding in intramuscular lipomas. Skeletal Radiol. 1999;28:145–52.
5. Pfenninger JL, Fowler GC. Procedures for primary care. 3rd ed. Philadelphia: Elsevier; 2011. p. 69–84.
6. Nishida J, Morita T, Ogose A, Okada K, Kakizaki H, Tajino T, et al. Imaging characteristics of deep-seated lipomatous tumors: intramuscular lipoma, intermuscular lipoma, and lipoma-like liposarcoma. J Orthop Sci. 2007;12:533–41.

Index

A

Abdominoperineal resection
(APR)
  anesthesia, 432–433
  indications, 430–431
  patient positioning, 432
  post-operative care, 446
  pre-operative imaging and
    procedures, 431–432
  procedure
    anococcygeal ligament,
      441, 442
    anterior dissection plane,
      442, 444
    elliptical incision, 441
    perineal incision, 442, 445
  robotic, 445–446
Abscess drainage
  anesthesia, 761–762
  antibiotic therapy, 759
  complications, 766
  indications, 760
  patient positioning, 761
  post-procedure
    instructions, 766
  pre-procedure evaluation,
    760–761
  procedure
    abscess cavity, loculations
      of, 764, 765

anesthetization, 763
incision, 763, 764
informed consent, 762
packing abscess cavity,
  764, 765
potential risks, disclosure
  of, 762
protective equipment, 762
skin preparation, 763
ACC. *See* Adrenocortical cancer
  (ACC)
Achalasia. *See* Esophageal
  achalasia
Adjustable gastric banding
  (AGB), 237, 244–245
Adrenalectomy
  indications for, 62
  laparoscopic (*see*
    (Laparoscopic
    adrenalectomy))
  open (*see* (Open
    adrenalectomy))
Adrenal incidentaloma, 63
Adrenocortical cancer (ACC)
  laparoscopic adrenalectomy
    (*see* (Laparoscopic
    adrenalectomy))
  open adrenalectomy (*see*
    (Open
    adrenalectomy))

H. Chen (ed.), *Illustrative Handbook of General Surgery*,
DOI 10.1007/978-3-319-24557-7,
© Springer International Publishing Switzerland 2016

818   Index

right gastric artery, 705
skin incision, 701, 702
subpancreatic tunnel, 704
superior mesenteric artery, 706
superior pancreaticoduodenal
    vein, 707, 709
ultrasound, 702

upper jejunum mobilization,
    706, 707
upper midline incision, 701
Whitehead's
    hemorrhoidectomy, 515
Wrist fistula. *See* Radiocephalic
    wrist fistula

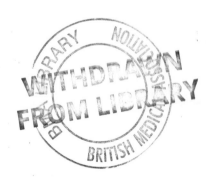